# Essays in Toxicology

# ESSAYS IN TOXICOLOGY

## EDITORIAL BOARD

MARY O. AMDUR
*Harvard University*

ROBERT E. GOSSELIN
*Dartmouth Medical School*

DONALD E. MORELAND
*North Carolina State University*

C. O. CHICHESTER
*University of Rhode Island*

WAYLAND J. HAYES, JR.
*Vanderbilt University*

GABRIEL L. PLAA
*University of Montreal*

THE PUBLICATION OF THIS BOOK WAS PARTIALLY SUPPORTED BY PUBLIC HEALTH SERVICE GRANT NO. ES-00265.

# ESSAYS IN TOXICOLOGY
# Volume 4

*Edited by* WAYLAND J. HAYES, Jr.

CENTER IN TOXICOLOGY
DEPARTMENT OF BIOCHEMISTRY
SCHOOL OF MEDICINE
VANDERBILT UNIVERSITY
NASHVILLE, TENNESSEE

1973

ACADEMIC PRESS    New York and London

Copyright © 1973, by Academic Press, Inc.
ALL RIGHTS RESERVED.
NO PART OF THIS PUBLICATION MAY BE REPRODUCED OR
TRANSMITTED IN ANY FORM OR BY ANY MEANS, ELECTRONIC
OR MECHANICAL, INCLUDING PHOTOCOPY, RECORDING, OR ANY
INFORMATION STORAGE AND RETRIEVAL SYSTEM, WITHOUT
PERMISSION IN WRITING FROM THE PUBLISHER.

ACADEMIC PRESS, INC.
111 Fifth Avenue, New York, New York 10003

*United Kingdom Edition published by*
ACADEMIC PRESS, INC. (LONDON) LTD.
24/28 Oval Road, London NW1

LIBRARY OF CONGRESS CATALOG CARD NUMBER: 69-18335

PRINTED IN THE UNITED STATES OF AMERICA

# Contents

LIST OF CONTRIBUTORS .................................................... vii
PREFACE ................................................................. ix
CONTENTS OF PREVIOUS VOLUMES ............................................ xi

## 1. Drug Dependence: Whither the Drug?
### James M. Fujimoto

| | | |
|---|---|---|
| I. | Introduction | 1 |
| II. | Mechanism of Tolerance to Barbiturates by Changes in Drug Metabolism | 3 |
| III. | Distribution of Barbiturates to the Central Nervous System | 8 |
| IV. | Urinary Excretion of Barbiturates | 9 |
| V. | Unmasking the Culprit—Heroin | 12 |
| VI. | Metabolism of Morphine | 17 |
| VII. | Metabolic Transformation of Codeine to Morphine | 21 |
| VIII. | Metabolism of Naloxone | 23 |
| IX. | Excretion of Narcotics and Metabolites in Urine | 26 |
| X. | Transport in Brain | 39 |
| XI. | Placental Transfer | 41 |
| XII. | Biliary Excretion | 43 |
| XIII. | Certain Aspects of Metabolism of $\Delta^9$-Tetrahydrocannabinol | 47 |
| | References | 49 |

## 2. Kinetics of Active-Site-Directed Irreversible Inhibition
### A. R. Main

| | | |
|---|---|---|
| I. | Introduction | 59 |
| II. | Trivial Names and Symbols | 62 |
| III. | Origins | 64 |
| IV. | Kinetics | 72 |
| | References | 102 |

3. **Recondite Toxicity of Trace Elements**

   *Henry A. Schroeder*

|      |                                                                                          |     |
|------|------------------------------------------------------------------------------------------|-----|
| I.   | Introduction                                                                             | 108 |
| II.  | Specific Considerations                                                                  | 112 |
| III. | General Conclusions                                                                      | 115 |
| IV.  | Recondite Toxicity in Terms of Growth                                                    | 115 |
| V.   | Effects on Body Weights of Aged Animals                                                  | 124 |
| VI.  | Effects of Trace Elements on Survival and Longevity                                      | 124 |
| VII. | Effects on Tumors                                                                        | 126 |
| VIII.| Longevity and Median Life-Span                                                           | 129 |
| IX.  | Other Manifestations of Recondite Toxicity                                               | 132 |
| X.   | Recondite Toxicity of Trace Elements as Expressed by Effects on Reproduction of Rats and Mice | 151 |
| XI.  | Some Clues to Mechanisms of Toxicity                                                     | 156 |
| XII. | Production of Chronic Diseases Stimulating Human Disorders                               | 174 |
| XIII.| Recondite Toxicity of Other Metals or Elements in Man                                    | 186 |
| XIV. | Innate Toxicity from Water                                                               | 188 |
| XV.  | Summary and Conclusions                                                                  | 193 |
|      | References                                                                               | 194 |

AUTHOR INDEX .................................................................. 201
SUBJECT INDEX ................................................................. 207

# List of Contributors

JAMES M. FUJIMOTO, Department of Pharmacology, Medical College of Wisconsin, Milwaukee, Wisconsin

A. R. MAIN, Department of Biochemistry, North Carolina State University, Raleigh, North Carolina

HENRY A. SCHROEDER,[*] Department of Physiology, Emeritus, Dartmouth Medical School, Hanover, New Hampshire

---

[*] Present address: Trace Element Laboratory-Dartmouth Medical School, Brattleboro, Vermont.

# Preface

The articles that have been published thus far in *Essays in Toxicology* have been papers invited by the Editorial Board, a practice we intend to continue. However, volunteered papers now will be considered by the Board, although any paper of this kind should be discussed with the Editor before it is submitted. We are grateful to the authors whose papers have already been published for their enthusiasm and workmanship, including their regard for detail which has helped to lighten the Editor's task.

This series of essays was started in 1969 to provide persons with scientific training with informative insights into toxicology. It is still our aim to publish papers that may be read for pleasure by the specialist and for profit by the senior student. We are now probing the limits of that specification.

This volume contains three essays. One is on habituating drugs, a subject of considerable popular interest. The second is on kinetics, a matter of great importance in toxicology that unfortunately does not lend itself to a simple, nonmathematical approach. The last essay in this volume is a summary of a long, vigorous investigation that has opened up a completely new phase of toxicology—the hidden effects of trace elements. This masterful summary is more detailed than any we have offered previously. In addition to thorough coverage of its subject, it contains some of those simple observations that mark great research and might furnish clues for new developments, for example, the suppression of tumors by cadmium, nickel, arsenic, germanium, and titanium and the simple observation that animals dying of old age autolyze rapidly.

We hope that the inclusion of material that is more technical or is presented in more detail will prove welcome.

Wayland J. Hayes, Jr.

# Contents of Previous Volumes

Volume 1

Poisons as Tools in Studying the Nervous System
  RICHARD D. O'BRIEN
Teratology
  R. S. MCCUTCHEON
The Significance of Methemoglobinemia in Toxicology
  ROGER P. SMITH
Lead Poisoning. An Old Problem with a New Dimension
  P. B. HAMMOND
*Author Index—Subject Index*

Volume 2

Fungal Toxins
  EIVIND B. LILLEHOJ, ALEX CIEGLER, AND ROBERT W. DETROY
Hyperbilirubinemia and Cholestasis, a Different Form of Liver Injury Produced in Animals
  GABRIEL L. PLAA
The Vanishing Zero: The Evolution of Pesticide Analyses
  GUNTER ZWEIG
*Author Index—Subject Index*

Volume 3

The Vital Sacs: Alveolar Clearance Mechanisms in Inhalation Toxicology
  LOUIS J. CASARETT
The Effect of Physical Environmental Factors on Drug Response
  JOHN DOULL
Tests for Detecting and Measuring Long-Term Toxicity
  WAYLAND J. HAYES, JR.
Molecular Aspects of Toxicants
  ROBERT W. NEWBURGH
*Author Index—Subject Index*

Chapter 1

# Drug Dependence: Whither the Drug?

JAMES M. FUJIMOTO

|  |  |  |
|---|---|---|
| I. | Introduction | 1 |
| II. | Mechanism of Tolerance to Barbiturates by Changes in Drug Metabolism | 3 |
| III. | Distribution of Barbiturates to the Central Nervous System | 8 |
| IV. | Urinary Excretion of Barbiturates | 9 |
| V. | Unmasking the Culprit—Heroin | 12 |
| VI. | Metabolism of Morphine | 17 |
| VII. | Metabolic Transformation of Codeine to Morphine | 21 |
| VIII. | Metabolism of Naloxone | 23 |
| IX. | Excretion of Narcotics and Metabolites in Urine | 26 |
|  | A. Glomerular Filtration | 27 |
|  | B. Modification of Excretion by the pH-Dependent Process of Nonionic Diffusion and Ionic Trapping | 27 |
|  | C. Secretory Mechanisms for Excretion of Narcotic Analgesics | 29 |
|  | D. Renal Tubular Transport and Metabolism of Morphine in the Chicken | 31 |
|  | E. Urine Monitoring for Drug Abuse | 35 |
| X. | Transport in Brain | 39 |
| XI. | Placental Transfer | 41 |
| XII. | Biliary Excretion | 43 |
| XIII. | Certain Aspects of the Metabolism of $\Delta^9$–Tetrahydrocannabinol | 47 |
|  | References | 49 |

## I. INTRODUCTION

The purpose of this essay is to examine certain dependence-producing drugs from a constrained yet hopefully unique perspective. At the outset, it must be stated that the term, drug dependence, will be used in this essay in place of the somewhat ambiguous term, drug addiction *(1)*. Drug dependence in its broadest sense need not be confined to drugs but may include inhalation of solvents, ingestion of plant products, and smoking and snuffing of materials, including those not usually thought of as drugs but certainly definable as toxicants. The toxicological nature of drug dependence has, in fact, been emphasized by Berjerot *(2)*, who felt that all drug dependence in one way or another involved intoxication. The approach in this essay, however, will not cover such broad areas, nor will it endeavor to include the frequently discussed topics of etiology, sociology, penology, and medical treatment. Rather, the self-imposed constraint may be easily stated.

This essay will discuss certain dependence-producing drugs from the perspective of what the organism does to the drug. Since the organism is a much more complex entity than the drug, this approach to understanding drug action has the merit of studying the simpler of the two interdependent systems. If the organism did not do anything to the drug, the drug would have an infinitely long persistence in the body. The body possesses mechanisms by which drugs are eliminated and action terminated. One major process is metabolic transformation of the toxicant. It is no accident that termination of action by metabolic transformation has been often called a detoxication process. A most extensive survey of such processes is given in a book, "Detoxication Mechanisms," by R. T. Williams *(3)*. One of the present purposes is to examine detoxication processes for certain dependence-producing drugs. Obviously, if the metabolic process for detoxifying the drug can be speeded up, a more rapid termination and overall reduced intensity of drug action could be obtained. Concrete examples from the barbiturates establish this one mechanism for development of tolerance. Since detoxication reactions are carried on by enzymes which do not possess omniscient toxicological knowledge, the product of the reaction is not always inactive. In this context, the essay will discuss the formation of morphine from heroin and codeine, and *N*-dealkylation to form normorphine and to reduce naloxone to another compound.

Another mechanism for terminating drug action is excretion. The kidney, by its ability to filter blood and transport drugs, is of paramount importance. Some new insights into renal transport mechanisms are provided by studies with morphine. The liver also has an excretory function as regards bile. Major products of morphine metabolism are excreted in bile, and some new information on biliary excretion will be examined. In the more general area of translocation of drugs from one tissue compartment to another, certain tissues possess mechanisms for delimiting drug action by controlling the ultimate accessibility of the drug to an organ. The barrier which exists to certain drugs in the central nervous system explains quantitative differences between such drugs as heroin and morphine. Some interesting studies have been reported on transport mechanisms in the central nervous system; transplacental transfer of narcotics will also be considered.

## II. MECHANISM OF TOLERANCE TO BARBITURATES BY CHANGES IN DRUG METABOLISM

Tolerance is measured quantitatively either in terms of the change in magnitude of *response* to a constant dose of the toxicant or the change in the *dose* necessary to produce a constant response. If several different responses to a given dose are measured, it is possible that the rate and magnitude of development of tolerance will be different for each of the responses. The individual may have become completely tolerant to the euphoric action of heroin while retaining an undiminished sensitivity to its pupillary constricting effect. Using another permutation, one response may be measured during separate administration of two different drugs. If this single response shows tolerance to both drugs, there is said to be *cross tolerance* between the two drugs for that response. If tolerance occurs to one drug but not to the other drug, there is no cross tolerance between the drugs. Thus, extensive cross tolerance can occur to the respiratory depressant effect of heroin and morphine, but little cross tolerance occurs to the the respiratory depressant effect of these drugs and that of pentobarbital. These preliminary statements are made because all drugs have more than one site of action, and it is well to remember that in the discussion to follow, an attempt has been made to isolate one mechanism of tolerance at a time. By manipulating the experimental parameters, a particular mechanism of tolerance may become overt, but extrapolations based on the experiments must be made with caution.

Basically there are two broad ways in which tolerance occurs. The first involves a dispositional phenomenon of tolerance referable to the drug where the absorption, fate, distribution, or excretion of the drug may be altered; this approach is the one under prime consideration in this essay. The second involves changes in the sensitivity of the organism, an approach which would ultimately be concerned with receptor phenomena. Tolerance mechanisms then may be examined by looking for changes in what the organism does to the drug or changes in what the drug does to the organism. With the barbiturates both tolerance mechanisms are seen.

Tolerance to barbiturates through a dispositional mechanism was clearly established by Remmer and his group *(4–6)*. As Remmer indicated, the stage had been set for his work by the findings of Brodie's laboratory *(7)* that various drugs are oxidized by microsomal enzymes in the liver and that barbiturates such as hexobarbital and pentobarbital lose their hypnotic effect after oxidation. Remmer reasoned that in animals which had developed tolerance to barbiturates, increased oxidation of the barbiturate might be occurring, and if so, such changes ought to be demonstrable *in vitro* and *in vivo*. Starting in 1958 *(5,6)* Remmer and his group successfully filled in the major details for this tolerance concept *(4,8–10)*.

In Figs. 1 and 2, several facets of tolerance by this enzymatic mechanism are seen. Rats treated with pentobarbital for 2 or 16 days manifested

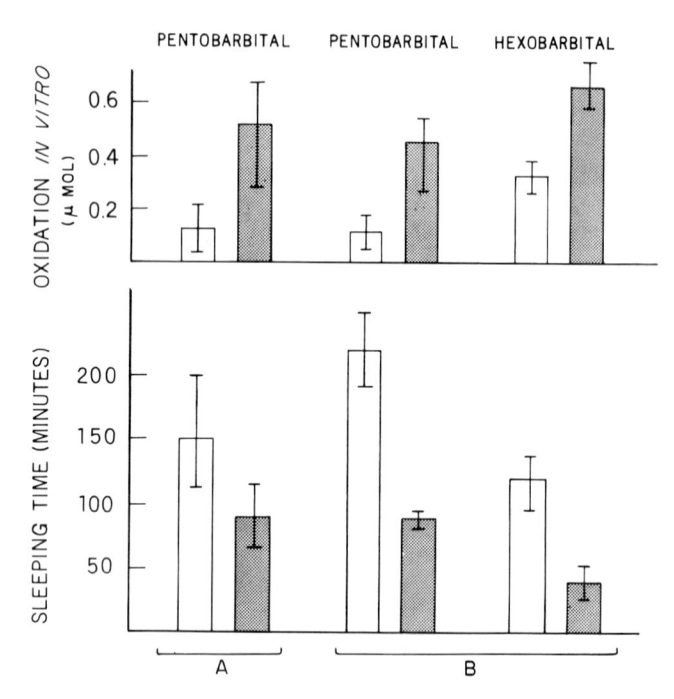

FIG. 1. The development of tolerance to pentobarbital in female rats. Open bars = controls; solid bars = experimental group. Bottom panel: in A, experimental rats were treated for 2 days with pentobarbital, in B for 16 days. Twenty-four hours after termination of the treatment, the sleeping time to another dose of pentobarbital or hexobarbital was measured. Top panel: corresponding measurements were made on ability of liver supernatant preparation from these rats to oxidize the drugs *in vitro*. Pentobarbital pretreated rats (A and B) showed tolerance to pentobarbital and hexobarbital by a decrease in sleeping time and an increase in ability to oxidize pentobarbital and hexobarbital. Modified and redrawn from Remmer *(4)* with permission of Little, Brown and Company.

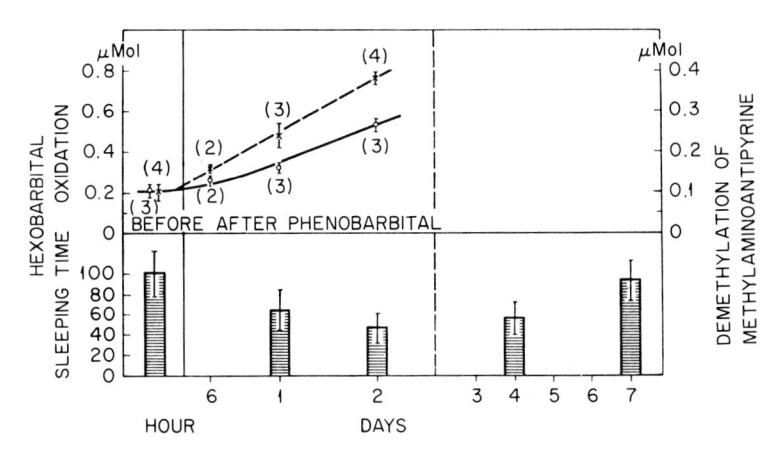

FIG. 2. Development of cross tolerance to hexobarbital by pretreatment with phenobarbital in rats. Abscissa: time after pretreatment with a single dose of phenobarbital in rats. Ordinate: the sleeping time response to hexobarbital and ability of *in vitro* liver preparation to oxidise hexobarbital (- - -) and demethylate methylaminoantipyrine (——) were measured. Phenobarbital pretreated rats were cross tolerant to hexobarbital as seen by a reduced sleeping time to hexobarbital with tolerance effects persisting for 4 days. Increased oxidation of hexobarbital and demethylation of methylaminoantipyrine occurred as well. Adapted from Remmer *(8)* with permission of Springer Verlag, Berlin.

tolerance to pentobarbital by a shortened sleeping time, that is, the effect of the same dose of pentobarbital was less in tolerant rats than in control rats. Correlated with this tolerance was an increased rate of oxidation of pentobarbital in the *in vitro* microsomal enzyme preparation. Interestingly, cross tolerance to another barbiturate, hexobarbital, occurred in rats tolerant to pentobarbital, an effect seen as a shortened sleeping time to hexobarbital; the microsomal enzyme fractions prepared from pentobarbital-treated rat liver oxidized hexobarbital more rapidly than did those from control rats. This same kind of cross tolerance may be seen in Fig. 2; a single dose of phenobarbital was shown to produce tolerance to hexobarbital at the same time that oxidation of hexobarbital was increased. The cross tolerance effect was characterized by a slow onset, starting at about 1 day after the phenobarbital pretreatment, and persisting for a number of days. Note that another microsomal enzyme activity, demethylation of methylaminoantipyrine, was also enhanced, as was the oxidation of hexobarbital. Table I shows the effect of 6 days of treatment with several short- and long-acting barbiturates. Regardless of the class of barbiturate, all reduced the biological half-life of hexobarbital. Thus, these experiments and those by others *(11)* established the concept that one mechanism for tolerance to barbiturates is increased oxidation of barbiturates by the liver.

TABLE I

THE EFFECT OF 6 DAYS OF PRETREATMENT WITH VARIOUS BARBITURATES (SUBCUTANEOUSLY) ON HALF-LIFE OF HEXOBARBITAL IN MICE[a]

| Pretreatment | Daily dose (mg/kg) | Hexobarbital half-life (minutes) |
|---|---|---|
| Saline | — | 81 |
| Hexobarbital | 100 | 41 |
| Butallylonal | 70 | 38 |
| Thiopenthal | 50 | 31 |
| Phenobarbital | 100 | 29 |
| Barbital | 100 | 19 |

[a] From Remmer (5).

Observations on the stimulatory effect of barbiturates on the hepatic microsomal metabolism of other drugs and the inducing effects of other drugs on barbiturate oxidation were quickly extended (11–14). One of the most exhaustive lists of both inducers and systems induced has been compiled by Mannering (14). Examination of any such list leads to the realization that both the inducing effect of the barbiturates on metabolism of other drugs and the inducing effect of other drugs on barbiturate metabolism have broad specificity as to the chemical nature of the substrate and inducer. This broad specificity harmonizes with the original concept that many drug metabolism reactions carried on by the microsomal enzymes are considered to be hydroxylation reactions requiring molecular oxygen and NADPH mediated by mixed function oxidase (15). The phenomenon of induction has had not only the practical effect of revealing a mechanism for tolerance to barbiturates but has opened up new approaches to studying the fundamental nature of many drug detoxication reactions. The discovery of the inducing effect has broached the mechanism not only for the synthesis of more enzyme protein but for synthesis and function of a closely associated system called cytochrome $P_{450}$. Also, comparison of differences in inducing action between the barbiturates and other agents has provided insights into the basic biochemistry of microsomal enzymes. These and other related areas are under intensive study but are not within the scope of the present discussion. The reader can gain a good general view of these areas from several excellent books which have recently been published (12,13,16).

In retrospect, some of the earliest studies (1947) on the basic mechanisms relating to action of inducing agents on the liver were performed by Brazda and his associates using a compound called nikethamide (17,18). They not only studied structure–activity relationships for stimulation of liver growth but also found effects on nucleic acid and protein metabolism *(19,20)*. It is interesting that although these early studies are rarely cited, subsequent studies have shown that nikethamide induces increased barbiturate metabolism *(21,22)*. These studies are mentioned because nikethamide was being used clinically as an analeptic agent in treating barbiturate poisoning, as it possessed moderate central nervous system stimulant actions. As it turned out, the finding that nikethamide favors enzyme production was of little consequence in the rationale of the treatment since the induction of enzymes is too slow to be of any value to a victim on the threshold of immediate death from acute barbiturate poisoning. On the other hand, the subsequent waning of the clinical use of nikethamide may have arisen in part from yet another discovery, namely, that the immediate action of nikethamide is to inhibit barbiturate metabolism *(21,23)*. Figure 3 shows that nikethamide had a diphasic effect on hexobarbital action. The enzyme-induction phase corresponds to the response, where shortening of hexobarbital sleeping time occurs. Profound prolongation of hexobarbital sleeping time corresponds to the phase of inhibition of barbiturate metabolism. Because of its initial inhibitory

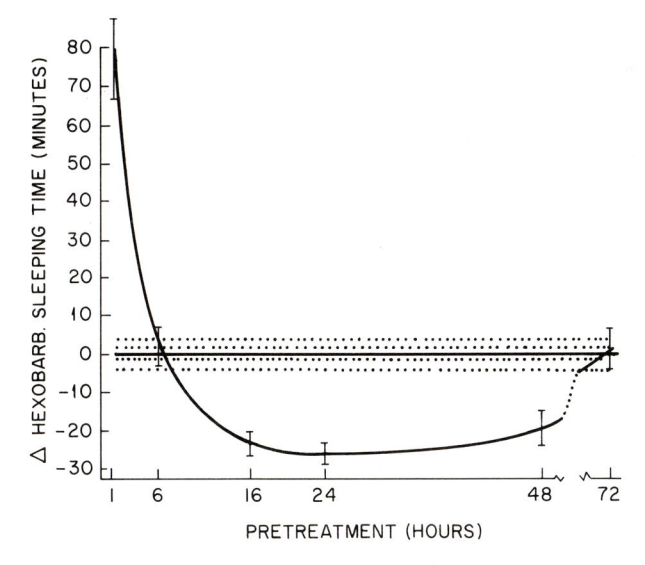

FIG. 3. The diphasic effect of nikethamide—relationship between hexobarbital sleeping time in mice and the period of pretreatment with nikethamide. The abscissa gives the interval in hours between the administration of nikethamide (200 mg/kg, p.o.) and the hexobarbital sodium (150 mk/kg, i.p.). The ordinate gives the change in mean hexobarbital sleeping time compared with the control. The control sleeping time is indicated by the horizontal line at zero; the actual control sleeping time was 63.8 minutes. The dotted area is the standard error for each control group. From Serrone and Fujimoto *(23)* with permission of Pergamon Press, Oxford.

effect, the clinical use of nikethamide for treating acute intoxication by certain barbiturates becomes questionable. The diphasic effect of nikethamide was found to occur with other microsomal enzyme inhibitors; compounds such as N-methyl-3-piperidyl-$N',N'$-diphenyl carbamate *(24)* and SKF 525A *(23,25)* initially inhibit and subsequently stimulate barbiturate metabolism.

Even though there has been an emphasis on the biochemical aspects of enzyme induction as evident from the volume of original research publications, more physiologically oriented investigations have not been overlooked. For instance, phenobarbital-induced mice cleared sulfobromophthalein *(26)* and indocyanine green *(27)* from the blood faster than did control mice. Since neither of these two drugs was metabolized by the microsomal enzyme system, the results suggested yet another effect of the phenobarbital on elimination of drugs. Work by Plaa and his associates *(28–30)* and by Klaassen *(31, 32)* systematically established that phenobarbital induction increases bile flow and biliary excretion of many drugs, including sulfobromophthalein and indocyanine green. These workers have provided some critically needed new approaches to studying the physiology of biliary excretion. The possibility that phenobarbital induction might increase the rate of delivery of drugs to the liver had been entertained *(27,33)*; recent work by Ohnhaus et al. *(34)* and Brodeur and Marchand *(35)* demonstrates clearly an increase in blood flow to the liver in phenobarbital-induced animals. Thus, the work which started out to seek clear explanation of one mechanism of tolerance by studying the oxidation of barbiturates has cascaded into areas of new research; it appears that barbiturate effects may have far-reaching consequences for further research.

## III. DISTRIBUTION OF BARBITURATES TO THE CENTRAL NERVOUS SYSTEM

Even though enzyme induction is clearly involved in the mechanism of tolerance to barbiturates, the central nervous system itself develops tolerance by a mechanism independent from that of enzyme induction in the liver. As intimated in the previous section, enzyme induction would play a greater role in tolerance to those barbiturates that depend on metabolism by the liver to terminate their action. For other barbiturates, particularly the long-acting, more slowly metabolized ones, enzyme induction does not explain tolerance. Here, the sensitivity of the central nervous system has been found to decrease. In this situation, studying the disposition of the barbiturate to the central nervous system has given some critical answers. The work on barbital, a compound whose action is terminated more by excretion than by metabolism, will serve to illustrate the point. Ebert, Yim, and Miya *(36)* showed that at a time when the mean brain concentrations of barbital were identical, the tolerant group manifested less barbiturate action than did the control group. Remmer, Siegert, Nitze and Kirsten *(37)* showed that, at the time when both tolerant and nontolerant rats awoke from barbital, the tolerant group had brain concentrations of barbital 35–50% higher than did the nontolerant group. The results from both studies lead to the conclusion that animals tolerant to barbital must have a specific decreased sensitivity of the central nervous system. The validity of this conclusion rests in turn upon the fact that the action of barbital is correlated normally with the concentration and persistence of the barbiturate in the central nervous system, a correlation derived by Butler *(38)*.

A well-known reverse tolerance phenomenon to thiopental was also elucidated by studying drug disposition. Even though thiopental had a short duration of action after a single dose, repeated doses were known to produce longer and longer effects *(39)*, that is, instead of tolerance, the drug produced unpredicted cumulative effects. Several groups provided the answer to this phenomenon *(39–41)*. The rapid disappearance of the thiopental in the initial dose was found to be due to redistribution of the thiopental to other tissues, primarily skeletal muscle. On repetition of the dose, this source of storage of thiopental became less and less efficient in redistributing thiopental away from the brain. Also, storage in fat depots became a factor. Thus, repeated injections produced longer- and longer-lasting effects. By following the kinetics of what was happening to the drug, an explanation was found to what otherwise might have been a mysterious phenomenon.

## IV. URINARY EXCRETION OF BARBITURATES

Some measure of control could be exercised on excretion of certain barbiturates in the urine if the rate of excretion of the particular barbiturate were sensitive to changes in urinary pH. Then, the simple expedient of changing the urinary pH would serve to enhance excretion of the barbiturate for therapeutic treatment of barbiturate poisoning. Even though all the commonly used barbiturates are filtered at the glomerulus, they are efficiently reabsorbed through the renal tubular cells as the glomerular filtrate courses down the tubular lumen. Large amounts of the water in the filtrate are reabsorbed by the tubules in the normal course of conserving body water, and the urine is usually acidified. Both processes

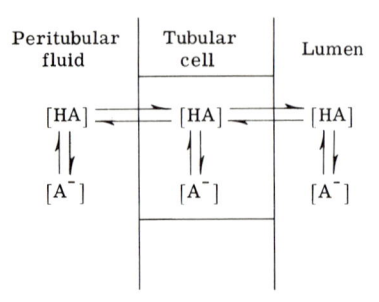

```
Peritubular  | Tubular  | Lumen
   fluid     |  cell    |
             |          |
  [HA]   ⇌   [HA]   ⇌   [HA]
   ⇅          ⇅          ⇅
  [A⁻]       [A⁻]       [A⁻]
```

FIG. 4. Urinary excretion of an acid (HA) by nonionic diffusion and pH gradient ionic trapping mechanism in the kidney. For explanation see text.

work in favor of reabsorption of the barbiturates so that with many barbiturates urinary excretion of the free barbiturate is low. If, however, the barbiturate has a $pK_a$ such that large changes in its dissociation can be imposed by changes in the urinary pH, a means of obtaining enhanced excretion is available. The general concept is illustrated in Fig. 4. Phenobarbital has a $pK_a = 7.2$ and can be represented as an acid dissociation where HA $\rightleftarrows$ H⁺ + A⁻ and $pK_a$ = pH − log (A⁻)/(HA). As pictured, the undissociated form (uncharged form) penetrates through the tubular cell whereas the anionic form does not. The undissociated form is relatively nonpolar, and this lipophilic property confers on phenobarbital the ability to penetrate biological membranes having lipid properties. The anion is, on the other hand, highly polar, hydrophilic, and not lipophilic, so it does not readily penetrate the renal tubular cells. Under these conditions, it can be seen that if the urine has a lower pH than the plasma, the phenobarbital will be reabsorbed. If, however, the urinary pH can be made less acid by administering a urinary alkalinizing agent such as sodium bicarbonate, a large shift in the ratio of (A⁻)/(HA) in favor of (A⁻) in the urine can be achieved. Thus, by this pH-dependent ionic trapping mechanism, increased excretion of phenobarbital is achieved. The practical application of alkalinizing agents for treating phenobarbital poisoning is thereby apparent. The work by Waddell and Butler *(42)* and Milne *et al.* *(43)* dealt with this concept in greater depth. The early work of Clowes *et al.* *(44)* at the cellular level was amazing for the clarity with which pH effects on barbiturate distribution were presented. Others applied the same concepts to absorption of barbiturates from the gastrointestinal tract *(45)*.

Another facet of the same phenomenon is seen in Fig. 5. It will be noted that the excretion of phenobarbital follows a circadian (approximately

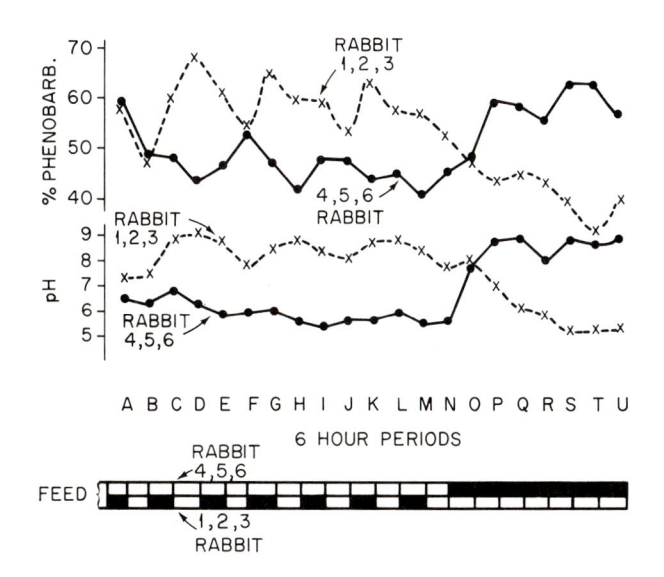

FIG. 5. Relationship of the feeding schedule to the pH of the urine and the excretion of phenobarbital. Phenobarbital-2-$^{14}$C was given intravenously at A to 6 rabbits. Urine samples were collected every 6 hours. Rabbits were fed (dark area) and fasted (blank area) according to the schedule shown at the bottom. The middle panel shows the pH of the 6-hour urine samples and the top panel shows phenobarbital excretion expressed as percentage of total radioactivity in each urine sample accounted for as phenobarbital. Note the close parallelism between pH and excretion of phenobarbital. From Fujimoto and Donnelly (46) with permission of Marcel Dekker, New York.

daily) cycle. The circadian character of the excretion of phenobarbital was seen to be correlated with diurnal changes in pH of the urine of the rabbits. Furthermore, Fig. 5 shows that the schedule of feeding and fasting influenced the results. In the fasting state, the urinary pH was constantly low, excretion of phenobarbital decreased, and the circadian rhythm in excretion was hard to see. When a schedule of fasting and feeding was instituted, large oscillations in pH of the urine were obtained, and increased phenobarbital excretion occurred during the times when pH was high. This schedule did not override the circadian rhythm since two cycles of feeding and fasting resulted in one cycle of pH changes. This particular study emphasized the fact that a very simple explanation was available for the circadian effect, namely, the pH changes. But, on the whole, circadian phenomena are highly complex and difficult to explain (47). Further examples of urinary pH–drug excretion correlations are given in a subsequent section on excretion of narcotic analgesics.

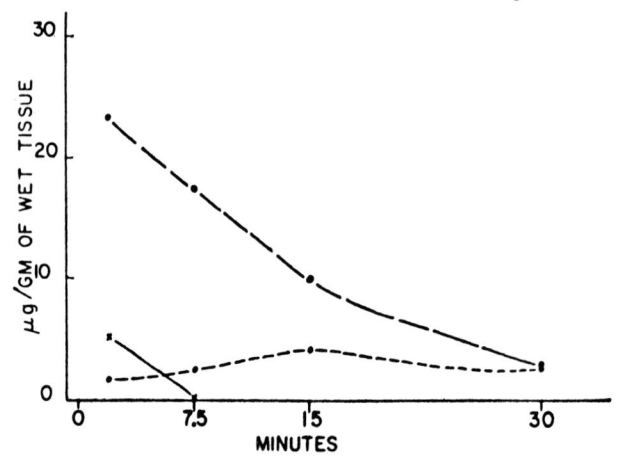

FIG. 6. Brain levels of heroin (X—X), 6-monoacetylmorphine (●—●), and morphine (●— —●) at specific time intervals following administration of 37.5 mg/kg heroin intravenously in mice. From Way et al. *(51)* with permission of Williams & Wilkins, Baltimore.

## V. UNMASKING THE CULPRIT—HEROIN

A drug may be changed by the organism into a compound which is the active form of the administered drug. A case in point is heroin, where the effects appear to be derived from hydrolysis products formed within the organism. Just as unmasking the culprit is one step closer to solving the crime, recognition of an active product is one step closer to understanding the action of the drug. On the other hand, unmasking an active product may for a time create a problem in itself. The fact that all the urinary excretion products of heroin are identical to those of morphine had for a long time created a paradox: It appeared that heroin should be identical in potency to morphine, but it really is more potent. Let us see how the paradox recently was resolved.

More than 40 years ago, reports began to appear that heroin may be excreted in the urine as morphine. Subsequent work has confirmed these reports *(48–50)*. In 1942, Wright *(49)* proffered arguments based on substantial experimental data that the conversion of heroin to morphine by the liver was fast enough to account for all the action of heroin, being mediated by the morphine formed. Though the arguments were persuasive, certain anomalies could not be explained. In man, heroin was generally known to be more potent than morphine. For this very reason, morphine is converted chemically to heroin for the illicit drug market. In mice, heroin was about four times more potent than morphine by subcutaneous injection and about seven times more potent than morphine by

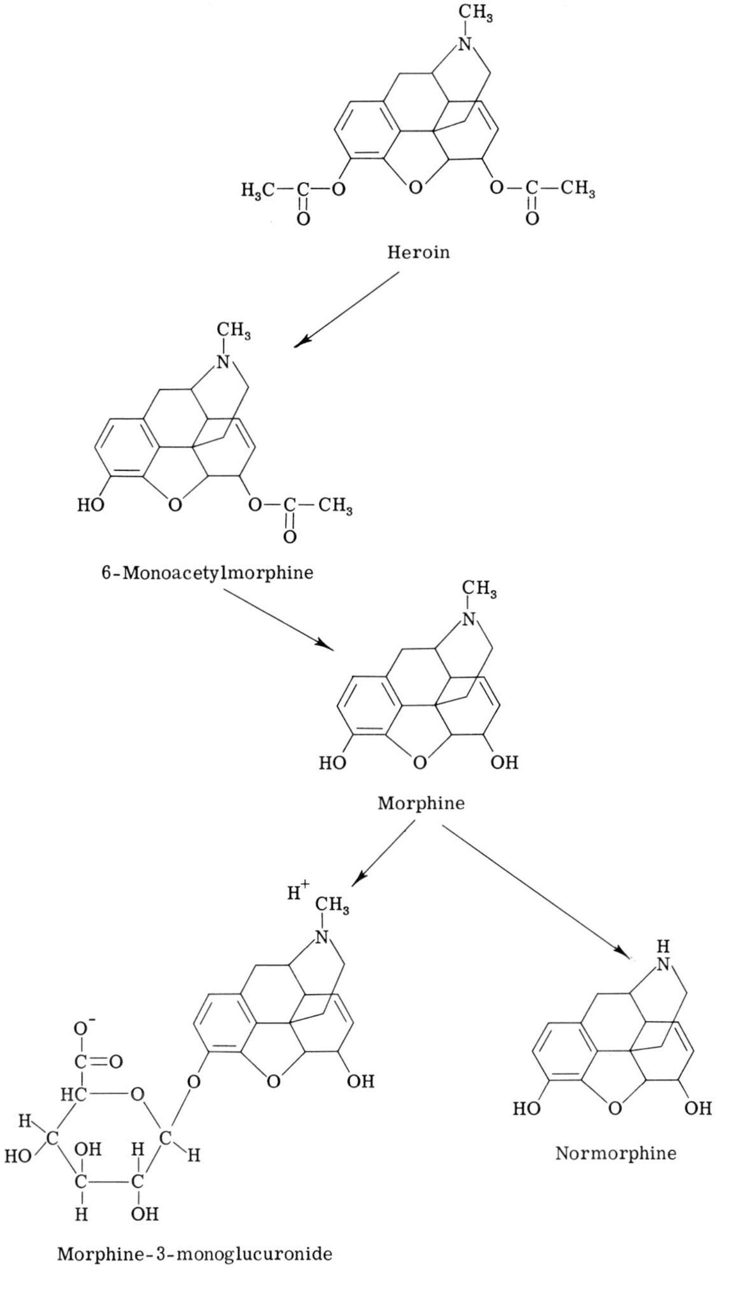

FIG. 7. Major pathways for metabolism of heroin.

intravenous administration *(51)*. If all the action of heroin were due to morphine, it would seem that the potency of heroin should be identical to that of morphine or even less if the metabolism were sufficiently slow. Way and his colleagues resolved this paradox and provided the critical analysis based on the distribution and metabolism of heroin.

Figure 6 illustrates the data from Way *et al. (51)* on the brain concentrations of heroin, 6-monoacetylmorphine, and morphine after intravenous administration of heroin to mice. Note that the concentration of heroin in the brain was low and that it disappeared rapidly from the brain within 10 minutes. Since the pharmacologic action of the drug was sustained well beyond 10 minutes, the results suggested that heroin, if active at all, contributes only to a short initial action and that the more sustained effect must be due to the other compounds formed. Hydrolysis of the 3-acetyl group from heroin (Fig. 7) led to formation of 6-monoacetylmorphine; the concentration of this metabolite in the brain was impressively high initially and declined at a relatively fast rate. Formation of morphine occurred by hydrolysis of both acetyl groups from the heroin through the pathway shown in Fig. 7. Morphine concentrations built up slowly in the brain but were more persistent than either heroin or 6-monoacetylmorphine concentrations. The next important step in establishing the hypothesis that these metabolites are the compounds responsible for the pharmacologic action was the comparison of the toxicity of these compounds by various routes of administration as seen in Table II. After intravenous administration, heroin was the most potent (lowest $LD_{50}$) and morphine the least potent drug. The same order of activity held upon subcutaneous administration. However, application of these compounds directly to the central nervous system (where the drugs act) led to a completely different order. Notice that morphine had the lowest $LD_{50}$ by intracerebral administration!

Taking a relative potency of 1 for heroin by intracerebral administration, the relative potencies of morphine and 6-monoacetylmorphine be-

TABLE II

Toxicity ($LD_{50}$) of Heroin, 6-Monacetylmorphine (MAM) and Morphine in Mice with Different Routes of Administration[a]

| Compound | Intravenous (mg/kg) | Intracerebral (mg/kg) |
|---|---|---|
| Heroin | 38 (33–43) [b] | 15 (10–22) |
| MAM | 93 (81–105) | 35 (25–49) |
| Morphine | 258 (217–307) | 6.1 (4.1–9.1) |

[a] Adapted from Way *et al. (51)* with permission of Williams & Wilkins, Baltimore.
[b] Figures in parentheses represent 19/20 confidence limits for the $LD_{50}$.

come, respectively, $16/6.1 = 2.46$, and $13/35 = 0.43$ times that of heroin. Therefore, these relative potencies had to be taken into account when assessing the importance of the metabolite concentration in the brain. At a relative potency of 2.46, the contribution of morphine to the total pharmacologic activity is represented by an area 2.46 times greater than that under the morphine curve pictured in Fig. 6. The relative contribution of 6-monoacetylmorphine would be reduced to 0.43 times that indicated in Fig. 6, and the area for heroin would be unchanged. Then, as Way and his colleagues concluded, it becomes evident that the greatest part of the action of heroin is due to the morphine, some is due to the 6-monoacetylmorphine, and only a small initial amount of the action is due to the heroin itself.

The problem of the difference in potency between heroin and morphine was also considered. It appeared that there exists a greater barrier to the passage of morphine into the central nervous system than for heroin. Morphine is less potent than heroin by intravenous administration because of the presence of this barrier to passage of morphine into the central nervous system. In essence then, the greater potency of heroin by usual modes of administration and also as a street drug is due to easier penetration of heroin into the central nervous system than morphine. Once in the brain, heroin is rapidly hydrolyzed to 6-monoacetylmorphine

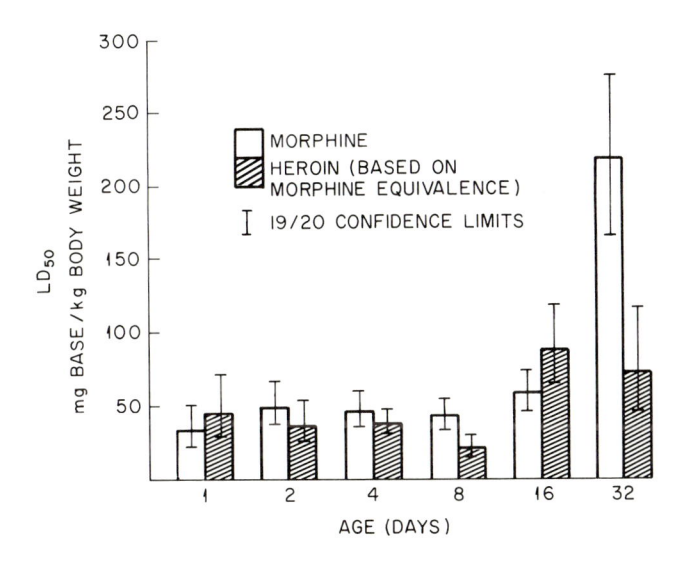

FIG. 8. Lethality of morphine and heroin in rats of varying age after intraperitoneal administration. From Kupferberg and Way (53) and Way (52) with permission of Williams & Wilkins, Baltimore.

and morphine, the two metabolites of heroin, which are responsible for the action.

The postulate that a blood–brain barrier exists for morphine but not for heroin was advanced further by the work of Kupferberg and Way *(53)* on the age dependency of $LD_{50}$ values for morphine and heroin. Note in Fig. 8 that up to 16 days of age, the $LD_{50}$ values for heroin and for morphine by intraperitoneal injection are similar. But, between the 16th and 32nd day of age, a drastic increase in $LD_{50}$ for morphine occurs, whereas the $LD_{50}$ for heroin remains about the same. This sudden increase in $LD_{50}$ for morphine corresponds to development of the blood–brain barrier for morphine as shown in Fig. 9, which depicts the brain and blood concentrations of morphine in 16- vs. 32-day-old rats. The 50- and 150-mg/kg doses were the equitoxic ones ($LD_{30}$) for the 16- and 32-day-old rats, respectively. At these equitoxic doses the brain concentration of morphine is about the same in the two groups, indicating that the brain in the 16-day-old rat has about the same sensitivity to morphine as in the 32-day-old rat. Yet, three times more morphine on a unit-body-weight basis has to be given in the 32-day-old rat than in the 16-day-old rat to achieve similar biological brain concentrations. In order to achieve these parallel concentrations in the brain, greater concentra-

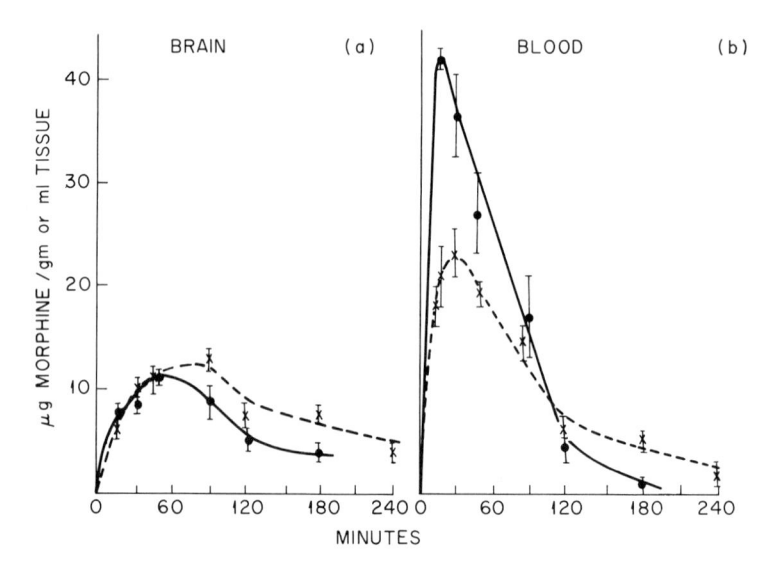

FIG. 9. (a) Brain and (b) blood concentrations of morphine in 16- and 32-day-old rats given morphine intraperitoneally. Comparisons are based on dosages that are equitoxic ($LD_{30}$). X—-X, 16 day old, 50 mg/kg; ●—●, 32 day old, 150 mg/kg. Adapted from Kupferberg and Way *(53)* with permission of Williams & Wilkins, Baltimore.

tion gradients have to exist from the blood to the brain in older than in younger rats. This need for higher concentration gradients means that in the older rat, there is a functional blood–brain barrier to passage of morphine into the central nervous system. In the younger rats a smaller gradient is necessary because less barrier exists. For heroin, no such barrier exists in either the young or older rats; the $LD_{50}$ therefore does not change with age. The implications of these studies were that, as the brain develops, a mechanism of resistance to morphine develops. Obviously, where this resistance mechanism is not present, as for instance in the fetus *in utero*, problems of morphine toxicity arise, a subject covered in Section XI.

## VI. METABOLISM OF MORPHINE

Some detailing of the metabolism of morphine is of interest because morphine serves as the prototype for the narcotic analgesics. Also, heroin is converted into morphine, and certain of the changes in metabolism of morphine per se have been investigated as a possible source of explanation for development of tolerance.

The major part of the dose of morphine is metabolized to morphine-3-glucuronide in man *(54,55)* and in commonly used laboratory animals such as the dog *(56,57)*, guinea pig, mouse, rat, and rabbit *(58–60)*. This metabolite is inactive by systemic administration, so that this conjugation of morphine with glucuronic acid leads to detoxication. At first it appeared that changes in this major pathway for detoxication might explain the development of tolerance to morphine *(61)*, but evidence indicates that only minimal changes occur and that they are not commensurate with the large degree of tolerance obtained with morphine *(62,63)*. Unlike tolerance to barbiturates, tolerance to morphine cannot be explained by enzyme induction occurring in the major pathway for metabolism.

A recent turn of events has demonstrated why it is so important to have unequivocal identification of metabolites. The major metabolite, morphine-3-glucuronide, is inactive but a minor metabolite, morphine-6-glucuronide, has been found to possess activity *(64)*. Synthetic morphine-6-glucuronide, when injected subcutaneously, is three to four times more potent and twice as long-lasting in duration of analgesic action than is morphine. Thus, it does make a big difference whether the conjugation with glucuronic acid occurs at the 3 or the 6 position of morphine. Fortunately, it has been established that morphine-3-glucuronide is the major metabolite and morphine-6-glucuronide is a minor metabolite *(58,59,60,64,65)*, so that discovery of high activity for morphine-6-glucuronide has not resulted in any confusion of the relationship of metabolism to pharmacologic activity. Another minor pathway appears to be methylation of the 3-OH group of morphine to form codeine *(66)*.

Studies on the metabolism and distribution of narcotic analgesics have provided two concepts which have attempted to unify the approach to understanding the mechanism of action and development of tolerance to narcotic analgesics. If one looks at the different narcotic analgesics for common features about their metabolism, a single process stands out above all else. That process is *N*-dealkylation to form NOR compounds. The portion remaining after removal of the alkyl group is designated as a NOR compound, *N*itrogen *o*hne (without) *R*adical. Evidence cited in several review articles *(62,67)* amply indicates that dealkylation of meperidine, codeine, methadone, and morphine occur. Lesser known analgesics as well as nalorphine, a narcotic antagonist possessing some morphine-like activity, are also dealkylated.

The two hypotheses that incorporate this feature, *N*-dealkylation, were propounded in the mid-1950s. The one by Beckett's group *(68,69,70)* proposed that *N*-dealkylation is an important first step in the production of analgesia. The proposal by Axelrod *(71)* relates a decrease in *N*-dealkylation to development of tolerance to narcotic analgesics.

Chronicling of the events leading up to these two hypotheses and the marshaling of arguments for and against the two hypotheses are thoughtfully reviewed by Way and Adler *(62)*. Because of the heuristic aspects of Beckett's hypothesis, the main thoughts behind the proposal will be presented without involvement in the arguments against the hypothesis. Beckett's group pictured narcotic analgesics such as morphine combining with receptors in the central nervous system by making a 3-point attachment to the receptor surface. This 3-point attachment confers stereospecificity to the drug–receptor interaction. In this interaction, they visualized the receptor being activated as the drug on the receptor is dealkylated. This hypothesis immediately brings up the possibility that the NOR compounds are the active intermediates. Because Miller *et al. (72)* had found that normorphine, the possible intermediate, possesses low analgesic activity on systemic administration, the hypothesis might have been short lived. Lockett and Davis *(73)*, in a timely report, found that normorphine, applied directly to the central nervous system by intracisternal administration, does have analgesic activity. Furthermore, the action of normorphine develops a little more rapidly than that of morphine. The practical value of Beckett's hypothesis was demonstrated when this work stimulated others to look for the required process of normorphine formation right in the brain. Milthers *(74)* presented *in vivo* evidence that normorphine is formed in the brain itself and added the precautionary note that although this finding supported Beckett's hypothesis, the hypothesis was still far from proved. Elison and Elliott *(75)* incubated brain slices with $N^{14}CH_3$ morphine, codeine, and meperidine and observed liberation of $^{14}CO_2$, thus demonstrating that there are enzymes present in the brain to carry on the dealkylation.

Another tenet to the hypothesis is that, as the alkyl group on the nitrogen increases in size from methyl to ethyl to allyl, the attraction between the receptor and the drug increases but the rate of dealkylation of the drug on the receptor decreases. This idea of increased binding to the receptor with decreased rate of dealkylation agrees with the fact that narcotic agonist action decreases and narcotic antagonist action increases in going from methyl substitution of morphine to the allyl substitution as found in nalorphine (*N*-allylnormorphine) *(76,77)*. Thus nalorphine, as was already known, is an antagonist to morphine. Interestingly this tenet of the hypothesis predicts that formation of normorphine from nalorphine should be slower than formation of normophine from morphine. That normorphine should be formed at all appears to be consistent with the fact that nalorphine, even though it is an antagonist in the presence of morphine, possesses by itself some morphine-like agonist activity. Milthers *(74)* did find that dealkylation of nalorphine in the brain is slower than that of morphine. In this context, the recent observation by Weinstein *et al.* *(78)* that naloxone, a potent narcotic anatagonist, undergoes dealkylation of the allyl group, provokes consideration of the hypothesis. If one extrapolates from the previous analogies, then the dealkylated product, nornaloxone, would be expected to have some morphine-like activity. Up to now, in mammalian species, naloxone appears to have "pure antagonist" action, but the existence of the hypothesis does suggest the need to look deeper into this "pure antagonist" action. The discovery of endoetheno–oripavine-type compounds such as etorphine, which has more than 1000 times the analgesic potency of morphine *(79)*, offers a new challenge to the dealkylation hypothesis. If the dealkylation of etorphine is the first step in analgesia and only a small amount of etorphine is dealkylated in the brain, then the active form of etorphine must indeed be present there in minute quantities. This intermediate must be extremely potent, and we would be approaching a highly specific drug receptor interaction where the usual surfeit of drug over that of the receptor would be reduced.

Like Beckett's hypothesis, the hypothesis put forward by Axelrod is amenable to direct experimental scrutiny. Axelrod *(71)* proposed that the *N*-demethylating system in the liver microsomal fraction might be a model system which is exemplary of the way in which the receptor sites in the CNS might change as tolerance develops to narcotic analgesics. Thus, chronic treatment of the rat with morphine is shown to depress the $N$-demethylating activity of the liver enzyme system, much as may be happening to the receptors in the CNS. The strongest piece of supporting evidence for demethylation playing a role in tolerance is that specificity exists for the depression of demethylation. Demethylation of cocaine is not depressed, whereas demethylation of morphine as well as of certain of the other narcotic analgesics is depressed in morphine-tolerant rats. These observations are consonant with the fact that cross tolerance does not occur between morphine and cocaine but does occur between individual drugs within the narcotic analgesic group. Subsequent work by many others has shown the kind of specificity envisaged by Axelrod for the $N$-dealkylating system could not be retained *(62,67)*. Even though the model has been found to be imperfect at this stage of knowledge of the molecular processes and receptor mechanisms, it may be wise not to discard the model too early. If one takes the broad point of view that tolerance is a manifestation of an allosteric change in the morphine receptor *(80)*, Axelrod's hypothesis may yet have redeeming value. The susceptibility of the $N$-dealkylating enzyme activity to endocrine and nutritional influences, to sex differences, and to species variability *(67)* may likewise involve allosteric changes in the morphine receptor perhaps not unlike those which might occur during development of tolerance. It appears now that any primary hypothesis on tolerance to narcotic analgesics should involve considerations on receptor phenomena.

The possibility exists that the development of tolerance and physical dependence could be due to still another product formed by the metabolism of morphine. In a recent report, Misra, Mitchell, and Woods *(81)* gave witness to the occurrence of a long persistence in the brain of radioactive material formed from morphine-$N$-$^{14}CH_3$. The material persisted for at least 3 weeks after a single subcutaneous dose of radioactive morphine to rats and was shown not to be free morphine or morphine-3-glucuronide. Since the radioactivity remained "bound" to tissue constituents, the authors felt that the radioactive material was associated with or incorporated into proteins or nucleic acids; they cited work by others *(67,82)* which implicated proteins and ribonucleic acids in the tolerance process. However, a word of caution is necessary. March and Elliott *(83)*, working with morphine-$N$-$^{14}CH_3$, had shown that much of the $^{14}CO_2$ formed from the $N$-demethylation was excreted by the lungs, but this excretion of $^{14}CO_2$ lasted 4 or 5 days after drug administration. Thus, it appeared to them that the $^{14}CH_3$ group may have been incorporated into metabolic pools from which $^{14}CO_2$ was slowly liberated. Thus, it is possible that Misra et al. *(81)* were measuring the incorporation of just the labile portion of the morphine molecule, the $^{14}CH_3$ group, into metabolic pools, and not dealing with the disposition of the main portion of the morphine molecule.

## VII. METABOLIC TRANSFORMATION OF CODEINE TO MORPHINE

A discussion of the metabolism of morphine would not be complete without mentioning the problem associated with the formation of morphine after administration of codeine. Even though the ether bond in codeine, linking the $CH_3$ group to the 3-OH of morphine (Fig. 10), was known to be chemically very stable, Adler and Shaw *(84)* conclusively proved that this bond is broken and morphine is formed from codeine in rats. Subsequently, Mannering et al. *(85)* and Adler et al. *(86)* confirmed the occurrence of this biotransformation in man. This, as well as

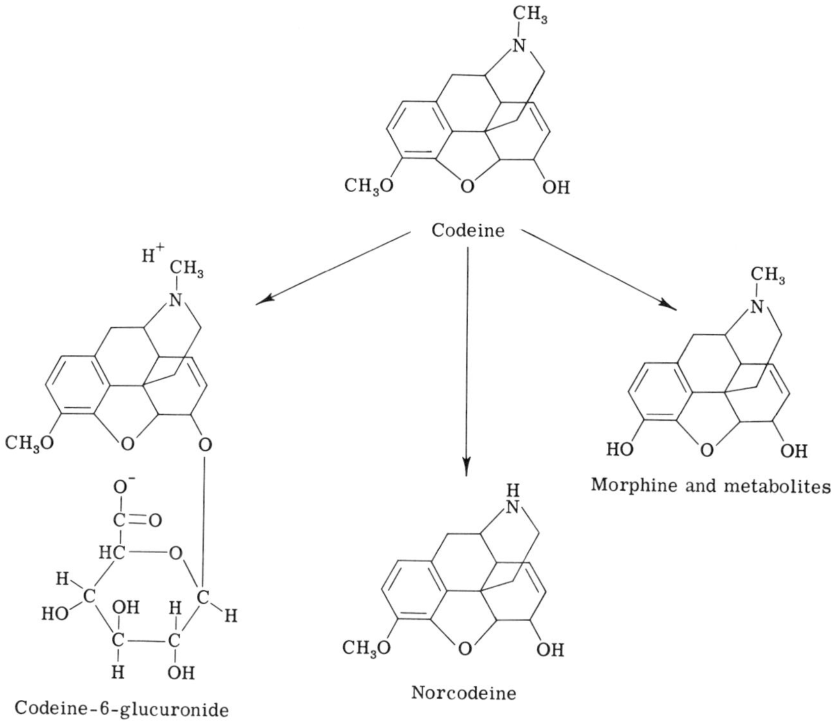

FIG. 10. Major pathways of codeine metabolism.

some of the other biotransformation pathways for codeine, is shown in Fig. 10. The reader may have anticipated the occurrence of many of these pathways from our preceding discussion on the metabolism of morphine. The question at hand, however, is how important is the liberation of morphine in the overall action of codeine? Mannering et al. (85) posed an interesting medicolegal question: "The finding of morphine in a toxicologic specimen may raise grave suspicions, the finding of codeine usually does not, but, in view of the observations of Adler and Shaw, what are the implications when both alkaloids are found?" One obvious requirement for answering such questions is to determine exactly how much morphine is formed from codeine. Adler et al. (86) found in six human volunteers that 5–17% of the dose of codeine was excreted as morphine in the urine. A crucial example may be that of the subject who was given 282 mg of codeine over a 4-hour period. He excreted 22.2 mg of total morphine in the urine in 24 hours. This excretion value could be equated to a dose of morphine which when administered would yield the same amount of morphine in the urine. Assuming that about 60% of administered morphine is excreted in urine (62), 22.2 mg of morphine in the urine would be equivalent to administering about 37 mg of morphine. Administering this calculated dose of morphine to man would indeed have given pharmacologic effects. Somewhat analogous calculations applied to experiments with monkeys (87) indicate that at least part of the pharmacologic effect of codeine is attributable to the liberated morphine. However, in the monkey, the pharmacologic action of codeine in production of dependence and abstinence effects is not identical to "equivalent" doses of morphine; it appeared that the morphine liberated from codeine is less effective than injected morphine. In the rat, as much as 55–71%

TABLE III

Major Metabolite of Morphine and Naloxone Isolated and Characterized in Certain Species

| Species[a] | Parent compound administered | | | |
|---|---|---|---|---|
| | Morphine | | Naloxone | |
| Man | Morphine-3-glucuronide | (54)[b] | Naloxone-3-glucuronide | (94) |
| Rabbit | Morphine-3-glucuronide | (59) | Naloxone-3-glucuronide | (91) |
| Cat | Morphine-3-ethereal sulfate | (92, 93) | Naloxone-3-ethereal sulfate | (95) |
| Chicken | Morphine-3-ethereal sulfate | (93) | ?[c] | |

[a] This list does not include all species in which the major metabolite of the morphine has been unequivocally identified.

[b] Numbers in parentheses are reference citation numbers.

[c] The question mark has been placed here so that the reader might predict what the metabolite ought to be.

of a dose of codeine is $O$-demethylated *(88)*. On the other hand, the dog possesses very little of this capacity, but codeine is still active in this species *(87)*. In the mouse, morphine is 100 times more potent than codeine when these drugs are injected directly into the central nervous system by intraventricular administration *(89)*. These species differences in amount of conversion to morphine, the large potency difference between codeine and morphine by intraventricular administration, and the somewhat different intensity of pharmacologic action between codeine and "equivalent" doses of morphine liberated from codeine still leave doubt as to the quantitative aspects. It cannot be denied that in man part of the action of codeine appears to be mediated by morphine. However, until more research is done, a precise, quantitative assignment cannot be made.

## VIII. METABOLISM OF NALOXONE

Because of its potent antagonistic actions against morphine effects, naloxone is a compound of great theoretical interest *(77)*. Although many have considered naloxone to be a pure antagonist devoid of any agonist actions (actions like morphine), it is interesting that in birds naloxone has been found to have agonist actions *(90)*. Perhaps the answer to this species difference lies in the manner in which the bird metabolizes naloxone compared to those other laboratory animals in which naloxone appears to have only antagonist actions. Now, as an exercise, the reader may wish to make a prediction. Table III shows some of the information already discussed on morphine as well as some further information. What would you predict that the metabolite of naloxone ought to be in the chicken? The question posed is a reasonable one in that much of this type of work is predicated on extrapolations from one species to another and from one compound to another. The formulas of naloxone and naloxone-3-glucuronide are given in Fig. 11. Since species differences such as those shown in the table exist, it is obvious that it may be erroneous to extrapolate from one species to another. On the other hand, consistency seems to be apparent for a particular species in going from one compound to the other. A reasonable guess would be that the chicken, like the cat, will metabolize naloxone to naloxone-3-ethereal sulfate. This surmise would be wrong on two counts. The metabolite found was not an ethereal sulfate nor was the parent half of the molecule unchanged naloxone! It was through the analytical power of infrared absorption spectrometry that the precise answer was obtained *(91)*. Figure 12 gives the infrared spectra of the unknown metabolite from both the chicken, spectrum 1, and from naloxone-3-glucuronide, spectrum 2. The new metabolite might have been identical to naloxone-3-glucuronide except that the strong absorption band at 5.8 $\mu$ for the C = O group at position 6 of naloxone was altered. This observation suggests that the parent portion of the naloxone had been altered; it was then an easy task to prove this point. Both the naloxone-3-glucuronide and the unknown glucuronide were hydrolyzed to remove the glucuronic acid moiety; the base portions of the metabolites were extracted into organic solvents and isolated. Infrared spectra were obtained on these two isolated portions and compared to naloxone and a compound called EN 2265 (Fig. 11). The IR (infrared) spectra in Fig. 13 showed that the base portion of the metabolite from the chicken was identical to EN 2265. Thus, the metabolite of naloxone in the chicken was established as N-allyl-14-hydroxy-7,8-dihydronormorphine-3-glucuronide (EN 2265 glucuronide, Fig. 11).

The presence of a residual absorption band for the chicken metabolite at 5.8 $\mu$ in the IR spectra (Figs. 12 and 13) requires further explanation.

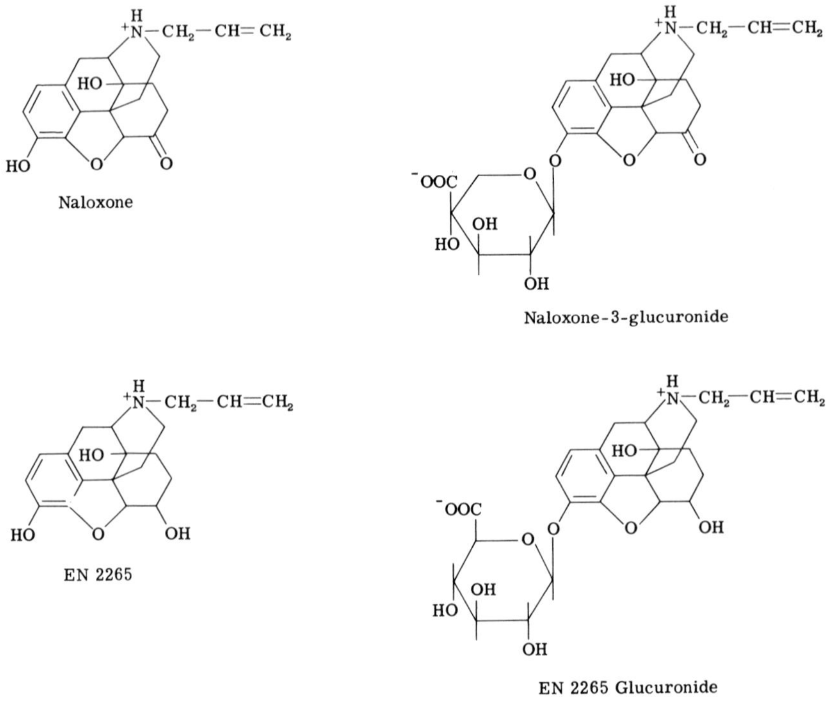

FIG. 11. Formulas for naloxone, EN 2265 (N-allyl-14-hydoxy-7,8-dihydronormorphine), naloxone glucuronide, and EN 2265 glucuronide. From Fujimoto (91) with permission of the publisher.

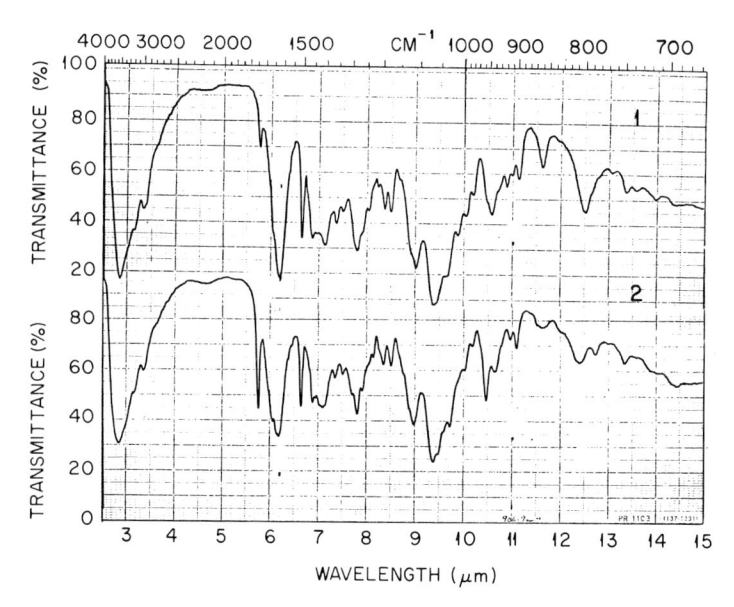

FIG. 12. Infrared spectra of two metabolites isolated from the urine of the chicken (1) and rabbit (2). Note difference at 5.8 $\mu$ wavelength. Adapted from Fujimoto *(91)* with permission of the publisher.

Although the analytical thin-layer chromatography technique used in our laboratory was not sensitive enough to detect the small amount of naloxone-3-glucuronide in the EN 2265 glucuronide, Weinstein et al. *(78)* demonstrated that the presence of the residual absorption band at 5.8 $\mu$ was due to small amounts of naloxone-3-glucuronide. This finding explained the spectral data in both Figs. 12 and 13 down to the minutest detail.

Returning to the pharmacological action of naloxone in birds *(90)*, it may very well be that EN 2265, formed as an intermediate in metabolism, conferred some morphine-like actions on naloxone. In the other species so far examined, man *(94)* and rabbit *(91)*, naloxone appeared not to be converted to any great extent to EN 2265. These findings imply that if EN 2265, the intermediate, is administered, it must have at least some agonist activity even in species in which naloxone has no agonist activity. In 1969, Dayton and Blumberg *(96)* did indeed report that EN 2265 had agonist actions, so that the hypothesis seems to be valid. However, a more recent observation [McMillan et al. *(90)*], does need to be taken into account. These workers found that, in the pigeon, naloxone is more potent as an agonist than was EN 2265. This difference in potency militates against the hypothesis since naloxone appears to have its own

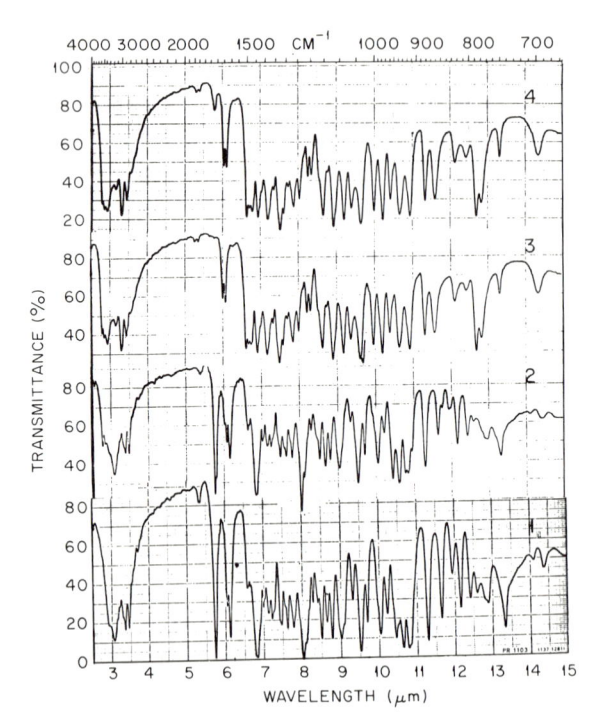

FIG. 13. Infrared spectra of free bases: (1) naloxone, (2) derived from the naloxone metabolite of the rabbit, (3) EN 2265 (N-allyl-14-hydroxy-7,8-dihydronormorphine), (4) derived from the naloxone metabolite of the chicken. Note similarity of spectra (1) and (2). The close similarity of (3) and (4) was evident; the differences seen in these spectra are discussed in the text. From Fujimoto (*91*) with permission of the publisher.

action beyond that of EN 2265 formed *in vivo*. These latter findings indicate that more work is necessary, particularly on the localization of drugs in the central nervous system, if not at the receptor level, to ultimately establish the hypothesis.

## IX. EXCRETION OF NARCOTICS AND METABOLITES IN URINE

The urine is the most important route of excretion, on a quantitative basis, for the narcotics and many of their metabolites. Urinalysis is therefore a useful approach for monitoring drug abuse. A review of some of the mechanisms at work in transferring these compounds from blood into urine may be of some use in understanding this complex process. Many narcotics have not been studied thoroughly in this regard because their pharmacologic potency frequently precluded their use in the doses necessary to obtain quantitative data in studying such mechanisms. The work by Baker and Woods *(97)* illustrated the kind of care necessary in overcoming some of these difficulties. They devised a morphine treatment protocol which did not reduce glomerular filtration rate of the kidney. Radioactively labeled narcotics have in part ameliorated this problem, but their general availability remains limited. Therefore, this section is written to illustrate some concepts based on studies of a few compounds. No evidence exists to indicate that narcotic analgesics are handled any differently by the kidney than are other organic bases. On the other hand, conjugation of these bases with glucuronic or sulfuric acid converts them to compounds readily transported by the renal tubular system. The metabolism of narcotics by the kidney will be included as it relates to the transport mechanisms. Many excellent reviews have been published that serve as broad background material; a few will be mentioned. Weiner *(98)* gives comprehensive coverage of the excretory mechanisms by which drugs are processed; papers by Peters *(99)* and Cafruny *(100)* are particularly useful for methodology.

## A. Glomerular Filtration

Glomerular filtration may be assumed to occur for all the narcotics and their metabolites. Baker and Woods *(97)* found that the clearance rate for free morphine and also for conjugated morphine (formed in the animal from morphine) equaled the glomerular filtration rate. Therefore, they concluded that morphine and the conjugated metabolite were both excreted by glomerular filtration. Since as much as 25% of morphine in the plasma may be bound to proteins, correcting for this factor raised the clearance value for morphine to above the value for inulin. This suggested that some tubular secretion was occurring. Unequivocal experimental evidence for tubular secretion was provided subsequently by experimenters working with dihydromorphine.

## B. Modification of Excretion by the pH-Dependent Process of Nonionic Diffusion and Ionic Trapping

If a narcotic possesses high lipid solubility, it is likely that little of it will be excreted in the urine. Even in the face of glomerular filtration, this lipophilic property leads to reabsorption of the drug from the lumen of the renal tubules because the renal tubular membrane is permeable to lipophilic compounds. As the glomerular filtrate becomes concentrated by removal of water in its course down the tubular lumen, a concentration gradient is created for the lipophilic compound from the tubular lumen toward the blood. Reabsorption then occurs by diffusion. If a pH gradient exists between the urine and the blood and the narcotic can be made to exist more in an ionized form in the fluid of the tubular lumen, then reabsorption can be reduced by trapping of this ionized species. Ionization makes the narcotic more hydrophilic and less lipophilic. Milne et al. (101) discuss the various conditions which determine whether an organic base with a given $pK_a$ value will be excreted by this pH-dependent ionic trapping process. This process has been clearly involved for the excretion of meperidine, levorphanol, and methadone.

The essential portion of the concept of nonionic diffusion and ionic trapping was discussed earlier in the section on urinary excretion of barbiturates. The same concepts apply to the excretion of diffusible basic drugs. If the free base form of the drug, for instance, meperidine, is represented by B, then the acid salt form, meperidine hydrochloride, can be represented as the conjugate acid, $BH^+$ (Fig. 14). The acid dissociation may be written $BH^+ \rightleftharpoons B + H^+$ where $K_a = (B)(H^+)/(BH^+)$. Then $pK_a = pH - \log(B)/(BH^+)$. If the tubular lumen is more acid than pH 7.4, it will be seen that the concentration of $BH^+$ in the tubular lumen will be greater than in the peritubular fluid. If the lumen is more alkaline than pH 7.4, the concentration of $BH^+$ will be less in the lumen than peritubular fluid.

Asatoor et al. (102) studied the excretion of meperidine and one of its metabolites, normeperidine, in humans. In patients who received sodium bicarbonate and who were excreting highly alkaline urine, the total excretion of meperidine and normeperidine in 48 hours was less than 5% of the subcutaneously administered dose of meperidine. In patients whose urines were highly acidic due to ammonium chloride ingestion, the total

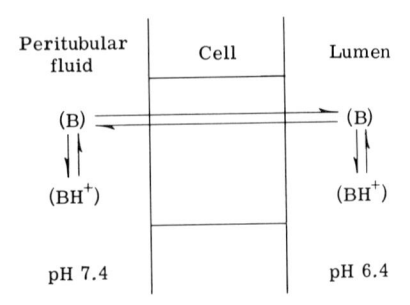

FIG. 14. Urinary excretion of a base (B) by nonionic diffusion and pH gradient ionic trapping mechanism in the kidney. For explanation see text.

excretion of meperidine and normeperidine in 48 hours was about 50% of the administered dose of meperidine. Since the $pK_a$ of meperidine was 8.6 and that of normeperidine was 9.7, relatively more of the ionized forms of these compounds was trapped in the lumen of the tubules when the pH there was low. The pH sensitivity and the magnitude of the effect in going from 5 to 50% excretion provides assurances that nonionic diffusion and ionic trapping by a pH gradient play an important role in meperidine excretion. Asatoor's experiments were further instructive in showing what happens to excretion of certain acidic metabolites with changes in pH. Metabolic hydrolysis of meperidine and normeperidine yield meperidinic and normeperidinic acid, respectively. Excretion of these two carboxylic acids was greater when the urine was relatively more alkaline. More ionization and thereby less reabsorption occurs in alkaline than acid urine. Conversion of the bases meperidine and normeperidine to acidic metabolites reverses the effect of acidification and alkalinization of urine.

Beckett et al. *(103, 104)* and Baselt and Casarett *(105)* studied the metabolism of metadone and correlated excretion with changes in urinary pH. Methadone with a $pK_a$ of 8.6 was excreted in larger amounts in acid than in alkaline urine. The excretion of the metabolite 2-ethylidene-1,5-dimethyl-3,3-diphenylpyrrolidine, with a $pK_a$ of 10.4, was related to urine flow more than pH of the urine. Baselt and Casarett make the cogent point that this "dependency of methadone excretion on pH of the urine is of considerable importance in methadone maintenance therapy. Patients are maintained at a dosage designed to block heroin euphoria while permitting reasonable normal function. Changes in diet, occupational exposure to other chemicals, other medications, and other factors may alter the pH of the urine, upsetting the steady state of the established methadone dose regimen." It is clear that understanding this phenomenon has practical applications. In carrying out studies of this type, the rabbit should prove to be a most useful animal model since simple feeding and fasting produce large shifts in urinary pH in a circadian fashion, shifts which have been correlated with drug excretion *(46)*.

## C. Secretory Mechanisms for Excretion of Narcotic Analgesics

Hug, Mellet, and Cafruny *(106)*, using the method of stop-flow analysis *(100)*, demonstrated that dihydromorphine was secreted by the proximal tubules in the dog and monkey. They identified the apparent renal tubular segment where radioactively labeled dihydromorphine was transported from blood into urine. After collecting free-flow urine samples as in conventional clearance experiments the ureteral cannulas were occluded for a short time. During this period glomerular filtration came to a stop, but tubular secretion of p-aminohippuric acid (PAH) and tubular reabsorption of $Na^+$ and $Cl^-$ continued. Volume changes for water within the tubules were monitored with inulin since once inulin entered the tubular lumen by glomerular filtration it was not reabsorbed. After release of the occlusion of the cannula, serial urine samples were collected rapidly. In this procedure, samples collected first represented fluid from the collecting ducts and distal portions of the tubules. The later samples represented the more proximal portions of the tubules up to a point where new glomerular filtrate started to enter. Once the measured concentrations were corrected for volume changes of water by the inulin factor, troughs in the concentration in the serial samples for $Na^+$ and $Cl^-$ delineated more distal portions of the nephron, whereas proximal tubular portions were indicated by the peak for PAH. The important finding was that dihydromorphine shows a peak at the same location as PAH, indicating that dihydromorphine is secreted at the level of the proximal tubules. The secretory transport system for dihydromorphine is further characterized by responsiveness to inhibitors. Classically, drugs that are actively secreted are transported either by an organic anion or cation transport system, each of which is independent of the other. Transport of drug by the anion system can be blocked by an acid, probenecid, and cation system transport can be blocked by a variety of bases including cyanine 863, mepiperphenidol, and quinine. In the experiments by Hug's group, both mepiperphenidol and cyanine 863 blocked transport of dihydromorphine as indicated by diminution of the proximal tubular secretory peak. Probenecid, on the other hand, had no effect on dihydromorphine transport. Therefore, dihydromorphine was transported by the cation and not the anion transport system. The results were consistent with the fact that dihydromorphine would exist as a cation under these conditions. Also, diffusion of the nonionzed form into the tubular fluid followed by trapping of the ionized species by the pH gradient mechanism appears to be highly unlikely under the conditions of their experiments.

In addition, they investigated the transport of a metabolite of dihydromorphine presumed to be a conjugate with glucuronic acid. This endogenously formed metabolite also showed a secretory peak in the proximal tubules. This active proximal tubular secretion was blocked by both mepiperiphenidol and probenecid. Because it appeared that this metabolite was the glucuronide conjugate, they suggested that this conjugate was transported by both the anion and cation systems since dihydromorphine glucuronide should exist in the zwitterion form at physiologic pH. The zwitterion structure had been previously shown for morphine-3-glucuronide *(107)*. Since the anion and cation transport systems were independent systems, transport of the dihydromorphine metabolite by both systems was a rare example of a compound simultaneously handled by both systems. If the two transport systems were not coupled to each other, it is puzzling why dihydromorphine glucuronide would not continue to be effectively transported when one or the other transport system was blocked; blockage of one system should automatically lead to the other system's taking over the transport function. More work remains to be done with this type of metabolite.

### D. Renal Tubular Transport and Metabolism of Morphine in the Chicken

The chicken differs from the rodent and other mammalian species commonly used in the laboratory in possessing a renal portal system. Sperber recognized the usefulness of this feature for experimental purposes and developed a technique for studying renal tubular transport of drugs *(108–111)*. We have recently coupled renal metabolism and renal transport studies for morphine with this system, and this coupling has provided some unique answers about the site of action of certain drugs. The technique as we use it today *(112)* will be described along with a simplified version of its conceptual basis, as illustrated in Fig. 15.

If an agent is infused into the saphenous vein of one leg, venous blood from that leg passes through the ipsilateral renal portal system without being filtered by the glomeruli. The agent first comes into contact with the tubular cells before the agent passes into the general circulation. Any part of the infused material not excreted in one pass reaches the systemic

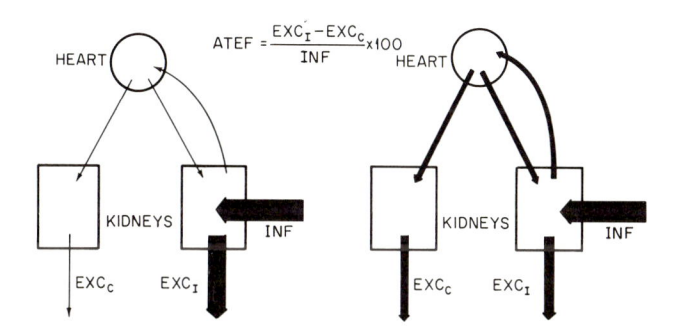

FIG. 15. Schematic illustration of the concept of the Sperber preparation *(108)* for renal tubular excretion of drugs in the hen. Case 1 (left panel) shows active transport for a compound having a high apparent tubular excretion fraction, ATEF. Case 2 (right panel) occurs where the ATEF is near zero.

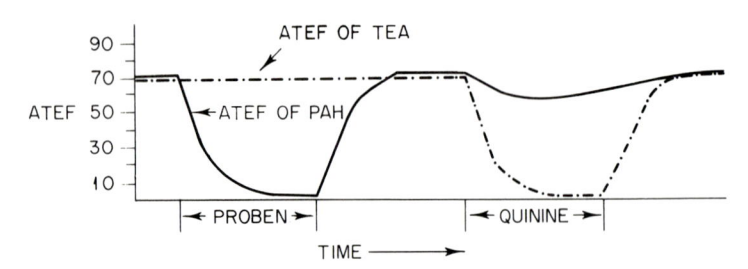

FIG. 16. Example of an experiment in the Sperber preparation (*108*) where the anion (PAH) and cation (TEA) transport systems can be independently blocked by probenecid and quinine respectively. From Watrous (*113*).

circulation and then returns to both kidneys in equal concentration. Thus an entity called the "apparent tubular excretion fraction" (ATEF) shows how much drug was excreted by the tubules on the first pass. ATEF = (EXC$_I$ − EXC$_C$)/INF · 100, where EXC$_I$ is the amount excreted in the urine from the ipsilateral kidney, EXC$_C$ is the amount from the contralateral kidney, and INF is the amount infused during the same period as the urine collection.

In effect, the ATEF is an expression of the percent of the infused dose that has been excreted by the ipsilateral kidney on the first pass. A high ATEF indicates active secretory transport of the drug from blood to tubular lumen. In the left-hand panel of Fig. 15, Case I, it is seen that the infused compound is excreted rapidly into the urine on its first pass through the ipsilateral kidney. In this example, the ATEF is large and indicates active tubular transport of the drug. The situation illustrated in the right-hand panel, Case II, leads to an ATEF near zero—obviously net tubular secretion of drug does not occur.

Figure 16 illustrates the way in which an experiment is performed. Two drugs known to be transported actively (high ATEF) are infused simultaneously into the saphenous vein. PAH (*p*-aminohippuric acid), is secreted into the urine by an organic anion transporting system which, as can be seen, is blockable by probenecid, itself an acid compound. TEA (tetraethylammonium), is excreted by an organic cation transporting system which is blocked by quinine, one of a number of bases effective in blocking the cation transport system. Note that the two transport systems are independent of each other in that each can be blocked without effect on the other. Morphine can then be substituted for one of these standard agents to study its excretory mechanism.

Morphine excretion fits into Case I of Fig. 15. When morphine-$^{14}$C was infused, the ATEF for $^{14}$C excretion was high (*114*), thereby indicating that renal tubular secretion was occurring. Furthermore, this ATEF was drastically reduced by quinine while not affected by probenecid *(114, 115)*. Therefore, morphine was determined to be transported by the cation secretory system, a finding which agreed with the earlier conclusion of Hug *et al. (106)* with dihydromorphine transport in the dog and monkey. These confirmatory findings were followed by more exciting observations. By countercurrent distribution analysis, the $^{14}C$ material in the urine was separated into morphine $^{14}C$- and $^{14}C$ metabolite fraction. Analyses of urine samples from the ipsilateral and contralateral kidneys showed that a large excess of both metabolite and morphine occurred on the ipsilateral side. This excess of metabolite meant that the ipsilateral kidney was metabolizing morphine *(114)*, and part of the picture seen in Fig. 17 emerged. At this point the metabolite was isolated by using a new resin, Amberlite XAD-2 *(93)*. The resin is mentioned here because it was to become the basis for a widely used urine screening method for drug abuse as discussed in the next section. The isolated metabolite was identified to be morphine-3-ethereal sulfate (MES), a sulfuric acid ester

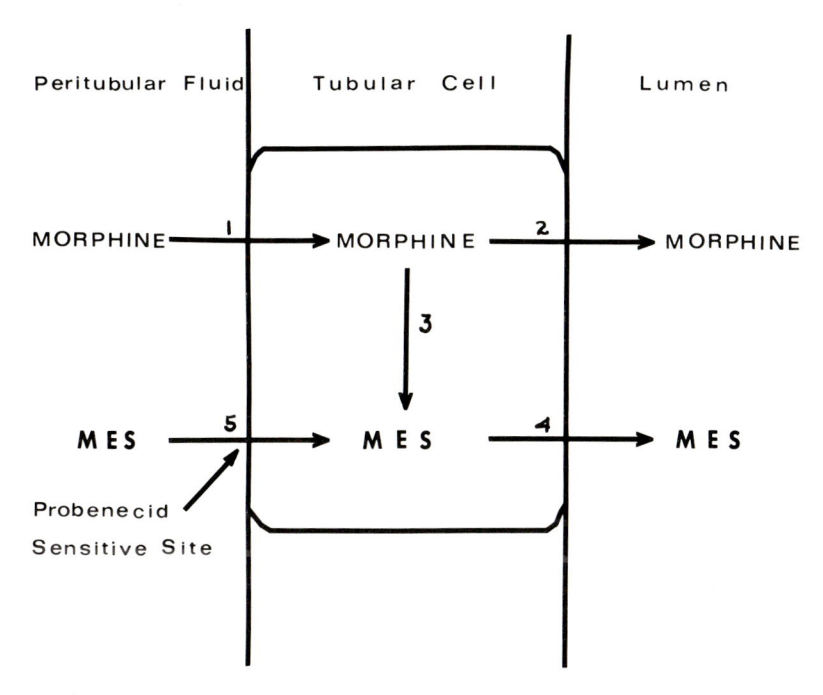

FIG. 17. The morphine–morphine ethereal sulfate (MES) model system for transport and metabolism in the Sperber preparation. Adapted from Watrous *et al. (115)* with permission of the publisher.

TABLE IV

EFFECT OF BLOCKING AGENTS ON MEAN MES-¹⁴C, AND PAH ATEF DURING MES-¹⁴C INFUSION[a,b]

| Blocking agent | Molar ratio | No. of periods | ¹⁴C | ATEF %Δ | PAH | %Δ |
|---|---|---|---|---|---|---|
| None | — | 4 | 23.2 | | 28.0 | |
| Mepiperphenidol | 1 | 4 | 23.1 | 0 | 27.2 | 0 |
| None | — | 6 | 58.2 | | 58.2 | |
| Probenecid | 10 | 6 | 2.7 | −95 | 11.3 | −80 |

[a] Rate of infusion of MES-¹⁴C was 0.2 μmol/kg/minute. The molar ratio is the concentration of blocking agent infused to the molar concentration of MES-¹⁴C in the infusion solution.

[b] From Watrous et al. (115) with permission of the publishers.

of morphine at the 3-OH position (93). The presence of the sulfate group conferred a strong negative charge on the molecule, and, in fact, at physiological pH values the molecule would be expected to be in zwitterion form, that is, to carry both a + and − charge. The immediate question was by which system, anion or cation, would this zwitterion be transported in the chicken? To investigate this question the isolated MES-¹⁴C was infused into the Sperber preparation to study its transport independent of that of morphine (115). Results in Table IV show that MES was transported well by the renal tubules; its ATEF was high and like that of PAH. Its transport as well as that of PAH was blocked by probenecid, but mepiperphenidol had no effect. Therefore, MES was secreted by the anion transport system and the cation system was not involved. After MES transport was studied independently, the knowledge gained was applied to the morphine system, and a complete picture evolved, as shown in Fig. 17. Morphine is actively transported across the renal tubular cell (steps 1 and 2), it is metabolized in the cell to MES (step 3) and excreted (step 4). The striking finding involves step 5. Even though probenecid blocks the transport of intravenously administered MES, probenecid does not block the excretion of MES which was formed within the cell from morphine. This finding means that the site of action of probenecid is at step 5, the transport of MES across the peritubular border of the renal tubular cell. By inference, the transport system for anions other than MES must also be located on the peritubular side, at least for secretory transport. Evidence for at least one other anion supported this prediction (116).

If indeed, the morphine-MES system functioned as pictured in Fig. 17, additional experiments could be devised. If we were able to find a compound that blocked step 3, the metabolism of morphine, then there should be a decrease in MES excretion at the same time that an exactly compensatory increase in morphine-$^{14}$C excretion occurred, providing that step 1, transport across the peritubular membrane, remained constant. The required inhibitor for step 3 was found in catechol *(117)*. Sperber had shown that catechol was conjugated with sulfate *(111)*. In a timely report, Quebbemann and Rennick *(118)* had found that catechol was transported by the renal tubules. Therefore, we reasoned that catechol must get into the cell and be a substrate for the sulfokinase enzyme system, and thereby catechol might serve as an inhibitor of morphine conjugation with sulfate. Our results *(117)* showed that catechol has no effect on the amount of $^{14}$C transported into urine during morphine-$^{14}$C infusion. Although the ATEF for $^{14}$C was unchanged, the amount of metabolite, MES-$^{14}$C, decreased to zero on the ipsilateral side. There was a compensatory rise in excretion of free morphine-$^{14}$C. Therefore all the morphine-$^{14}$C that was transported across the renal tubular cell was being excreted without being metabolized. The prediction had been fulfilled.

Since catechol had worked well in inhibiting morphine metabolism, it was possible to test other, more classical, inhibitors of drug metabolism reactions, namely, the SKF 525A-type compounds mentioned earlier *(11,119)*. The results of these studies were unexpected in that SKF 525A, *N*-methylpipyridyldiphenyl carbamate (MPDC), and Lilly 18947 did not inhibit the metabolism of morphine but blocked the transport of morphine *(120,121)*. The results indicate that all of these compounds act as inhibitors of morphine transport at the peritubular membrane, step 1, by virtue of being organic bases. This nonspecific effect was found also with diethylaminoethanol, the portion of the SKF 525A and Lilly 18947 molecule that makes these compounds basic. Therefore, the morphine–MES system is useful not only in studying transport and metabolism of morphine but also in localizing sites of action of other drugs on the kidney.

### E. Urine Monitoring for Drug Abuse

Under the Narcotic Addict Rehabilitation Act of 1966 *(122)*, the monitoring of urine samples for dependence-producing drugs in patients on methadone maintenance and rehabilitation programs has become common practice. Also, urine monitoring is one way to detect drug abuse for individual, medical, or legal needs. Today's research laboratories are equipped with many sophisticated analytical instruments and one would think that it would be a simple task to devise a good method for monitoring urine samples for drugs of abuse. However, devising a universally acceptable method has been a challenging and even frustrating problem in the clinical or toxicological laboratory. The reason lies in the difficulty of getting the right combination of some of the following requirements for an ideal method.

1. Economy

The method must be inexpensive enough for a laboratory to run only a few or as many as several hundred urine samples in a day. Not only must the materials be inexpensive, but technical and professional labor costs must be minimal. For instance, it is not practical as a screening procedure to run gas chromatograms on several hundred urine samples or to run very many mass or infrared spectra in a day, particularly as many of the samples would contain no drug. Nor would it be wise to invest in an expensive analytical instrument just to run a few samples per day if cost is a factor.

2. Specificity

Many highly specific methods exist. However, if a given method is useful for detecting only a few compounds, then many additional methods must be run to cover the wide spectrum of agents that are abused. Narcotic analgesics, barbiturates, amphetamines, and cocaine are some of the major drugs that the monitoring method must detect, differentiate, and identify. Elegant methods, such as the radioimmunossay for morphine *(123,124)*, and the commercially available, highly sensitive FRAT (Free Radical Assay Technique) *(125)*, lack breadth of applicability. Fluorometric assay *(126)* suffers from the same disadvantage.

3. Sensitivity

This requirement does not appear to be as critical as the first two in that most methods now in use appear to approach realistic levels of sensitivity. Radioimmunoassay, FRAT, fluorometric assay, and gas–liquid chromatography possess more than the required sensitivity.

To a large extent these requirements dictate the nature of the methods in common use today for urine monitoring. As a basic method, thin-layer chromatography enjoys the widest use because of its simplicity, economy, and broad applicability. However, preparation of the urine sample for thin-layer chromatography has been a problem, and has been handled in several ways. Since our method *(127)*, or modifications thereof, is notable for simplicity and is being widely used, a brief description of the method, including thin-layer chromatography, follows. The basic steps of the

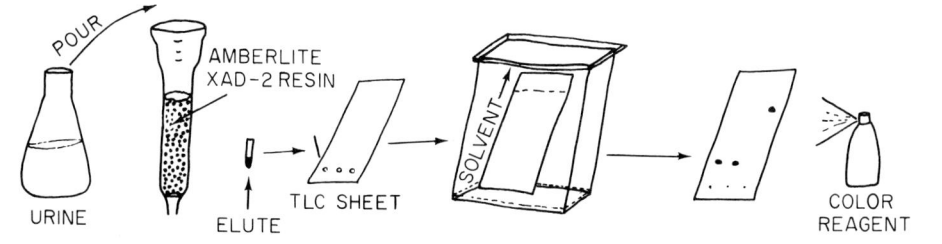

FIG. 18. Major steps in the Fujimoto–Wang method *(127)* for detecting drugs of abuse. See text for explanation.

Fujimoto–Wang method are illustrated in Fig. 18. Urine is poured rapidly through a column of Amberlite XAD-2 resin. The drugs are adsorbed onto the resin as the urine passes through the column. The adsorbed drugs are eluted from the resin with an organic solvent such as methanol and condensed to a small volume. This collected eluate is spotted on a thin-layer chromatogram sheet and the chromatogram developed in an organic solvent system. After development, the chromatogram is dried briefly, and then sprayed with appropriate color-producing reagents to

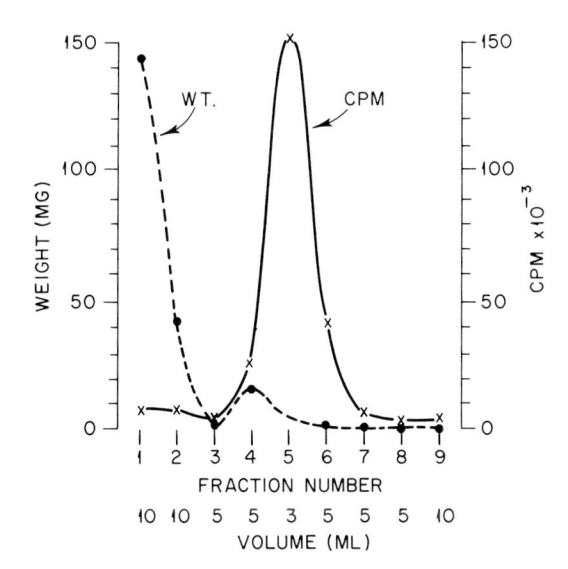

FIG. 19. Separation of morphine-$N$-$^{14}CH_3$ and contaminants from urine by an Amberlite XAD-12 resin column. Ten milliliters of urine containing $230 \times 10^3$ cpm of morphine was processed through the column with 10 ml of water and eluted with methanol. The radioactivity and dry weight content of each fraction was determined. From Fujimoto and Wang *(127)* with permission of the publisher.

visualize the spot of drug. Identification of the drug is done by comparing the chromatogram with known standards. A useful innovation in the method involves the resin adsorption step, as shown in Fig. 19.

When urine was flushed through the column, note that most of the impurities (determined as residue weight) came right through the column without being adsorbed. Morphine, on the other hand (morphine-$^{14}$C was used here to facilitate quantitative evaluation of the method) was adsorbed onto the resin. The adsorbed morphine could then be easily eluted from the resin with methanol. The morphine, now in the methanol eluate, was present in purified form and in a much more concentrated form than originally present in the urine sample. A further concentrating effect could be achieved by partially evaporating the solution before spotting on the TLC. With the advent of prepackaged Amberlite XAD-2 resin in disposable columns in improved forms as described by Quame *(128)*, and the availability of complete kits including thin-layer chromatography materials *(129,130)*, this approach to urine monitoring has become even more practical. Parts of one kit being used to analyze batches of urine samples are illustrated in Fig. 20. The method is applicable to narcotic analgesics, amphetamines, barbiturates, and cocaine.

In another commonly used method, paper impregnated with a different resin is used for sample preparation before thin-layer chromatogra-

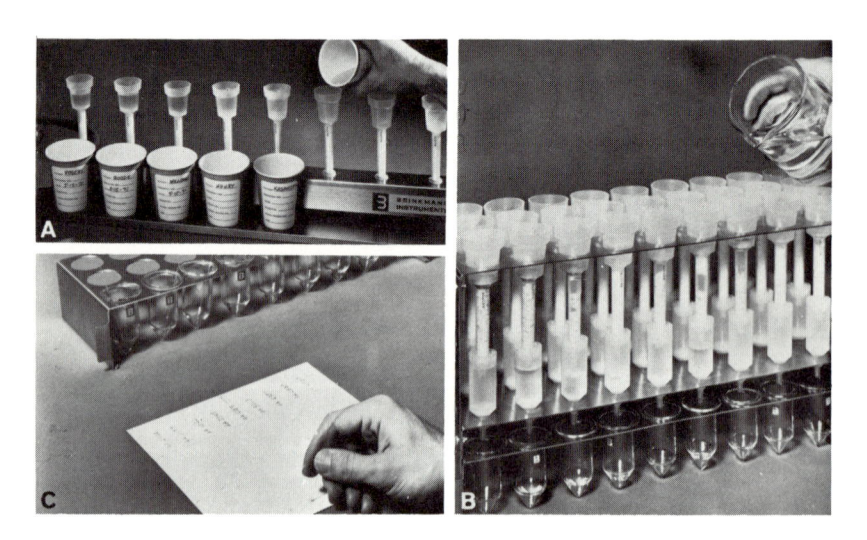

Fig. 20. Example of the use of a commercially available kit for urine monitoring for drugs of abuse. (a) Pouring the urine through the column to adsorb drugs on the resin. (b) Elution of the adsorbed drugs from the column with a polar organic solvent. (c) Spotting the concentrate on a thin-layer plate. Courtesy of Brinkmann Instrument Co.

phy. Drugs are extracted from the resin paper by adjusting the pH and using several organic solvents so that again narcotic analgesics, amphetamines, etc., can easily be determined by thin-layer chromatography. This method developed by Dole et al. *(131)* must be accorded special acknowledgment because it clearly set forth at a very early stage some of the requirements as well as some of the practical solutions for carrying on a successful urine monitoring program. It is not possible in this essay to mention modifications of the Dole method or to describe the variety of other methods in use today. The reader should consult the review by Taylor *(126)* for a more thorough discussion of methodology in this field. Less technical reviews are also available *(132)*.

## X. TRANSPORT IN BRAIN

Earlier we discussed the presence of an apparent barrier to penetration of morphine into the brain. One mechanism which may contribute to this blood–brain barrier is the presence of a transport system in the choroid plexus. The choroid plexus, located in the lateral, third, and fourth ventricles of the brain, is a vascular membranous tissue, which forms cerebrospinal fluid. The choroid plexus may function to remove certain compounds from the cerebrospinal fluid *(133)*. The first indication of the morphine concentrating function of the choroid plexus was given by Miller and Elliott *(134)*. Autoradiographs of sections of the brain from rats given morphine-$^{14}$C showed high localization of radioactive material in the choroid plexus. In recent *in vivo* perfusion experiments in rabbits, Asghar and Way *(135)* found that morphine is extracted from cerebrospinal fluid by an active transport process. The existence of such a removal process is consistent with the rapid disappearance of the drug observed after morphine administration into the ventricle *(89)*. Insights into the mechanism of transport have been obtained *in vitro* by excising the choroid plexus and studying the accumulation and outflow of narcotic analgesics from this tissue (usually obtained from the rabbit). The accumulation process for these narcotics was measured by the buildup of a high concentration gradient of the drugs in the tissue beyond that in the medium in which the tissue was immersed. Takemori and Stenwick *(136)* and Hug *(137)* found that the accumulation process fulfilled many of the criteria for an active transport process such as inhibition by metabolic poisons, competition with other organic bases, and stimulation of transport by a countertransport mechanism. The general concept of the active transport process was much like that described already for the cation transport system in the kidney. There were, however, finite differences from the renal tubular system in that probenecid and ouabain blocked the active transport process in the brain. Tolerance did not alter the uptake process *(138)* to morphine. Also, morphine-3-glucuronide was not transported *(139)*. It is tempting to speculate that the transport process in the choroid plexus may be oriented toward removing morphine-type compounds from the cerebrospinal fluid into the blood. Such an orientation would indeed contribute to the blood–brain barrier phenomenon.

One compelling reason for investigating the localization of drugs within the organism has been the feeling that the specific sites of localization may well explain particular actions of each drug. There have been many such studies on distribution of narcotic analgesic agents [see Way and Adler *(62)* and Clouet *(67)*]. Even though grossly observable differences have been found in localization of morphine in certain areas in the central nervous system, correlations with probable sites of action of the drug have not been possible. This lack of correlation has also been reflected in studies of the mechanisms for tolerance; no great changes in localization of the narcotics in the central nervous system have been found in spite of the development of large degrees of tolerance *(140)*. Another approach to the same problem has been to use narcotic antagonists. Since narcotic antagonists such as nalorphine appear to owe their specific pharmacological effectiveness to their ability to compete with the narcotic drugs for receptor sites in the central nervous system, some efforts have been made toward demonstrating that competition at receptor sites does indeed reduce the amount of narcotic present in the central nervous system. Negative correlation has been obtained with nalorphine; concentrations of morphine in the CNS increased in the presence of nalorphine *(141)*. In another study, no effect on subcellular distribution of morphine in brain was obtained with nalorphine treatment *(142)*. Perhaps in all of these studies the pharmacologically effective portion of the narcotic that combined with the receptors was such a minute part of the narcotic present in the central nervous system that occupation of these receptors by the antagonist may not measurably change the gross drug concentrations. Wuepper *et al.* *(143)* found, contrary to this concept of surfeit of drug and paucity of receptor, that nalorphine lowered the concentration of radioactively labeled levorphanol in dogs. Dobbs *(144)* similarly studied the combination of etorphine-$^3$H and cyprenorphine. Brain and spinal cord concentrations of etorphine-$^3$H were reduced for considerable periods of time in cyprenorphine-treated as compared to untreated controls. Since etorphine was about 1000 times more potent than morphine as an analgesic *(79)* and cyprenorphine was 35 times more potent than nalorphine as an antagonist, these increased potencies may reflect a more selective localization at active receptor sites. Thus, the reduction in excess of both narcotic and narcotic antagonist relative to the receptor achieved by Dobbs enhances the feasibility of studying localization at cellular and subcellular levels.

## XI. PLACENTAL TRANSFER

Although there is a paucity of information on the mechanisms of placental transfer of narcotics, there is no doubt that opiates reach the fetus when they are administered to the mother. Drug effects such as respiratory depression and even drug dependence have been seen in the human neonate and in a few instances drug levels have been measured in the newborn (145). The unique situation exists where two individuals, the mother with a well-developed blood–brain barrier, and the fetus with a poorly developed blood–brain barrier, coexist separated by the placenta. In the experimental animal this situation has been shown to lead to distinctively different distributions of the narcotic in the mother and in the fetus. Sanner and Woods (146) administered dihydromorphine-$^3$H (DHM) subcutaneously to pregnant rats near term. In Fig. 21, it can be

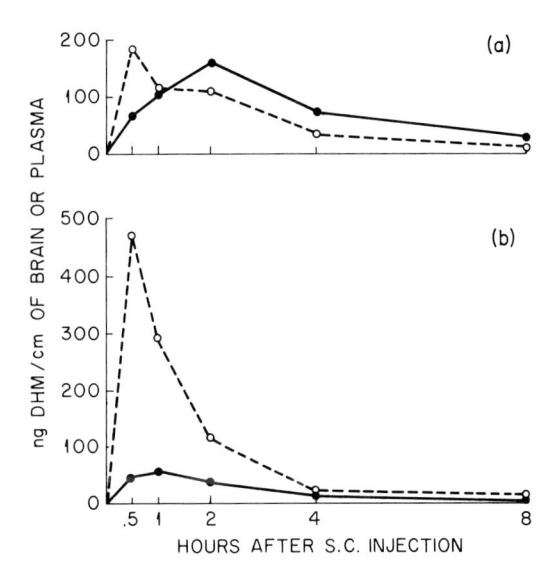

FIG. 21. A comparison of dihydromorphine-$^3$H concentrations in (a) fetal and (b) maternal brains (●) and plasma (○) after the subcutaneous administration of 2 mg/kg of the labeled drug to pregnant rats. From Sanner and Woods (146) with permission of the publisher.

seen that the fetal plasma concentrations of DHM were considerably below the maternal plasma concentration for as much as 2 hours; therefore, the placenta initially served as a barrier to rapid transit of the drug into the fetus. After 2 hours the plasma concentrations equilibrated between fetus and mother. Upon examination of the brain-to-plasma ratio of DHM in the mother, it was strikingly evident that a blood–brain barrier existed in the adult animal; in the fetus, however, no such sustained difference occurred–there appeared to be no blood–brain barrier. Most important, the concentrations of DHM in the brain of the fetus were, as a result, much higher than the brain concentrations in the mother. Detectable brain concentrations persisted in the fetus longer than in the mother. These findings are in accord with our previous discussion of the consequences of the existence of the blood–brain barrier to morphine in the adult rat and the lack of a blood–brain barrier to morphine in young rats. Likewise, the fetus *in utero* had not yet developed a blood–brain barrier to morphine. The consequences of such findings for humans deserve our consideration.

Since it is known that the fetus *in utero* can become dependent on the heroin that the mother abuses, there seems to be the distinct possibility that the fetus is being exposed to continually higher levels of the drug than is the mother. Obviously, physical dependence in the newborn could be a more severe problem than in the mother.

The involvement of a time factor in attaining the steady state between dam and fetus has its practical counterpart in man. Marx *(145)* has reviewed the evidence supporting the view that, if morphine is given to the mother at term, the time interval between administration of the morphine and delivery is crucial in determining whether toxicity occurs in the neonate. If the interval is short, effects are minimal. As the interval increases to several hours, more morphine effects appear in the neonate as complications of drug treatment of the mother. In other words, if the interval is short, little transplacental transfer of morphine seems to occur, while at longer intervals, more morphine appears to be transferred to the fetus. Therefore, one method of minimizing morphine toxicity to the fetus is to use morphine only in situations where the time of administration would be immediately prior to time of delivery of the baby. In more recent years, the problem has been circumvented in part by using meperidine.

The clinical impression had long existed that meperidine produced much less respiratory depression of the newborn than did morphine. This impression was hard to reconcile with the known pharmacology of the two agents in nonpregnant subjects, where there was little evidence to suggest that meperidine should be any better than morphine. The two drugs under ordinary circumstances produce about the same degree of respiratory depression in subjects when used in equianalgesic doses. Why then does meperidine not cause as much respiratory depression of the fetus as does morphine? Since no special placental barrier exists to meperidine, there seems to be no simple explanation. Recently, Way and his group provided the answer *(52,147)*. The answer lies in the fact that in the adult, no blood–brain barrier exists to meperidine as it does to morphine. Therefore, at near *equianalgesic doses* of the two drugs in the mother, a much higher pharmacologically active equivalent of morphine than of meperidine reaches the fetus. In other words, the existence of the barrier to morphine in the mother makes the mother relatively more resistant to morphine at the expense of the fetus. It is therefore evident why meperidine would be preferable to morphine in the second stage of labor for obstetrical analgesia.

Then the question arises whether a narcotic analgesic which has enhanced access to the central nervous system in the adult might not be the ideal analgesic, exactly in contrast to morphine. Etorphine is an agent which has been considered for some of these special attributes. Blane and Dobbs *(148)* found that in rats etorphine was concentrated in the brain rather than in the blood. Under similar conditions, they found that the ratio of brain-to-blood concentration for dihydromorphine was 0.16, a ratio indicative of the presence of the blood–brain barrier for dihydromorphine, as reported by Sanner and Woods *(146)*. The eminently interesting finding was that in the fetus, the relative concentration of etorphine was half as high as that of dihydromorphine. Therefore, etorphine has the desirable characteristic of reaching the brain of the mother much more easily than dihydromorphine while at the same time not reaching the fetus in as high a concentration as dihydromorphine. We will have to wait to see whether etorphine does indeed have advantages as an analgesic for obstetrical use. A narcotic analgesic is yet to be discovered which produces as much analgesia in the mother as does morphine or meperidine and yet has no depressant effect on respiration in the newborn. But some immediate answers to certain questions are necessary. Does methadone traverse the placenta to enter the fetus in large concentrations? Does a pregnant patient on large doses of methadone for maintenance therapy expose her unborn baby to large amounts of methadone? Is methadone really less of a risk to the baby than is heroin, or is it perhaps even worse?

## XII. BILIARY EXCRETION

Work by Oberst *(149)* and by Elliott *et al. (150)* indicated that in man morphine is excreted into bile as a conjugated metabolite. This me-

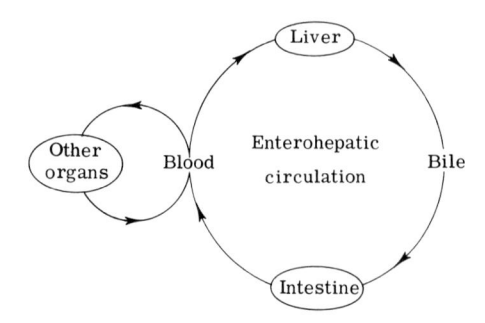

FIG. 22. Enterohepatic circulation of morphine. Morphine in the blood is metabolized to morphine-3-glucuronide in the liver and the latter is excreted into bile. The bile carries the metabolite into the intestine where bacteria hydrolyze the metabolite to free morphine. The latter is reabsorbed from the intestine and returns to the blood.

tabolite is nearly completely hydrolyzed by bacterial flora in the intestinal tract, so that what appears in the feces is free morphine. Even though only about 7% of the administered dose of morphine appears to follow this pathway, it is of interest in that, compared with other species, man seems to have an exceptionally low morphine excretion in bile. The figures in man belie the observations that very large amounts of morphine metabolite are excreted in bile in many animals. For instance, by cannulating the bile duct in the rat, March and Elliott *(83)* found that in 6 hours 62.6% of the administered dose of morphine was found in this collected bile! In the urine, only 18.1% of the dose was found. This latter figure rose to 63.6% urinary excretion in the intact rat where the bile was not collected but allowed to flow normally into the intestine. Clearly, urinary excretion of 63.6% of the dose could only be possible if the material that is excreted in bile is reabsorbed from the intestine. An enterohepatic circulation of the material was occurring. This meant that, as we usually do excretion studies by measuring urinary and fecal output of drugs and metabolites, enterohepatic circulation would be overlooked. The enterohepatic circulation process is diagrammed in Fig. 22. For the dog, a similar enterohepatic circulation was found for morphine by Woods *(56)*. Twelve hours after administration of morphine, 37.7% of the dose was collected in bile. Since the usual fecal excretion was less than 10% in dogs in which bile was not collected *(151)*, Woods concluded that a large amount of morphine underwent enterohepatic circulation. He further identified the main constituent excreted in the bile of the dog and rat as morphine-3-glucuronide. This discovery meant that morphine-3-glucuronide was probably hydrolyzed in the intestine to free morphine and the latter was reabsorbed by the intestine. That enterohepatic circulation was not peculiar to the glucuronide metabolite or to the rat and dog was shown by using the cat in which the biliary metabolite was morphine-3-ethereal sulfate *(92)*. In a fine piece of work, Dobbs *et al. (152)* showed that etorphine underwent enterohepatic circulation in the rat. This cycle of biliary excretion and reabsorption could be interrupted by sterilizing the intestinal tract of certain bacteria by use of an antibiotic. They conclusively demonstrated that bacteria hydrolyze the etorphine-3-glucuronide. Because etorphine-3-glucuronide itself is not reabsorbed, and sterilizing the intestine effectively inhibits the hydrolysis of this glucuronide, no free etorphine is available for reabsorption in the antibiotic-treated animals.

Since biliary excretion involves such a large percentage of the dose of some narcotics, studying these examples may provide insights into what mechanisms are involved in this excretory process. Is the fact that man does not excrete much of these narcotics into bile an indication of a lack of an excretory mechanism for the narcotic? Part of this answer will come from studying humans more thoroughly. Are the mechanisms for biliary secretion in the liver similar to the mechanisms which exist in the kidney for secretion of the same compounds?

Superficially, there appears to be a close similarity of the hepatic and renal "active" excretory mechanism. In the liver, one system handles anions such as bromosulfophthalein, phenol red, and chlorothiazide; another system handles cations such as procainamide ethobromide, mepiperphenidol, benzomethamine, and certain other quaternary nitrogen compounds. By an imperfect analogy to the renal systems, the systems in the liver also appear to involve active transport processes or at least carrier-mediated processes since they show: (a) saturation of transport capacity with increasing concentration of compound, (b) competition for transport between compounds within each system, (c) inhibition by compounds which poison the metabolic processes of the cell, (d) transport from blood plasma to bile frequently against a concentration gradient. See reviews by Sperber *(153)*, Shanker *(154)*, Brauer *(155)*, and Stowe and Plaa *(156)*, among others, for further details. A third system which transports neutral compounds such as ouabain has been described by Kupferberg and Schanker *(157)*. Even though mechanisms of biliary excretion are broadly classified and are being studied intensively at the present time, very little work has been done specifically on the mechanism of biliary excretion of morphine and its metabolites. Some recent information from our laboratory which indicates the complexity of the problem and at the same time gives some new insights will be presented.

Table V shows that the rat excreted administered morphine as morphine-3-glucuronide to a greater extent than the cat excreted administered morphine as morphine-3-ethereal sulfate. Was this species difference in biliary excretion of morphine due to different excretory capacities

**TABLE V**

BILIARY EXCRETION OF RADIOACTIVITY IN RENAL-LIGATED ANIMALS AFTER ADMINISTRATION OF MORPHINE-$N^{14}CH_3$, MORPHINE-3-GLUCURONIDE (MG), OR MORPHINE-3-ETHEREAL SULFATE (MES). THE COMPOUNDS WERE ADMINISTERED INTRAVENOUSLY AND BILE WAS COLLECTED FOR 3 HOURS.[a]

| Compound Given | Percentage of dose recovered ± S.E. | |
|---|---|---|
| | Rat | Cat |
| Morphine | 64 ± 5[b] | 23 ± 1[c] |
| MG | 81 ± 4 | 17 ± 4 |
| MES | 29 ± 5 | 20 ± 3 |

[a] From Peterson et al. (158).
[b] Mostly morphine-3-glucuronide with small amount of morphine.
[c] Mostly morphine-3-ethereal sulfate with some morphine-3-glucuronide. In all other cases the compound excreted was that which was administered.

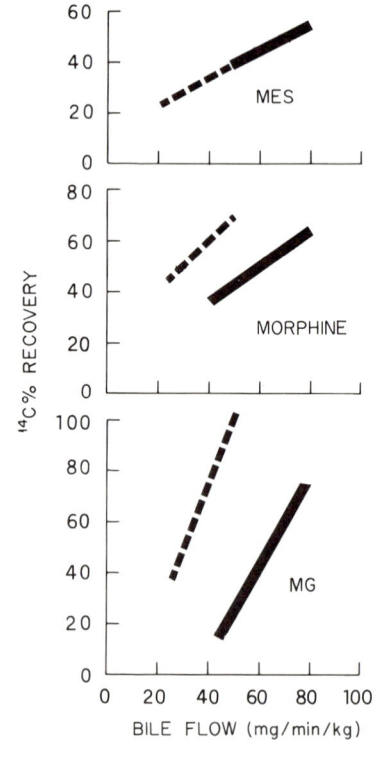

FIG. 23. The biliary excretion of $^{14}C$ after intravenous administration of morphine-$N^{14}CH_3$ ethereal sulfate (MES), morphine, or morphine glucuronide (MG) to rats and relation to bile flow. Control rats – – –; phenobarbital pretreated rats ——. Phenobarbital pretreatment consisted of daily doses of 70 mg/kg of phenobarbital sodium given intraperitoneally for 3 days. The rats were used on the fourth day. Note that phenobarbital pretreatment has different effects depending on the compound administered; morphine and MG or MES. Adapted from Peterson and Fujimoto (159).

of the rat and cat or due to the different biliary metabolites excreted in each species? To answer this question, the rat metabolite, morphine-3-glucuronide, was administered to both species. The results in the table show that this administered morphine glucuronide was excreted to a greater extent in the rat than the cat. This result closely paralleled the total recoveries when morphine was given in each species. In direct contrast, when the cat metabolite, morphine ethereal sulfate, was administered, it was excreted to the same extent in both species. Thus, the biliary excretion of morphine ethereal sulfate in the rat and cat was similar while the excretion values after morphine and morphine glucuronide were different in these species. These results indicate that different factors govern the excretion of morphine glucuronide as compared to those that govern the biliary excretion of morphine ethereal sulfate.

Further evidence for this last statement has been provided by Peterson and Fujimoto *(159)* in phenobarbital-induced rats. Figure 23 shows that when bile flow was enhanced by phenobarbital induction, the increase in excretion of morphine ethereal sulfate was parallel to the increase in bile flow. On the other hand, the biliary excretion of morphine glucuronide, whether exogenously administered or formed from morphine within the animal, was not enhanced by phenobarbital treatment even though bile flow was greatly increased. Thus, a linear continuity related to bile flow was seen in excretion of morphine ethereal sulfate between control and phenobarbital-induced animals. A discontinuity was evident for morphine glucuronide in going from control to phenobarbital-treated rats. Therefore, phenobarbital induction affected biliary excretion of morphine ethereal sulfate in a distinctly different fashion from morphine glucuronide. Although both the ethereal sulfate and glucuronide are organic anions, the systems involved in their excretion into bile are separable. The mechanisms for transport in the liver are not analogous to those found in the kidney. We are optimistic that our initial studies on excretion of these compounds into bile may be one approach which will help us understand the general physiology of biliary excretion and later perhaps tell us why the system in man is so different from that in certain animals.

## XIII. CERTAIN ASPECTS OF METABOLISM OF $\Delta^9$- TETRAHYDROCANNABINOL

Because the primary active constituent of marihuana has been established to be L-$\Delta$-9-*trans*-tetrahydrocannabinol, $\Delta^9$-THC, *(160,161)*, much research has been done recently on the metabolism of this substance. One major metabolite, 11-hydroxy-$\Delta^9$-THC (Fig. 24), was independently discovered by Nilsson *et al. (162)* and Wall *et al. (163)*. Other metabolites have been described by these and other groups, but the 11-hydroxy metabolite has been the most interesting of those discovered

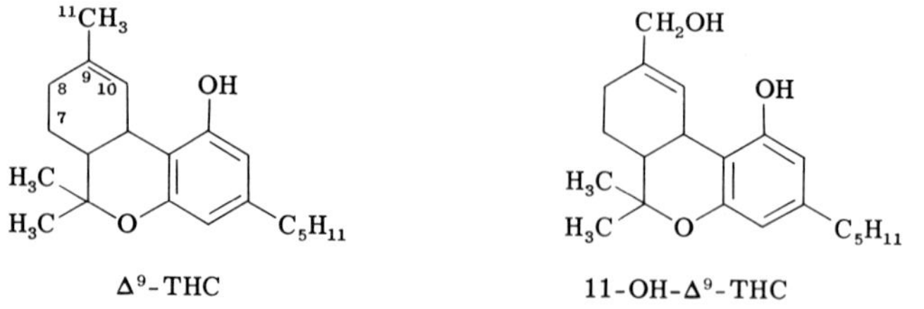

FIG. 24. Formula of $\Delta^9$-tetrahydrocannabinol and a major metabolite, 11-hydroxy-$\Delta^9$-tetrahydrocannabinol.

because it possesses high biological activity *(164)*. This metabolite, when injected intravenously into the mouse, was twice as active as the parent compound, $\Delta^9$-THC. Even more important, administered directly into the central nervous system by intracerebral administration, 11-hydroxy-$\Delta^9$-THC was 18 times more potent than $\Delta^9$-THC. These findings support the suggestion that a metabolite rather than the parent compound may be responsible for the pharmacological activity of $\Delta^9$-THC *(165, 166)*. Since this hydroxylation of $\Delta^9$-THC was carried on by the mixed function oxidase system of the liver *(162,163)*, there was an immediate flurry of research activity involving attempts to test the active metabolite hypothesis. For example, Nakazawa and Costa *(167)* found enhanced effects of $\Delta^9$-THC on motor activity of rats pretreated with 3-methylcholanthrene. The 3-methylcholanthrene pretreatment had induced microsomal enzymes for increased metabolism of $\Delta^9$-THC in the lung, so that a metabolite was implicated for the enhanced effects. On the other hand, there are reports that support an opposite point of view. Matilla-Plata and Harbison *(168)* found that in phenobarbital-induced mice $\Delta^9$-THC lethality is reduced and SKF 525A (diethylaminoethyl-2,2-diphenylvalerate), a compound frequently used as an inhibitor of microsomal drug metabolism, increases the lethality of $\Delta^9$-THC. Sofia and Barry *(169)* found that SKF 525A prolongs the effect of $\Delta^9$-THC on barbital sleeping time in mice. Thus, these latter studies appear to show that $\Delta^9$-THC rather than a metabolite is the active compound. From a predictive point of view it is difficult to know what to expect when the metabolism of $\Delta^9$-THC is altered by inhibitors and inducers of microsomal enzymes. Metabolism of $\Delta^9$-THC involves more than just the single step of the formation of the 11-hydroxy metabolite. Other pathways of metabolism as well as the subsequent steps of degradation of the 11-hydroxy-$\Delta^9$-THC might be affected by inducers and inhibitors of microsomal enzymes. Preliminary evidence for such effects exists *(167)*. To confound the situation even more, some of the effects attributed to changes at the microsomal enzyme-$\Delta^9$-THC metabolism level may involve interactions at another site, as shown by our work (170). In mice pretreated with phenobarbital, where microsomal enzymes had been induced, the responses to $\Delta^9$-THC were blocked. Superficially, these results were consistent with the thought that $\Delta^9$-THC itself rather than a metabolite was the active compound. However, further experiments showed that this conclusion was not valid because the interaction of phenobarbital with $\Delta^9$-THC could be shown to occur in the central nervous system rather than in relation to the microsomal enzyme system in the liver. In order to localize this interaction to the central nervous system, a small dose of phenobarbital was injected intracerebrally to the mice. Under this condition, no phenobarbital induction of microsomal enzymes occurred in the liver. Yet, the subsequent effects of $\Delta^9$-THC administration were blocked just as in the previous experiments. From these findings, the only reasonable conclusion was that induction of hepatic microsomal enzyme has little to do with the interactions observed in the experiment. It therefore appears that altered receptor sensitivity in the central nervous system rather than altered metabolism is responsible for the observed findings. It seems appropriate to end here on a somewhat cautious note because we have circuitously returned from considering what the organism does to the drug to the realm of what the drug does to the organism.

## ACKNOWLEDGMENT

The author wishes to acknowledge with gratitude the invaluable assistance of Richard Peterson and David Smith in preparing this manuscript.

## REFERENCES

1. Eddy, N., Halbach, H., Isbell, H., and Seevers, M. H. (1965). Drug dependence: its significance and characteristics. *Bull W. H. O.* **32**, 721–733.
2. Berjerot, N. (1970). "Addiction and Society." Thomas, Springfield, Illinois.
3. Williams, R. T. (1959). "Detoxication Mechanisms," 2nd ed. Wiley, New York.
4. Remmer, H. (1962). Drug tolerance. *In* "Enzymes and Drug Action" (J. L. Mongar and A. V. S. de Reuck, eds.), pp. 276–300. Little, Brown, Boston, Massachusetts.
5. Remmer, H. (1958). Die Beschleunigung des Evipanabbaues unter der Wirkung von Barbituraten. *Naturwissenschaften* **45**, 189–190.
6. Remmer, H., and Alsleben, B. (1958). Die Aktivierung der Entgiftung in den Lebermikrosomen wahrend der Gewohnung. *Klin. Wochensch.* **36**, 332–333.
7. Brodie, B. B. (1956). Pathways of drug metabolism. *J. Pharm. Pharmacol.* **8**, 1–17.
8. Remmer, H. (1959). Der beschleunigte Abbau von Pharmaka in den Lebermikrosomen unter dem Einfluss von Luminal. *Arch. Exp. Pathol. Pharmakol.* **235**, 279–290.
9. Remmer, H. (1963). Die Ursache der Gewohnung an oxydable Barbiturate. *Arch. Exp. Pathol. Pharmakol.* **244**, 311–333.

10. Remmer, H., and Siegert, M. (1964). Beschleunigter Arzneimittelabbau durch Enzyminduktion beim Hunde nach Behandlung mit Phenobarbital. *Arch. Exp. Pathol. Pharmakol.* **247**, 522–543.
11. Conney, A. H., and Burnes, J. J. (1962). Factors influencing drug metabolism. *Advan. Pharmacol.* **1**, 31–58.
12. Hodgson, E., ed. (1968). "Enzymatic Oxidation of Toxicants." North Carolina State Univ., Raleigh, North Carolina.
13. Gillette, J. R., Conney, A. H., Cosmides, G. J., Estabrook, R. W., Fouts, J. R., and Mannering, G. J., eds. (1959). "Microsomes and Drug Oxidations." Academic Press, New York.
14. Mannering, G. J. (1968). Significance of stimulation and inhibition of drug metabolism in pharmacological testing. *In* "Selected Pharmacological Testing Methods" (A. Burger, ed.), pp. 51–119. Dekker, New York.
15. Brodie, B. B., Gillette, J. R., and La Du, B. N. (1958). Enzymatic metabolism of drugs and other foreign compounds. *Annu. Rev. Biochem.* **27**, 427–454.
16. La Du, B. N., Mandel, H. G., and Way, E. L., eds. (1971). "Fundamentals of Drug Metabolism and Drug Disposition." Williams & Wilkins, Baltimore, Maryland, 1971.
17. Coulson, R. A., and Brazda, F. G. (1947). Effect of feeding pyridine derivatives to young rats on a high protein diet. *Proc. Soc. Exp. Biol. Med.* **65**, 1–5.
18. Brazda, F. G. (1948). The influence of coramine on the liver of the young rat. *Proc. Soc. Exp. Biol. Med.* **67**, 37–40.
19. Dessaur, H. C., and Brazda, F. G. (1955). Effect of coramine on liver and plasma protein. *Proc. Soc. Exp. Biol. Med.* **89**, 676–678.
20. Foster, W. R., and Brazda, F. G. (1958). Effect of nikethamide on incorporation of radioactive phosphate into rat liver deoxypentosenucleic acid. *Cancer Res.* **18**, 289–293.
21. Brazda, F. G., and Baucum, F. G. (1961). The effect of nikethamide on the metabolism of pentobarbital by liver microsomes of the rat. *J. Pharmacol. Exp. Ther.* **132**, 295–298.
22. Brazda, F. G., Hudingsfelder, S., and Martin, M. (1965). Effect of nikethamide on pentobarbital sleeping time in various animal species. *Comp. Biochem. Physiol.* **14**, 239–244.
23. Serrone, D., and Fujimoto, J. M. (1962). The effect of certain inhibitors in producing shortening of hexobarbital action. *Biochem. Pharmacol.* **11**, 609–615.
24. Serrone, D. M. and Fujimoto, J. M. (1961). The diphasic effect of N-methyl-3-piperidyl-N',N'-diphenylcarbamate HCl (MPDC) on the metabolism of hexobarbital. *J. Pharmacol. Exp. Ther.* **133**, 12–17.
25. Kato, R., Chiesara, E., and Vassanelli, P. (1962). Stimulating effect of some inhibitors of drug metabolism (SKF 525A, Lilly 18947, Lilly 32391 and MG 3062) on excretion of ascorbic acid and drug metabolism. *Med. Exp.* **6**, 254–260.
26. Fujimoto, J. M., Eich, W. F., and Nichols, H. R. (1965). Enhanced sulfobromophthalein disappearance in mice pretreated with various drugs. *Biochem. Pharmacol.* **14**, 515–524.
27. Fujimoto, J. M. (1965). Enhanced (indocyanine green) liver function produced by drug pretreatment in mice. *23rd Int Congr. Physiol. Sci.* p. 503.
28. Roberts, R. J., and Plaa, G. L. (1967). Effect of phenobarbital on the excretion of an exogenous bilirubin load. *Biochem. Pharmacol.* **16**, 827–835.
29. Klaassen, C. D., and Plaa, G. L. (1968). Studies on the mechanism of phenobarbital-enhanced sulfobromphthalein disappearance. *J. Pharmacol. Exp. Ther.* **161**, 361–366.

30. Klaassen, C. D., and Plaa, G. L. (1969). Plasma disappearance and biliary excretion of indocyanine green in rats, rabbits and dogs. *Toxicol. Appl. Pharmacol.* **15**, 374–384.
31. Klaassen, C. D. (1969). Biliary flow after microsomal enzyme induction. *J. Pharmacol. Exp. Ther.* **168**, 218–223.
32. Klaassen, C. D. (1970). Plasma disappearance and biliary excretion of sulfobromphthalein and phenol-3,6-dibromphthalein disulfonate after microsomal enzyme induction. *Biochem. Pharmacol.* **19**, 1241–1249.
33. Whitsett, T. L., Dayton, P. G., and McNay, J. L. (1971). The effect of hepatic blood flow on the hepatic removal rate of oxyphenbutazone in the dog. *J. Pharmacol. Exp. Ther.* **177**, 246–255.
34. Ohnhaus, E. E., Thorzeirsson, S. S., Davies, D. S., and Breckenridge, A. (1971). Changes in liver blood flow during enzyme induction. *Biochem. Pharmacol.* **20**, 2561–2570.
35. Brodeur, J., and Marchand, C. (1971). Effect of splenectomy on the activity of drug-metabolizing enzymes in the liver of rats. *Can. J. Physiol. Pharmacol.* **49**, 161–166.
36. Ebert, A. G., Yim, G. K. W., and Miya, T. S. (1964). Distribution and metabolism of barbital [14]C in tolerant and nontolerant rats. *Biochem. Pharmacol.* **13**, 1267–1274.
37. Remmer, H., Siegert, M., Nitze, H. R., and Kirsten, I. (1962). Die Gewohnung an langwirkend Barbiturate. *Arch. Exp. Pathol. Pharmakol.* **243**, 468–478.
38. Butler, T. C. (1950). The rate of penetration of barbituric acid derivatives into the brain. *J. Pharmacol. Exp. Ther.* **100**, 219–226.
39. Brodie, B. B., Bernstein, E., and Mark, L. C. (1952). The role of body fat in limiting the duration of action of thiopental. *J. Pharmacol. Exp. Ther.* **105**, 421.
40. Price, H. L., Kovnot, P. J., Safer, J. N., Conner, E. H., and Price, M. L. (1960.) The uptake of thiopental by body tissues and its relation to the duration of narcosis. *Clin. Pharmacol. Ther.* **1**, 16–22.
41. Goldstein, A., and Aronow, L. (1960). The durations of action of thiopental and pentobarbital. *J. Pharmacol. Exp. Ther.* **128**, 1–6.
42. Waddell, W. J., and Butler, T. C. (1957). The distribution and excretion of phenobarbital. *J. Clin. Invest.* **36**, 1217–1227.
43. Milne, M. D., Scribner, B. H., and Crawford, M. A. (1958). Nonionic diffusion and the excretion of weak acids and bases. *Amer. J. Med.* **24**, 709–729.
44. Clowes, G. H. A., Keltch, A. K., and Krahl, M. E. (1940). Extracellular and intracellular hydrogen ion concentration in relation to anesthetic effects of barbituric acid derivaties. *J. Pharmacol. Exp. Ther.* **68**, 312–329.
45. Schanker, L. S. (1962). Passage of drugs across body membranes. *Pharmacol. Rev.* **14**, 501–530.
46. Fujimoto, J. M., and Donnelly, R. A. (1968). Effect of feeding and fasting on excretion of phenobarbital in the rabbit. *Clin. Toxicol.* **1**, 297–307.
47. Reinberg, A., and Halberg, F. (1971). Circadian chronopharmacology. *Annu. Rev. Pharmacol.* **11**, 455–492.
48. Way, E. L., and Adler, T. K. (1962). "The Biological Disposition of Morphine and Its Surrogates." World Health Organization, Geneva, Switzerland.
49. Wright, C. I. (1942). The deacetylation of heroin and related compounds by mammalian tissue. *J. Pharmacol. Exp. Ther.* **75**, 328–337.
50. Way, E. L., Young, J. M., and Kemp, J. (1965). Metabolism of heroin and its pharmacologic implications. *Bull. Narcotics* **17**, 25–33.

51. Way, E. L., Kemp, J. W., Young, J. M., and Grasetti, D. R. (1960). The pharmacological effects of heroin in relationship to its rate of biotransformation. *J. Pharmacol. Exp. Ther.* **129**, 144–154.
52. Way, E. L. (1971). Effects of narcotics and local anesthetics. In "Implications to Teratology," Proc. Conf. on Toxicology (R. Newburgh, ed.), pp. 234–256.
53. Kupferberg, H., and Way, E. L. (1963). Pharmacologic basis for the increased sensitivity of the newborn rat to morphine. *J. Pharmacol. Exp. Ther.* **141**, 105–112.
54. Fujimoto, J. M., and Way, E. L. (1957). Isolation and crystallization of "bound" morphine from urine of human addicts. *J. Pharmacol. Exp. Ther.* **121**, 340–346.
55. Fujimoto, J. M., and Way, E. L. (1958). Studies on the structure of "bound" morphine. *J. Amer. Pharm. Ass.* **47**, 273–275.
56. Woods, L. A. (1954). Distribution and fate of morphine in nontolerant and tolerant dogs and rats. *J. Pharmacol. Exp. Ther.* **112**, 158–175.
57. Oka, T. (1967). A simple method for the isolation of morphine glucuronide from urine. *Keio J. Med.* **16**, 31–36.
58. Oguri, K., Ida, S., Yoshimura, H., and Tsukamato, H. (1970). Metabolism of drugs. LXIX. Studies on the urinary metabolites of morphine in several mammalian species. *Chem. Pharm. Bull.* **18**, 2414–2419.
59. Yoshimura, H., Oguri, K., and Tsukamoto, H. (1969). Metabolism of drugs. XLII. Isolation and identification of morphine glucuronides in urine and bile of rabbits. *Biochem. Pharmacol.* **18**, 279–286.
60. Yoshimura, H., Mori, M., Oguri, K., and Tsukamoto, H. (1970). Metabolism of drugs. LXV. Studies on the urinary conjugated metabolities of codeine. *Biochem. Pharmacol.* **19**, 2353–2360.
61. Krueger, H., Eddy, N. B., and Sumwalt, M. (1941). Absorption and fate by Margaret Sumwalt. In "The Pharmacology of the Opium Alkaloids," Public Health Rep. Suppl. 165. pp. 759–811. U. S. Gov't. Printing Office, Washington, D. C.
62. Way, E. L., and Adler, T. K. (1960). The pharmacologic implications of the fate of morphine and its surrogates. *Pharmacol. Rev.* **12**, 383–446.
63. Mulé, S. J. (1971). Physiological disposition of narcotic agonists and antagonists. In "Narcotic Drugs: Biochemical Pharmacology" (D. Clouet, ed.), pp. 91–12. Plenum, New York.
64. Shimomura, K., Kamata, O., Ueki, S., Ida, S., Oguri, K., Yoshimura, H., and Tsukamoto, H. (1971). Analgesic effect of morphine glucuronides. *Tohoku J. Exp. Med.* **105**, 45–52.
65. Misra, A. L., Yeh, S. Y., and Woods, L. A. (1970). Morphine conjugates in the dog. *Biochem. Pharmacol.* **19**, 1536–1539.
66. Elison, C., and Elliott, H. W. (1964). Studies on the enzymatic N- and O-demethylation of narcotic analgesics and evidence for the formation of codeine from morphine in rats and dogs. *J. Pharmacol. Exp. Ther.* **144**, 265–275.
67. Clouet, D. H., ed. (1971). "Narcotic Drugs: Biochemical Pharmacology." Plenum, New York.
68. Beckett, A. H. (1956). Analgesics and their antagonists: some steric and chemical considerations. Part I. The dissociation constants of some tertiary amines and synthetic analgesics; the conformation of methadone-type compounds. *J. Pharm. Pharmacol.* **8**, 848–859.
69. Beckett, A. H., Casy, A. F., Harper, N. J., and Phillips, P. M. (1956). Analgesics and their antagonists: some steric and chemical considerations. Part II. The influence of the basic group on physicochemical properties and the activity of methadone and thiambutene-type compounds. *J. Pharm. Pharmacol.* **8**, 860–873.

70. Beckett, A. H., Casy, A. F., and Harper, N. J. (1958). Some steric and chemical considerations. Part III. The influence of the basic group on the biological response. *J. Pharm. Pharmacol.* **8**, 874–883.
71. Axelrod, J. (1956). Possible mechanism of tolerance to narcotic drugs. *Science* **124**, 263–264.
72. Miller, J. W., Anderson, H.H., and Hamilton, H. (1954). The effect of N-demethylation on certain pharmacologic actions of morphine, codeine and meperidine in the mouse. *J. Pharmacol. Exp. Ther.* **112**, 191–196.
73. Lockett, M. F., and Davis, M. M. (1958). The analgesic action of normorphine administered intracisternally to mice. *J. Pharm. Pharmacol.* **10**, 80–85.
74. Milthers, K. (1962). The *in vivo* transformation of morphine and nalorphine into normorphine in the brain of rats. *Acta Pharmacol. Toxicol.* **19**, 235–240.
75. Elison, C., and Elliott, H. W. (1963). N- and O-demethylation of some narcotic analgesics by brain slices from male and female Long-Evans rats. *Biochem. Pharmacol.* **12**, 1363–1366.
76. Woods, L. A. (1956). The pharmacology of nalorphine (N-allylnormoprhine). *Pharmacol. Rev.* **8**, 175–198.
77. Martin, W. R. (1967). Opioid antagonists. *Pharmacol. Rev.* **19**, 463–521.
78. Weinstein, S. H., Pfeffer, M., Schor, J. M., Indindoli, L., and Mintz, M. (1971). Metabolites of naloxone in human urine. *J. Pharm. Sci.* **60**, 1567–1568.
79. Blane, G. F., Boura, A. L. A., Fitzgerald, A. E., and Lister, R. E. (1967). Actions of etorphine hydrochloride (M99), a potent morphine-like agent. *Brit. J. Pharmacol. Chemother.* **30**, 11–22.
80. Belleau, B. (1965). Conformational perturbation in relation to the regulation of enzyme and receptor behavior. *Advan. Drug Res.* **2**, 89–125.
81. Misra, A. L., Mitchell, C. L., and Woods, L. A. (1971). Persistence of morphine in central nervous system of rats after a single injection and its bearing on tolerance. *Nature (London)* **232**, 48–50.
82. Smith, A. A. (1971), Inhibitors of tolerance development. *In* "Narcotic Drugs: Biochemical Pharmacology" (D. Clouet, ed.), p. 424. Plenum, New York.
83. March, C. H., and Elliott, H. W. (1954). Distribution and excretion of radioactivity after administration of morphine-N-methyl-C$^{14}$ to rats. *Proc. Soc. Exp. Biol. Med.* **85**, 494–497.
84. Adler, T. K., and Shaw, F. H. (1951). The biological liberation of morphine from codeine in the rat. *J. Pharmacol. Exp. Ther.* **104**, 1–10.
85. Mannering, G. J., Dixon, A. C., Baker, E. M., and Asami, T. (1954). The *in vivo* liberation of morphine from codeine in man. *J. Pharmacol. Exp. Ther.* **111**, 142–146.
86. Adler, T. K., Fujimoto, J. M., Way, E. L., and Baker, E. M. (1955). The metabolic fate of codeine in man. *J. Pharmacol. Exp. Ther.* **114**, 251–262.
87. Woods, L. A., Muehlenbeck, H. E., and Mellett, L. B. (1956). Plasma levels and excretion of codeine metabolites in the dog and monkey. *J. Pharmacol. Exp. Ther.* **117**, 117–125.
88. Yeh, S. Y., and Woods, L. A. (1969). Physiologic disposition of N-$^{14}$C-methylcodeine in the rat. *J. Pharmacol. Exp. Ther.* **166**, 86–95.
89. Adler, T. K. (1963). The comparative potencies of codeine and its demethylated metabolites after intraventricular injections in the mouse. *J. Pharmacol. Exp. Ther.* **140**, 155–161.
90. McMillan, D. E., Wolf, P. S., and Carchman, R. A. (1970). Antagonism of the behavioral effects of morphine and methadone by narcotic antagonists in the pigeon. *J. Pharmacol. Exp. Ther.* **175**, 443–458.

91. Fujimoto, J. M. (1969). Isolation of two different glucuronide metabolites of naloxone from urine of rabbit and chicken. *J. Pharmacol. Exp. Ther.* **168**, 180–186.
92. Yeh, S. Y., Chernov, H. I., and Woods, L. A. (1971). Metabolism of morphine by cats. *J. Pharm. Sci.* **60**, 469–471.
93. Fujimoto, J. M., and Haarstad, V. B. (1969). The isolation of morphine-ethereal sulfate from urine of the chicken and cat. *J. Pharmacol. Exp. Ther.* **165**, 45–51.
94. Fujimoto, J. M. (1970). Isolation of naloxone-3-glucuronide from human urine. *Proc. Soc. Exp. Biol. Med.* **133**, 317–319.
95. Ober, K., and Fujimoto, J. M. (1972). Isolation of naloxone-3-ethereal sulfate from urine of the cat. *Proc. Soc. Exp. Biol. Med.* **139**, 1068–1070.
96. Dayton, H. B., and Blumberg, H. (1969). A comparison of the narcotic antagonist naloxone and its 6-hydroxy analog EN 2265. *Fed. Proc.* **28**, 736.
97. Baker, W. P., and Woods, L. A. (1957). A study in the dog on the renal clearance of morphine and the effect of morphine on p-aminohippurate clearance. *J. Pharmacol. Exp. Ther.* **120**, 371–374.
98. Weiner, I. M. (1971). Excretion of drugs by the kidney. In "Handbuch der experimentellen Pharmakologie. Part I. Concepts in Biochemical Pharmacology" (B. B. Brodie, J. R. Gillette, Helen S. Ackerman, eds.), p. 328. Springer-Verlag, Berlin and New York.
99. Peters, L. (1960). Renal tubular excretion of organic bases. *Pharmacol. Rev.* **12**, 1–35.
100. Cafruny, E. J. (1971). Renal excretion of drugs. In "Fundamentals of Drug Metabolism and Drug Disposition" (B. N. La Du, H. G. Mandel, and E. L. Way, eds.), p. 119. Plenum, New York.
101. Milne, M. D., Scribner, B. H., and Crawford, M. A. (1958). Non-ionic diffusion and the excretion of weak acids and bases. *Amer. J. Med.* **24**, 709–729.
102. Asatoor, A. M., London, D. R., Milne, M. D., and Simenhoff, M. L. (1963). The excretion of pithidine and its derivatives. *Brit. J. Pharmacol.* **20**, 285–298.
103. Beckett, A. H., Boyer, R. N., and Tucker, G. T. (1968). Use of the analogue computer to predict distribution and excretion of drugs under conditions of fluctuating urinary pH. *J. Pharm. Pharmacol.* **20**, 277–278.
104. Beckett, A. H., Taylor, J. F., Casy, A. F., and Hassan, M. M. A. (1968). The biotransformation of methadone in man: synthesis and identification of a major metabolite. *J. Pharm. Pharmacol.* **20**, 754–762.
105. Baselt, R. C., and Casarett, L. J. (1972). Urinary excretion of methadone in man. *Clin. Pharmacol. Ther.* **13**, 64–70.
106. Hug, C. G., Mellett, L. B., and Cafruny, E. J. (1965). Stop-flow analysis of the renal excretion of tritium-labeled dihydromorphine. *J. Pharmacol. Exp. Ther.* **150**, 259–269.
107. Fujimoto, J. M., and Way, E. L. (1958). Studies on the structure of "bound" morphine. *J. Amer. Pharm. Ass.* **47**, 273–275.
108. Sperber, I. (1946). A new method for the study of renal tubular excretion in birds. *Nature (London)* **158**, 131.
109. Sperber, I. (1948). Investigations of the circulatory system of the avian kidney. *Zool. Bidrag Uppsala* **27**, 429–448.
110. Sperber, I. (1948). The excretion of some glucuronic acid derivatives and phenol sulphuric esters in the chicken. *Lantbrucks-hoegsk. Ann.* **15**, 317–349.
111. Sperber, I. (1949). The formation of sulphuric esters of phenols in the chicken. *Lantbruks-Hoegskol. Ann.* **16**, 446–456.
112. Fujimoto, J. M. (1971). Chap. 17. V. Sites of action of narcotic analgesic drugs—the

kidney. *In* "Narcotic Drugs: Biochemical Pharmacology" (D. Clouet, ed.), p. 366. Plenum, New York.
113. Watrous, W. M. (1972). Personal communication.
114. May, D. G., Fujimoto, J. M., and Inturrisi, C. E. (1967). The tubular transport and metabolism of morphine-N-methyl-C$^{14}$ by the chicken kidney. *J. Pharmacol. Exp. Ther.* **157**, 626–635.
115. Watrous, W. M., May, D. G., and Fujimoto, J. M. (1970). Mechanism of renal tubular transport of morphine and morphine ethereal sulfate in the chicken. *J. Pharmacol. Exp. Ther.* **172**, 224–229.
116. Hakim, R., Watrous, W. M., and Fujimoto, J. M. (1970). The renal tubular transport and metabolism of serotonin (5 HT) and 5-hydroxyindoleacetic acid in the chicken. *J. Pharmacol. Exp. Ther.* **175**, 749–762.
117. Watrous, W. M., and Fujimoto, J. M. (1971). Inhibition of morphine metabolism by catechol in the chicken kidney. *Biochem. Pharmacol.* **20**, 1479–1491.
118. Quebbemann, A. J., and Rennick, B. R. (1968). Catechol transport by the renal tubule in the chicken. *Amer. J. Physiol.* **214**, 1201–1204.
119. Anders, M. W. (1971). Enhancement and inhibition of drug metabolism. *Annu. Rev. Pharmacol.* **11**, 37–56.
120. Hakim, R. and Fujimoto, J. M. (1971). Inhibition of renal tubular transport of morphine by beta-diethylaminoethyl diphenylpropylacetate in the chicken. *Biochem. Pharmacol.* **20**, 2647–2662.
121. Fujimoto, J. M., Hakim, R., and Zamiatowski, R. (1972). Inhibition of renal tubular transport of morphine by diethylaminoethanol in the chicken. *Biochem. Pharmacol.* **21**, 2877–2886.
122. Narcotic Rehabilitation Act of 1966. Public Law 89-793. 89th Congress, H. R. 9167.
123. Spector, S. (1971). Quantitative determination of morphine in serum by radioimmunoassay. *J. Pharmacol. Exp. Ther.* **178**, 253–258.
124. Von Vunakis, H., Wasserman, E., and Levine, L. (1972). Specificies of antibodies to morphine. *J. Pharmacol. Exp. Ther.* **180**, 514–521.
125. Syva Corporation. (1971) Bulletin. Free Radical Assay Technique. U. S. Patent 3,489,522. Palo Alto, California.
126. Taylor, J. F. (1971). Methods of chemical analysis. *In* "Narcotic Drugs: Biochemical Pharmacology" (D. Clouet, ed.), Chapter 2. pp. 17–77. Plenum, New York.
127. Fujimoto, J. M., and Wang, R. I. H. (1970). A new method of identifying narcotic analgesics in human urine after therapeutic doses. *Toxicol. Appl. Pharmacol.* **16**, 186–193.
128. Quame, B. A. (1971). Column for testing biological fluids. U. S. Patent 3,567,029.
129. Brinkmann Products. (1971) Bulletin. 141-C. Brinkmann Instruments Inc., Westbury, New York. 11590.
130. Eastman Kodak Products (1971). Bulletin. Eastman Kodak Company, Rochester, New York 14650.
131. Dole, V. P., Kim, W. K., and Eglitis, I. (1966). Detection of narcotic drugs, tranquilizers, amphetamines and barbiturates in urine. *J. Amer. Med. Ass.* **198**, 349–352.
132. Screening for abused drugs (1971). *Lab. Management* **9** (10), 14–20.
133. Davson, H. (1967). "Physiology of Cerebrospinal Fluid." Little, Brown, Boston, Massachusetts.
134. Miller, J. W., and Elliott, H. W. (1955). Rat tissue levels of carbon-14 labeled analgetics as related to pharmacological activity. *J. Pharmacol. Exp. Ther.* **113**, 283–291.

135. Asghar, K., and Way, E. L. (1970). Active removal of morphine from the cerebral ventricles. *J. Pharmacol. Exp. Ther.* 175, 75–83.
136. Takemori, A. E., and Stenwick, M. W. (1966). Studies on the uptake of morphine by the choroid plexus *in vitro*. *J. Pharmacol. Exp. Ther.* 154, 586–594.
137. Hug, C. C., Jr. (1967). Transport of narcotic analgesics by choroid plexus and kidney tissue *in vitro*. *Biochem. Pharmacol.* 16, 345–359.
138. Craig, A. L., O'Dea, R. F., and Takemori, A. E. (1971). The uptake of morphine by the choroid plexus and cerebral cortical slices of animals chronically treated with morphine. *Neuropharmacology* 10, 709–714.
139. Muraki, T. (1971). Uptake of morphine-3-glucuronide by choroid plexuses in vitro. *Eur. J. Pharmacol.* 15, 393–395.
140. Mulé, S. (1971). Physiological disposition of narcotic agonists and antagonists. *In* "Narcotic Drugs: Biochemical Pharmacology" (D Clouet, ed.), p. 99. Plenum, New York.
141. Mulé, S. T., Woods, L. A., and Mellett, L. B. (1961). Distribution of N-C$^{14}$-methyl labeled morphine. II. Effect of nalorphine in the central nervous system of nontolerant dogs and observation of metabolism. *J. Pharmacol. Exp. Ther.* 136, 242–249.
142. Mulé, S. J., Redman, C. M., and Flesher, J. W. (1967). Intracellular disposition of H$^3$-morphine in the brain and liver of nontolerant and tolerant guinea pigs. *J. Pharmacol. Exp. Ther.* 157, 459–471.
143. Wuepper, K. D., Yeh, S. Y., and Woods, L. A. (1967). Effect of nalorphine and levallorphan on brain concentrations of levorphanol in the dog. *Proc. Soc. Exp. Biol. Med.* 124, 1146.
144. Dobbs, H. (1968). Effect of cyprenorphine (M 285), a morphine antagonist, on the distribution and excretion of etorphine (M 99), a potent morphine like drug. *J. Pharmacol. Exp. Ther.* 160, 407–414.
145. Marx, G. F. (1961). Placental transfer and drugs used in anesthesia. *Anesthesiology* 22, 294–313.
146. Sanner, J. H., and Woods, L. A. (1965). Comparative distribution of tritium-labeled dihydromorphine between maternal and fetal rats. *J. Pharmacol. Exp. Ther.* 148, 176–184.
147. Way, W. L., Costley, E. C., and Way, E. L. (1965). Respiratory sensitivity of newborn infant to meperidine and morphine *Clin. Pharmacol. Ther.* 6, 454–461.
148. Blane, G. F., and Dobbs, H. E. (1967). Distribution of tritium labeled etorphine (M 99) and dihydromorphine in pregnant rats at term. *Brit. J. Pharmacol.* 30, 166–172.
149. Oberst, F. W. (1942). Studies on fate of morphine. *J. Pharmacol. Exp. Ther.* 74, 37.
150. Elliott, H. W., Tolbert, B. M., Adler, T. K., and Anderson, H. H. (1954). Excretion of carbon-14 by man after administration of morphine-N-methyl-C$^{14}$. *Proc. Soc. Exp. Biol. Med.* 85, 77–81.
151. Cochin, J., Haggart, J., Woods, L. A., and Seevers, M. H. (1954). Plasma levels, urinary and fecal excretion of morphine in nontolerant and tolerant dogs. *J. Pharmacol. Exp. Ther.* 111, 74–83.
152. Dobbs, H. E., Hall, J. M., and Steiger, B. (19  ). Enterohepatic circulation of etorphine, a potent analgesic, in the rat. *Proc. Eur. Soc. Drug Toxicity* 11, 73–79.
153. Sperber, I. (1959). Secretion of organic anions in the formation of urine and bile. *Pharmacol. Rev.* 11, 109–134.
154. Schanker, L. S. (1965). Hepatic transport of organic cations. *In* "The Biliary System" (W. Taylor, ed.), pp. 469–480. Blackwell, Oxford.

155. Brauer, R. W. (1959). Mechanism of bile secretion. *J. Amer. Med. Ass.* **169**, 1462–1466.
156. Stowe, C. M., and Plaa, G. L. (1968). Extrarenal excretion of drugs and chemicals. *Annu. Rev. Pharmacol.* **8**, 337—356.
157. Kupferberg, H. J., and Schanker, L. S. (1968). Biliary secretion of ouabain-$^3$H and its uptake by liver slices in the rat. *Amer. J. Physiol.* **214**, 1048–1053.
158. Peterson, R. E., Smith, D. S., and Fujimoto, J. M. (1972). A comparison of the metabolism and biliary excretion of morphine, morphine-3-glucuronide and morphine-3-ethereal sulfate in the rat and cat. *Fed. Proc.* **31**, 2202.
159. Peterson, R. E., and Fujimoto, J. M. (1972). Bile flow: differential effects on morphine-3-ethereal sulfate and morphine-3-glucuronide excretion in the rat. *5th Int. Congr. Pharmacol., San Francisco,* p. 181.
160. Isbell, H., Gorodetzsky, C. W., Jasinski, D., Claussen, U., Spulak, F. V., and Korte, F. (1967). Effects of $(-)\Delta^9$-trans-tetrahydrocannabinol in man. *Psychopharmacologia* **11**, 184–188.
161. Mechoulam, R., Shani, A., Edery, H., Greenfeld, Y. (1970). Chemical basis of hashish activity. *Science* **169**, 611–612.
162. Nilsson, I. M., Agurell, S., Nilsson, J. L. G., Ohlsson, A., Sandberg, F., and Wahlquist, M. (1970). $\Delta^1$-Tetrahydrocannabinol: structure of a major metabolite. *Science* **168**, 1228–1229.
163. Wall, M. E., Brine, D. R., Brine, G. A., Pitt, C. G., Freudenthal, R. I., and Christensen, H. D. (1970). Isolation, structure and biological activity of several metabolites of $\Delta^9$-tetrahydrocannabinol. *J. Amer. Chem. Soc.* **92**, 3466–3468.
164. Christensen, H. D., Freudenthal, R. I., Gidley, J. T., Rosenfeld, R., Boegli, G., Testino, L., Brine, D. R., Pitt, C. G., and Wall, M. E. (1971). Activity of $\Delta^8$ and $\Delta^9$-tetrahydrocannabinol related compounds in the mouse. *Science* **172**, 165–167.
165. Grunfeld, Y., and Edery, H. (1969). Psychopharmacological activity of the active constituents of hashish and some related cannabinoids. *Psychopharmacologia* **14**, 200–210.
166. Mechoulam, R. (1970). Marihuana chemistry. *Science* **168**, 1159–1166.
167. Nakazawa, K., and Costa, E. (1971). The pharmacological implications of $\Delta^9$-tetrahydrocannabinol metabolism by lung: effects of 3-methylcholanthrene. *Ann. N.Y. Acad. Sci.* **191**, 216–221.
168. Matilla-Plata, B., and Harbison, R. D. (1971). Phenobarbital and SKF 525A effect on $\Delta^9$-tetrahydrocannabinol (THC) toxicity and distribution in mice. *Pharmacologist* **13**, 588.
169. Sofia, R. D., and Barry, H., III, (1970). Depressant effect of $\Delta^1$-tetrahydrocannabinol enhanced by inhibitors of its metabolism. *Eur. J. Pharmacol.* **13**, 134–137.
170. Fujimoto, J. M. (1972). Modification of the effects of $\Delta^9$-tetrahydrocannabinol by phenobarbital pretreatment in mice. *Toxicol. Appl. Pharmacol.* **23**, 623–634.

Chapter 2

# Kinetics of Active-Site-Directed Irreversible Inhibition*

*A. R. MAIN*

|      |                                                              |     |
| ---- | ------------------------------------------------------------ | --- |
| I.   | Introduction                                                 | 59  |
| II.  | Trivial Names and Symbols                                    | 62  |
|      | A. Trivial Names                                             | 62  |
|      | B. Symbols                                                   | 63  |
| III. | Origins                                                      | 64  |
|      | A. Stoichiometry and Early Kinetic Studies                   | 64  |
|      | B. Inhibitory Power                                          | 66  |
|      | C. First-Order Kinetics and the Inhibition Progress Curve    | 67  |
|      | D. The Kinetics Emerge                                       | 69  |
| IV.  | Kinetics                                                     | 73  |
|      | A. Inhibition Progress Curves                                | 73  |
|      | B. $K_a$ and $k_2$: Binding and Rates of Covalent Bond Formation | 84  |
|      | C. The Scope of the Present Treatment                        | 98  |
|      | References                                                   | 102 |

## I. INTRODUCTION

In 1964, when he introduced the term "active-site-directed irreversible inhibition" (1,2), Baker referred to "the jungles of the so-called active-

---

*Contribution of the Department of Biochemistry, School of Agriculture and Life Sciences, and School of Physical and Mathematical Sciences, North Carolina State University, Raleigh, North Carolina. Paper No. 3688 of the Journal Series of the North Carolina State University Agricultural Experiment Station, Raleigh, North Carolina.

site," in connection with the "frustrations" he had experienced in studying this subject (1). The emotion elicited by the words, "jungle" and "frustration," provide at least one point from which to view the kinetics of active-site-directed irreversible inhibition. But there are other and more promising aspects to the subject, and, while many difficulties remain, a central core has emerged around which a consistent and logical kinetic treatment can be developed. The core is the reaction scheme which describes, for kinetic purposes, the concept of active-site-directed irreversible inhibition:

$$E + AX \underset{}{\overset{K_a}{\rightleftharpoons}} EAX \overset{k_2}{\underset{X}{\searrow}} EA \quad\quad (I)$$

E is an enzyme, AX is the inhibitor with remaining group A and leaving group X, EAX is an enzyme–inhibitor binding complex of the Michaelis type, and EA is the irreversibly inhibited enzyme in which A is covalently linked to E. The equilibrium affinity constant governing formation of EAX is $K_a$, while the rate of covalent bond formation is governed by $k_2$.

This scheme leads to a relatively simple and unified kinetic treatment for a wide variety of inhibitors and enzymes, including (a) organophosphate, organosulfonate, and carbamate inhibitors of cholinesterase (3), and (b) alkylating antimetabolites such as azaserine and TPCK (4).

The present essay will be based primarily on experience with organophosphate and carbamate inhibitors, but the elements should apply to all active-site-directed irreversible inhibitors.

Baker described the interaction of DFP with cholinesterase as the first example of active-site-directed irreversible inhibition, and as a major milestone in the development of this concept (1). DFP was a milestone because its action with cholinesterases and other hydrolytic enzymes demonstrated for the first time and unequivocally that a covalent bond between enzyme and inhibitor could be formed. But the kinetic evidence with DFP did not until recently (5,6) indicate formation of a reversible "affinity" complex (7). The question of a reversible enzyme–inhibitor complex was thus left hanging despite the fact that it is an essential feature of the concept. Baker (1) stated, for example, that "initial complexing with the active site is an obligatory intermediate to the formation of an irreversible covalent bond." The question was how to demonstrate its existence.

The reversible affinity complex is almost as old as enzyme kinetics itself, and underlies our concept of enzyme specificity. The kinetic evidence for it is the rate-limiting velocity which is approached as the substrate concentration increases. Similarly, the kinetic evidence for a reversible complex in irreversible inhibition is the approach to a limiting rate of inhibition as the inhibitor concentration is increased. The kinetics of active-site-directed irreversible inhibition are then largely concerned with the equations and methods by which inhibition in this rate-limiting region can be studied. Although the principle of the rate-limiting step is the same in both the substrate and inhibition reactions, the kinetic approaches differ significantly. Substrate reactions are studied primarily with steady-state kinetics. Irreversible-inhibition kinetics combine the steady-state approach with chemical kinetics applied to elementary reactions. Although this mix has at times been confusing, the treatment has reached a stage where the elements can be described in a reasonably logical and straightforward manner. The present essay will use this approach, but it will not fully reflect the historical development. The historical development tended to be somewhat indirect and perhaps muddled. In order to place the kinetics in a more realistic perspective, an account of the origins will be given first.

Organophosphates and carbamates inhibit by a mechanism which appears to be strictly analogous with that of the substrate reaction (7). This does not seem to be generally true of the alkylating antimetabolites, particularly the exo-alkylating compounds. From the standpoint of a kinetic treatment, perhaps the most important consequence of the substrate analogy is the regeneration reaction. The phosphorylated and carbamylated forms of the enzyme may undergo significant dephosphorylation (8) or decarbamylation (9), respectively, to regenerate free enzyme. Regeneration is analogous with the deacylation phase of the substrate reaction (10,11). Carbamates in particular are characterized by relatively high regeneration rates and they are, in this sense, merely poor substrates (12,13). From the kinetic point of view, the crucial difference between a substrate and an inhibitor is in the relative values of their regeneration constants, for they react by the same sequence:

$$EH + AX \underset{k_{-1}}{\overset{k_1}{\rightleftarrows}} EHAX \overset{k_2}{\underset{HX}{\searrow}} EA + HOH \overset{k_3}{\longrightarrow} EH + AOH \qquad (II)$$

The inhibitors are characterized by much lower $k_3$ values than the substrates. When organophosphates and carbamates are considered, it is convenient to depict a protonated enzyme, EH (11); the H belongs to the hydroxyl group of the seryl residue at the active site, and it is this residue that is phosphorylated (14). Regeneration adds further complexities to the kinetic treatment of organophosphates and carbamates, complexities which are not usually associated with the treatment of alkylating antimetabolite inhibitors.

Before discussing the kinetic origins, something should be said about the remarkable toxicity of organophosphate and carbamate compounds which is undoubtedly, from a practical point of view, their most important characteristic. Some of them are of course widely used as insecticides, and others have potential use as war gases. Their toxicity is directly attributable to the high rates at which they inhibit cholinesterases. Consequently, the kinetics of inhibition is of direct toxicological significance. Among other things, kinetic criteria have been employed in the design of inhibitors through structure–activity studies. The concept of active-site-directed irreversible inhibition is of importance to such studies because it promises to lead to a clearer insight into the relationship between the structure of the inhibitor and its inhibitory power. The concept assigns two functions to the structure of the inhibitor. One is to bind reversibly to the active site, and the other is to form a covalent bond between the enzyme and inhibitor. The kinetic analysis provides a separate measure of each function. Inhibitory power is the product of the two. Previous treatments lumped the functions together and gave only a measure of overall inhibitory power. In providing separate measures, the kinetic analysis permits the structural features of the inhibitor involved in binding to be separated from those concerned with covalent bond formation. This in turn may lead to the design of more selective or more powerful inhibitors.

## II. TRIVIAL NAMES AND SYMBOLS

### A. Trivial Names

*DFP* (diisopropyl phosphorofluoridate)

$$(CH_3CHO)_2\overset{O}{\underset{\|}{P}}-F$$

*paraoxon* (diethyl *p*-nitrophenyl phosphate)

$$(C_2H_5O)_2-\overset{O}{\underset{\|}{P}}-O-\!\!\left\langle\;\right\rangle\!\!-NO_2$$

## 2. ACTIVE-SITE-DIRECTED IRREVERSIBLE INHIBITION

*malaoxon*   (*O,O*-dimethyl *S*-(1, 2-dicarboethoxy) ethyl phosphorothiolate)

$$(CH_3O)_2-\overset{O^-}{\underset{\parallel}{P}}-S-\underset{\underset{\underset{O}{\parallel}}{CH_2-C-O-C_2H_5}}{CH}-\overset{O}{\underset{\parallel}{C}}-O-C_2H_5$$

*tetram*   (*O,O*-diethyl *S*-2-diethylaminoethyl phosphorothiolate)

$$(C_2H_5O)_2-\overset{O}{\underset{\parallel}{P}}-S-CH_2CH_2-N(C_2H_5)_2$$

*eserine*   (physostigmine)

*neostigmine*   (prostigmine)   (3-trimethylaminophenyl *N,N*-dimethylcarbamate)

$$(CH_3)_2N-\overset{O}{\underset{\parallel}{C}}-O-\underset{}{\phantom{XX}}-\overset{+}{N}(CH_3)_3$$

*azaserine*

$$OH-\overset{O}{\underset{\parallel}{C}}-\underset{\underset{}{NH_2}}{CH}-CH_2-O-\overset{O}{\underset{\parallel}{C}}-CHN_2$$

*TPCK*   (L-1-chloro-4-phenyl-3-(*p*-tolylsulfonamido)-2-butanone)

## B. Symbols

E or EH, enzyme
AX, active-site-directed irreversible inhibitor with leaving group X and remaining group A
EA, covalently linked enzyme
EHAX or EAX, Michaelis-type binding complex
$k_1$, $k_{-1}$, $k_2$, $k_3$, elementary rate constants for the reaction Scheme (II)

$k_i$, bimolecular velocity constant
$K_a$, equilibrium affinity constant = $k_{-1}/k_1$ ($K_a$ has elsewhere been termed $K_i$ and $K_e$)
$\rho$, first-order inhibition rate constant ($\rho$ has elsewhere been termed $k_{obs}$ and $k_{app}$)
$v$, velocity of enzyme catalyzed substrate reaction
$v_0$, initial $v$
$S$, substrate
$s$, molar concentration of substrate
$e$, molar concentration of EH
$i$, molar concentration of AX (note that $i$ has a different meaning in Section IV,A)
$e_0$, initial $e$
$i_0$, initial $i$
$r$, molar concentration of EHAX
$q$, molar concentration of EA

## III. ORIGINS

### A. Stoichiometry and Early Kinetic Studies

Concepts about the kinetics of active-site-directed irreversible inhibitors may, with some justification, be traced to the discovery of cholinesterases (15). The justification lies with the fact that the inhibitory action of the naturally occurring carbamate, eserine (physostigmine), played a central role in this discovery. For present purposes, a paper by Easson and Stedman published in 1936 (16) provides a suitable, if somewhat arbitrary, point of departure, for it appears to have had a profound influence on the development of the kinetics of cholinesterase inhibition by carbamates and later organophosphates. Many of the elements of active-site-directed irreversible inhibition were set forth in this paper; in addition, some difficulties were made evident. In developing their analysis, Easson and Stedman assumed that "the drugs (e.g., prostigmine, see Section II) produce their inhibiting action by combining with the enzyme, that the mechanism of the combination is identical with that concerned in the combination between enzyme and substrate, and that consequently one molecule of drug will inhibit the activity of one unit or active center of enzyme by preventing the combination between the latter and the substrate." They were greatly impressed by the "extraordinary affinity of the inhibitor for the enzyme," and while assuming that the reaction was reversible as given by their scheme,

$$E + I \rightleftharpoons EI \qquad (III)$$

they stated further that "this great affinity must clearly mean that the rate of the reverse reaction is exceedingly slow relative to the direct one." They based their kinetics on the assumption that inhibition was of the reversible, noncompetitive type, but they also recognized that inhibition had a competitive component "in the sense that inhibitory action is developed more slowly in the presence than in the absence of substrate."

Their experimental approach emphasized the stoichiometry of the inhibition reaction rather than its rate. Indeed they made a remarkably accurate determination of their cholinesterase concentration, and with it, they calculated the turnover number of butyrylcholine at 30° C, pH 7.4 (3850 seconds$^{-1}$). Nevertheless, their kinetic treatment and those based on it that followed *(17–19)* are clearly at variance with present ideas of the kinetics of active-site-directed irreversible inhibition. The former is based on the assumption of *reversible, noncompetitive inhibition* [cf. Dixon and Webb *(20,* p. 332)] while the latter assumes a *competitive, irreversible* mechanism of inhibition.

Two features of early work are incorporated in the kinetics of active-site-directed irreversible inhibition. The first is "the fractional inhibition '$i$' produced by the inhibitor, a magnitude which can be *determined experimentally,* (and) is numerically equal to [EI]/[E]," where [EI] is the concentration of the enzyme–inhibitor complex, and [E] is "the original," or total concentration of enzyme. Thus, $i$ = [EI]/[E]. Others later designated $i$ as $\alpha$ *(20)* presumably to avoid confusion with the inhibitor concentration ($i$). To understand the present relevance of $i$, the experimental procedure must be examined.

Easson and Stedman incubated the enzyme and inhibitor together, for periods ranging up to 99 hours, *before* adding the substrate. (They recognized, incidentally, that cholinesterase slowly "decomposed" prostigmine and took this into account.) The long incubation periods and low inhibitor concentrations insured "equilibration;" or, more accurately, they allowed the reaction to go to completion. In this way, they titrated the enzyme with prostigmine. The extent of reaction was determined experimentally from the velocity of the substrate reaction catalyzed by the enzyme remaining uninhibited. Thus they recognized that

$$v \propto ([E] - [EI]) \qquad (1)$$

where $([E] - [EI])$ is the concentration of enzyme remaining uninhibited. Since the initial velocity of the control is given by $v_0 \propto [E]$ and $(v_0 - v) \propto [EI]$, then

$$i = \frac{(v_0 - v)}{v}. \tag{2}$$

Inhibition is still studied experimentally by incubating enzyme with inhibitor for some specified period and then *adding* substrate to the inhibition medium, and the progress of inhibition is still followed by measuring the velocity of the substrate reaction catalyzed by the uninhibited enzyme remaining.

Easson and Stedman also recognized that the inhibitor concentration of interest was the concentration in the incubation mixture *before* the addition of substrate.

## B. Inhibitory Power

The next step in developing present ideas of irreversible inhibition kinetics involved studies which led to criteria for evaluating the inhibitory power of carbamates (and later organophosphates) as opposed to the mole-for-mole stoichiometry of the reaction demonstrated by Easson and Stedman. Among these studies, one by Straus and Goldstein in 1943 *(18)* of the "zone" behavior of the cholinesterase–physostigmine system was preeminent. In zone A, the salient point is that the enzyme concentration is small relative to that of the inhibitor. The theoretical plot of the fractional inhibition, $i$, against the log of the concentration of the specific inhibitor was made, and this in turn led to an experimental plot of log *(M* physostigmine) against the percentage of activity remaining. The experimental method consisted of incubating inhibitor and enzyme together for only 18 minutes before adding substrate.

It remained only to adopt the $pI_{50}$, the negative log of the molar concentration of inhibitor giving 50% inhibition, obtained from zone A plots, as a criterion of inhibitory power. The $pI_{50}$, under the name p$C$ appears to have been used first by Mazur and Bodansky *(21)* some time during World War II in the course of studying cholinesterase inhibition by DFP and eserine.

Mackworth and Webb *(24)* employed the $pI_{50}$ criterion to characterize the inhibitory power of a series of structurally related alkyl fluorophosphonates. In their paper, a classical example is given of plots of percentage inhibition against $-\log$ (molarity of poison), from which $pI_{50}$ values are obtained.

The discovery that organophosphates inhibited cholinesterases appears to have been made before World War II by Gross, but the work was not published until later *(22)*. Two groups at Cambridge *(23,24)* discovered cholinesterase inhibition by DFP independently in the early years of World War II.

With the paper by Mackworth and Webb in 1948 *(24)*, the concept of active-site-directed irreversible inhibition could be clearly seen. They wrote, for example, "it is possible that the initial rapid inhibition is an equilibrium, but that it is followed by an irreversible destruction of the enzyme." Within a year (1949), the nature of the "irreversible destruction" had been identified by Boursnell and Webb *(25)* as phosphorylation of the active sites of both horse serum cholinesterase and horse liver carboxylesterase. Thus it was known before the decade of the 1940s ended that organophosphate inhibition was progressive, irreversible, and involved formation of a covalent bond. Inhibition by carbamates was similar, but was thought to differ in two important respects: inhibition was reversible, albeit slowly, and there was no evidence of covalent bond formation. Despite these differences and for obvious historical reasons, the inhibitory powers of both organophosphates and carbamates were measured by $pI_{50}$, a criterion which continues to be widely used.

## C. First-Order Kinetics and the Inhibition Progress Curve

Although it was known that inhibition by both DFP and eserine was progressive, the experimental method of determining the $pI_{50}$ involved incubating enzyme and inhibitor for a fixed time. In 1950, Aldridge *(26)* published a classical paper in which the incubation time was varied instead of being fixed. In this study, the progress of acetylcholinesterase inhibition by paraoxon was investigated. Enzyme and inhibitor were incubated for various times, and the reaction was stopped by addition of substrate in high concentration. The log of the percentage of activities remaining after incubation for the various times was then plotted against the corresponding times. The plots were linear, indicating that the reaction was first-order with respect to the enzyme concentration, "presumably because the concentration of inhibitor is in large excess compared with the concentration of enzyme." Aldridge correctly interpreted these results as indicating that "the 'slowest' reaction in the system is therefore bimolecular." The mechanism of inhibition suggested was, in essence, identical with Scheme (I), which describes the reaction of an active-site-directed irreversible inhibitor.

For present purposes, the salient feature of this work was the inhibition progress curve of the type shown in Fig. 1A. The inhibition progress curve, together with the experimental protocol by which it is obtained, are the foundations of the kinetics of active-site-directed irreversible inhibition. Although the mechanism suggested included a reversible intermediate, the kinetic results did not, in fact, support such a scheme. Instead they indicated the simple bimolecular reaction,

$$E + AX \xrightarrow{k_i} EA \atop X$$ (IV)

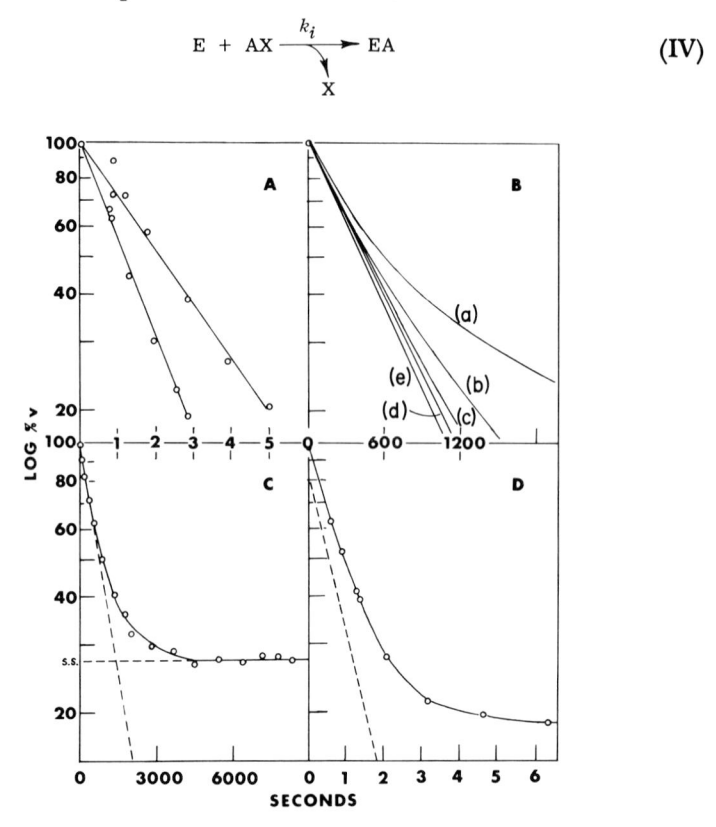

FIG. 1. Inhibition progress curves: (A) First-order rate plots for inhibition of bovine erythrocyte acetylcholinesterase by $2 \times 10^{-4}$ $M$ and $5 \times 10^{-4}$ $M$ di-$n$-propyl $p$-nitrophenyl phosphate ($n$-propyl paraoxon) at 5°C, pH 7.6. The first-order rate constants ($\rho$) were 20 minute$^{-1}$ and 33.6 minute$^{-1}$. (B) Theoretical inhibition progress curves illustrating curving as the initial inhibitor concentration, $i_0$, approaches the initial enzyme concentration $e_0$: $i_0 \to e_0$. The curves were calculated by assuming that $k_i = 1 \times 10^7$ $M^{-1}$minute$^{-1}$; that $i_0 = 1 \times 10^{-8}$ $M$, and that (a) $i_0 = e_0$, (b) $i_0 = 2e_0$, (c) $i_0 = 4e_0$, (d) $i_0 = 10e_0$, (e) $i_0 \gg e_0$. (C) Inhibition progress curve when regeneration is significant. The reaction reached a steady state at about 4500 seconds. The curve is for the inhibition of bovine erythrocyte acetylcholinesterase by $2 \times 10^{-4}$ $M$ phenyl $N$-methyl carbamate at 25° C, pH 7.6, $\rho = 0.056$ minute$^{-1}$. (D) Inhibition progress curve reflecting a multiple enzyme system. Inhibition of bovine erythrocyte acetylcholinesterase by $2 \times 10^{-4}$ $M$ tetram at 5° C, pH 7.0 is shown. The first-order rate constant of the first form (broken line) was 65.4 minute$^{-1}$.

Aldridge was convinced, nevertheless, that an affinity complex of significance was formed which preceded phosphorylation. An *irreversible* intermediate complex preceding phosphorylation was then proposed *(7,27)*

$$E + AX \xrightarrow{k_1} EAX \xrightarrow{k_2} EA \atop X \qquad (V)$$

Schemes (IV) and (V) cannot be distinguished by kinetic means alone; by mechanism (V), one could reconcile the simple bimolecular kinetics of (IV) with the intermediary complex. However, the problem of the existence of an intermediary complex remained, since reconciling Schemes (IV) and (V) does not demonstrate that an intermediary is formed. Aldridge *(27)* summed up his feelings about the reversible complex as follows: "The formation of the hypothetical reversible complex between inhibitor and enzyme, has not been demonstrated. . . . This failure to detect the reversible complex is not surprising, for enzyme substrate complexes have been detected only rarely."

It also was recognized that the phosphorylated enzyme was to some extent regenerated and that "it should be possible to find organophosphorous compounds which act like substrates" *(27)*. That carbamates might also react by a mechanism analogous with that of both organophosphates and substrates was recognized by Myers and Kemp *(12)*, when they wrote in early 1954 "the results described above suggest that dimethylcarbamyl fluoride and the alkanesulphonyl fluorides also inhibit esterases by the same mechanism as the diethyl phosphorofluoridates." This statement clearly implies that carbamates (and organosulfonates), like organophosphates, form a covalent bond with the active site. Perhaps the clearest statement of the concept of active-site-directed irreversible inhibition as it relates to organophosphates was made by O'Brien *(28)*. "There are two important factors deciding the *in vitro* anticholinesterase properties of an organophosphate. First, there is the affinity of the compound for the active site; secondly, there is the readiness with which the compounds, once arrived at the site, can phosphorylate it."

## D. The Kinetics Emerge

Following Aldridge's paper *(26)*, a number of approaches to the problem of developing a kinetics for active-site-directed irreversible inhibition emerged. One of them, curiously enough, appears to have evolved from the kinetics developed for studying the regeneration of the phosphorylated enzyme by oxime regenerating reagents such as pyridine-2-aldoxime methiodide. It happens that the scheme postulated for regeneration by Green and Smith in 1958 *(29)* is identical in form with Scheme (I) for active-site-directed irreversible inhibition

$$\text{EP} + \text{R} \underset{}{\overset{K_r}{\rightleftharpoons}} \text{EP:R} \xrightarrow{k_2} \text{E} + \text{PR} \tag{VI}$$

where EP is the phosphorylated enzyme, R is the reactivator (in this case, a 2-oxoaldoxime), EPR is a reversible intermediate binding complex, and $K_r$ is an equilibrium constant controlling its formation. Like the inhibitors, the regenerating reagents were regarded as active-site-directed. Green and Smith derived an equation from Scheme (VI) which was identical in form with that derived for active-site-directed irreversible inhibition *(5,10)*. In developing a kinetics for active-site-directed irreversible inhibition, one automatically has one for active-site-directed regeneration as well.

In 1960, Wilson, Hatch, and Ginsburg *(9)* derived an equation for Scheme (II) which included the regeneration step, and in which formation of the reversible complex under equilibrium conditions was also assumed. However, no effort was made to apply the equation to determination of the constants governing the separate binding and carbamylation rates, i.e., it was not applied to the kinetics of active-site-directed irreversible inhibition.

In 1963, a somewhat different approach emerged, that stemmed from an interest in a problem of long standing, namely irreversible inhibition in the presence of substrate. Mazur and Bodansky *(21)* had studied the effect of various DFP concentrations on the substrate progress curves and found them to be precisely linear. This suggested that no further inhibition occurred after addition of substrate to the enzyme inhibitor incubation mixture. Mackworth and Webb *(24)* confirmed this, and observed that varying the acetylcholine concentration had no effect on the degree of cholinesterase inhibition by DFP, but substrate did affect inhibition by eserine. Under their conditions, a graph of $(1/v)$ against $(1/s)$ made DFP appear as a classical noncompetitive reversible inhibitor, whereas eserine gave the classical competitive reversible inhibition plot *(20)*. (This had to be a little confusing in view of the noncompetitive reversible kinetics developed for inhibition by eserine and other carbamates.) Opinion seemed to have ranged from the idea that substrates gave almost complete protection to a recognition that the degree of protection depended on the relative inhibitor and substrate concentrations and on the particular inhibitor and substrate used *(28)*.

## 2. ACTIVE-SITE-DIRECTED IRREVERSIBLE INHIBITION

The point, however, was that a kinetic treatment for a system in which enzyme, inhibitor, and substrate reacted simultaneously had not been developed.

The problem of irreversible inhibition in the presence of substrate arose because of the cholinesterase inhibitor malaoxon (see Section II,A), which is the active form of the widely used and relatively safe insecticide malathion. Malathion and malaoxon are substrates for carboxylesterases, which catalyze the hydrolysis of one of the two ethyl esters on these compounds, thus detoxicating them *(30–32)*. In addition to acting as a substrate, malaoxon inhibits carboxylesterase by phosphorylating the active site. Here then was a compound which could act either as an inhibitor or as a substrate to carboxylesterase, and it was this problem which stimulated an interest in irreversible inhibition in the presence of substrate. The first step in developing a solution was to derive an equation for the system

$$EH + AX \xrightarrow{k_i} EA$$
$$\searrow$$
$$HX$$

$$E + S \underset{k_{-1}}{\overset{k_1}{\rightleftarrows}} ES \xrightarrow{k_2} E + \text{Products}$$

(VII)

in which a purely competitive irreversible inhibition by the organophosphate was assumed. The equation contained terms for both an irreversible step and a steady-state system *(33)*. The results obtained with a system in which acetylcholinesterase was inhibited by DFP in the presence of phenylacetate substrate were consistent with the equation derived and the assumptions made.

It was then just a step to an equation for an inhibition scheme in which the reversible complex was formed between the enzyme and inhibitor rather than with the substrate *(5)*. The crucial problem was how to test the equation.

For the better organophosphate inhibitors, such as DFP or paraoxon, testing the equation would have required inhibition times and inhibitor concentrations far beyond the ranges typically employed to determine inhibitory power by either the $pI_{50}$ or the bimolecular velocity constant. Fortunately, malaoxon is not a very good inhibitor of serum cholinesterase, so that the experimental methods then available, when pressed to their limits, succeeded in demonstrating the validity of the equation and the idea of reversible complex formation. These same experimental methods were tried, but failed to demonstrate a reversible complex between DFP and serum cholinesterase.

This work brought into sharp focus the fact that the principal problem in applying active-site-directed irreversible kinetics to organophosphate and carbamate inhibitors was experimental rather than theoretical. The psychological dimensions of the problem may be judged by the following quotation from Mackworth and Webb (24): "In preliminary experiments with diisopropylfluorophosphonate (DFP), it was found that concentrations above $10^{-7} M$ completely inhibited cholinesterase almost instantaneously." In determining the affinity and phosphorylation constants of DFP in reaction with the same cholinesterase, concentrations more than 200 times greater than that giving "instantaneous" inhibition were needed, and commensurately shorter inhibition times were employed (34). Determining the same constants with acetylcholinesterase required DFP concentration as high as $5 \times 10^{-3} M$, or 50,000 times greater (6). Thus the application of active-site-directed irreversible kinetics to

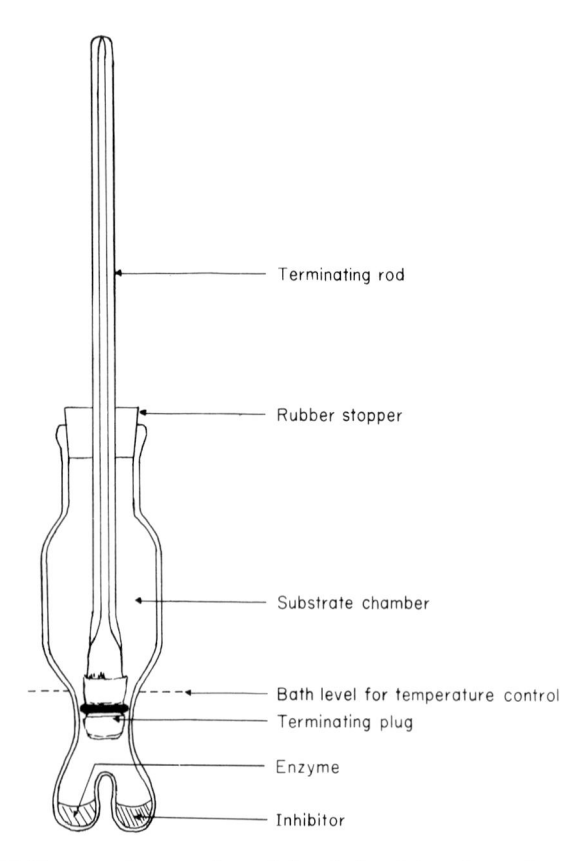

FIG. 2. Inhibition reaction vessel used for timing intervals as short as 0.8 seconds.

most of the organophosphates and carbamates of interest required developing procedures for measuring inhibition times in a range short enough to permit determination of valid inhibition progress curves. The high inhibitor concentrations present in the incubation mixture also led to problems after the addition of substrate. Unless appropriate measures were taken, inhibition continued in the presence of substrate at such high rates as to prevent valid estimates of residual velocities. These and related problems will be discussed in more detail in the following section.

The development of inhibition reaction vessels capable of measuring incubation times as short as one second at relatively low temperatures (Fig. 2) made it possible to examine the validity of active-site-directed irreversible inhibition kinetics as they apply to organophosphates and carbamates *(6)*. These studies clearly validated the concept, but the same studies produced new and unexpected complications related to the natures of both the enzyme and the reaction mechanism. The postulated mechanism seems valid, as far as it goes, but there is reason to believe that it does not adequately describe many systems of interest. For example, kinetic evidence of an allosteric site of significance to the inhibition reaction has been reported *(35)*.

The assumption that cholinesterase is a homogeneous enzyme also needs to be examined.

## IV. KINETICS

As studied experimentally, the kinetic analysis of active-site-directed irreversible inhibition can be divided for convenience into two parts. The first is concerned with following the time-course of enzyme inhibition at single-inhibitor concentrations. The second is concerned with the effect of various inhibitor concentrations on the rate constants governing inhibition.

The second approach leads to evaluation of the constants governing binding and rates of covalent bond formation. It also reflects on the number and order of the intermediates involved in the reaction sequence.

### A. Inhibition Progress Curves

Two experimental approaches have been used to obtain inhibition progress curves. One involves determining rates of inhibition continuously in the presence of substrate and will be considered later. Another, and by far the most common, method involves mixing an enzyme solution with an inhibitor solution to start the inhibition reaction. Inhibition is allowed to proceed for various measured times $(t)$, after which it is stopped by addition of substrate solution to the inhibition mixture. Timing begins when the enzyme and inhibitor are mixed and ends when the substrate is added. The enzyme which remains uninhibited after the measured time catalyzes a substrate reaction. The velocity of the substrate reaction is then measured. The volumes and initial concentrations of the enzyme, inhibitor, and substrate solutions are kept constant for any one progress curve—only time is varied. The temperature, pH, and ionic strength of the inhibition mixture are also kept constant during the measured time. Similarly, each substrate reaction is carried out at constant temperature, pH, and ionic strength, but these need not be the same as for the inhibition mixture. If the conditions in the substrate reaction differ greatly from those in the inhibition mixture, the possibility of complications may exist.

The inhibition progress curve is obtained by plotting $\log v$ against $t$. The plots may be straight or they may curve, depending on the system under study. Examples of both straight and curving plots are shown in Fig. 1, curves A, B, C, and D.

The conditions under which the plots will be straight, as well as some which lead to curving, will be considered. The basic assumption is made throughout that $v \propto e$. When the substrate reaction follows Michaelis kinetics

$$v = \frac{k \cdot e_0}{1 + (K_m/s)} \qquad (3)$$

the proportionality constant is then $k/[1 + (K_m/s)]$. However Michaelis kinetics need not be followed for the relationship, $v \propto e$ to hold.

### 1. The Linear Plot

A linear plot indicates a reaction which is first-order with respect to the enzyme concentration, since $i_0 \gg e_0$. The empirical equation for the straight line (Fig. 1A) is

$$\log v = - \rho' t + \log v_0. \qquad (4)$$

The first-order rate constant $\rho'$ is then the slope

$$\rho' = \frac{\log v_0/v}{t}. \qquad (5)$$

## 2. ACTIVE-SITE-DIRECTED IRREVERSIBLE INHIBITION

The simplest theoretical interpretation of $\rho'$ is obtained by assuming a bimolecular reaction between enzyme and inhibitor as given in Scheme (IV). Since $i_0 >> e_0$, $(i_0 - q) \simeq i_0$ and remains constant over the course of the reaction. The rate at which EH is inhibited is then

$$- de/dt = k_i i_0 e. \tag{6}$$

Arranging for integration

$$- \int (de/e) = k_i i_0 \int dt . \tag{7}$$

Integrating (7) between the limits $e = e_0$ when $t = 0$ and $e = e$ when $t = t$ gives

$$\ln (e_0/e) = ik_i t, \tag{8}$$

since $v_0 \propto e_0$ and $v \propto (e_0 - q)$

$$\ln (v_0/v) = ik_i t . \tag{9}$$

Changing from natural to ordinary logs, $\ln (v_0/v) = 2.3 \log (v_0/v)$, and

$$2.3 \log (v_0/v) = ik_i t. \tag{10}$$

The first-order rate constant $\rho$ governing the reaction is then

$$\rho = \frac{2.3 \log (v_0/v)}{t} = ik_i \tag{11}$$

so that $\rho = 2.3\rho'$. $\rho$ has an empirical and a theoretical interpretation. The empirical interpretation $[2.3 \log (v_0/v)]/t$ holds as long as the log $v$ against $t$ plot is straight. The theoretical interpretation $ik_i$ depends on the reaction scheme from which the equation was derived. The validity of the theoretical interpretation can be tested by determining how $\rho$ varies as $i$ is varied. In the case of Eq. (11) a plot of $\rho$ against $i$ would give a straight line going through the origin. Early experiments (27) indicated that inhibition by organophosphates and carbamates followed Eq. (11), indicating a simple bimolecular reaction.

If the log $v$ against $t$ plots are not linear or if they cannot be resolved into systems which are linear, the effect of varying $i$ cannot be tested in a way which will permit the validity or adequacy of the postulated reaction mechanism to be examined. In other words, the time-course of inhibition must either follow first-order kinetics or be resolved into components which do, in order to test the validity of the postulated reaction scheme.

A corollary is that linear log $v$ against $t$ plots do not, by themselves, reflect on the nature of the reaction scheme. They will be linear no matter how simple or complex the scheme. Remembering that these plots are obtained on the assumption that $i_0 \gg e_0$, it also follows that the nature and number of inhibitors present will not affect the linearity of the log $v$ against $t$ plots. The presence, for example, of two inhibitors, which would occur if the inhibitor consisted of steric isomers, would give a linear plot, just as does one inhibitor.

Since the nature and complexity of the reaction schemes as well as the possibility of multi-inhibitor systems are examined through the effect which varying $i$ has on the first-order rate constant, the experimental measurement of valid rate constants is of critical importance. Following is a brief description of some of the criteria and methods used.

2. Experimental Determination

Timing would ideally permit inhibitions ranging from 20 to 80% of completion to be measured routinely. In the initial phase of some studies, inhibition to 99% or more has been advisable *(34,36)*. At least four points, suitably spaced, are normally required to obtain a reasonable estimate of $\rho$ by regression fit. If the statistically fitted line does not pass through log $v_0$, or at least pass within the limits indicated by the precision of estimate (Fig. 1A), the validity of the first-order assumption is doubtful.

These criteria present no particular experimental difficulties for $\rho$ values of 2 minutes$^{-1}$ or less. The shortest time needed to obtain 20% inhibition is then about 10 seconds. However, intervals of 10 seconds are approaching the limits which can conveniently and reproducibly be measured with commonly available laboratory apparatus, so that when $\rho$ values exceeding 2 minutes$^{-1}$ are to be measured, special apparatus is required.

The design of such apparatus is in the early stages of development and much remains to be done. A device capable of measuring intervals as short as 0.8 seconds was designed by Main et al. *(6,36)*. A sketch of one model is shown in Fig. 2. The reaction vessel and terminating rod were of glass. The plug was an "O" ring male joint which sealed the inhibition chamber from the substrate chamber. The side arms held from 0.2 to 0.5 ml of solution. To measure inhibition, an appropriate volume of enzyme was pipetted into one arm and inhibitor was placed in the other. These were brought to the desired temperature by immersing the flask in a bath

## 2. ACTIVE-SITE-DIRECTED IRREVERSIBLE INHIBITION

to the level indicated in Fig. 2. Substrate, 20 ml, was placed in the substrate chamber just before starting inhibition. For cholinesterases, the colorimetric method of Ellman et al. *(37)* has proved convenient. Inhibition was started by tipping and sharply shaking to mix the contents of the side arms. A foot timer was started in the same instant. Inhibition was stopped by pulling up on the terminating rod, and the foot timer was stopped simultaneously. This flooded the inhibition mixture with substrate solution. The substrate solution served both to dilute the inhibitor and to complex the remaining free enzyme. The velocity of the substrate reaction was measured either by pH-stat *(6)* or colorimetrically *(37)*.

By measuring inhibition rates at lower temperatures (e.g., 5°C) an estimate of the rate constants governing inhibition by some of the more powerful organophosphates and carbamates could be made. At room temperatures, timing was still too slow.

### 3. THE PROBLEM OF INHIBITION IN THE PRESENCE OF SUBSTRATE

One other serious problem in addition to difficulty with timing is encountered when the procedure of incubating enzyme with inhibitor and then adding substrate is followed. This is the inhibition which occurs in the presence of substrate which complicates or may even prevent valid measurement of residual velocities. The problem may best be clarified by giving an example.

Paraoxon at $5 \times 10^{-4}$ $M$ inhibits 50% of acetylcholinesterase activity in about 1.5 seconds at 5°C, pH 7.6 (Fig. 1A). The volume of the inhibition solution was 1.0 ml and that of the added substrate 30 ml, so that the solution was diluted 31-fold. The measured $K_a$ was $4.1 \times 10^{-4}$ $M$ *(38)*. Substituting this value into Eq. (22) and calculating for a dilution of 31-fold, we find that the rate of inhibition was reduced 825 times by dilution. The acetylcholines substrate concentration was 3 m$M$ and $K_m$ was $1.2 \times 10^{-4}$ $M$. Accordingly, complexing with substrate reduced the concentration of free enzyme by 26 times. Addition of substrate reduced the rate of inhibition by about 21,450-fold (825-fold by dilution × 26-fold by complexing). At 5°C about 532 minutes would then have been required to inhibit the remaining acetylcholinesterase a further 50%. Since the substrate reaction was at 25°C, not 5°C, the time to 50% inhibition in the presence of substrate was much less, as shown in Fig. 3, curve 3. Log $v$ against $t$ plots obtained by taking tangents to curve 3 are shown by the broken line. With 3 m$M$ substrate inhibition in the presence of substrate was evidently too fast to permit valid estimates of $v$ to be made. Inhibition in the presence of substrate was reduced by increasing the concentration of acetylcholine to 30 m$M$ (curve 2). The velocity was then restored by adding 2% $n$-butanol (curve 1). The log $v$ against $t$

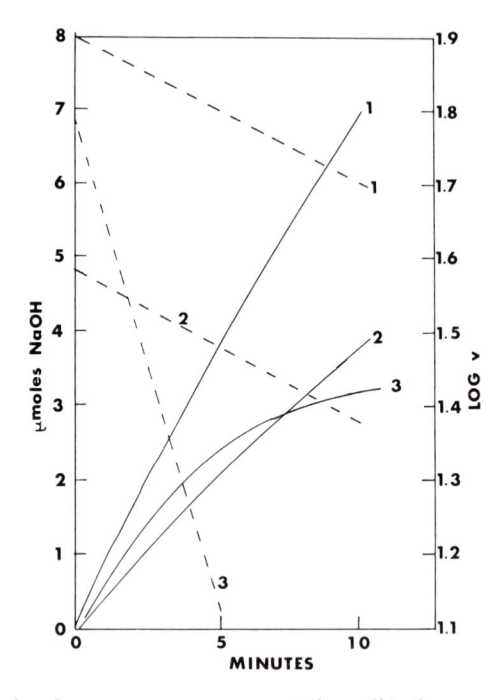

Fig. 3. Inhibited substrate progress curves. The solid lines are reproductions of recorder traces obtained with radiometer pH-stats. The rate of inhibition of acetylcholinesterase by $1.61 \times 10^{-5}$ $M$ paraoxon in 3 m$M$ acetylcholine (curves 3) was reduced in 30 m$M$ acetylcholine (curves 2), but the initial velocity was also reduced by 40%. The velocity was restored by adding 2% butanol to the 30 m$M$ substrate. Velocities were measured at 25°C, pH 7.6.

plots in Fig. 1A were then obtained using a 30 m$M$ acetylcholine substrate solution, which was 2% v/v in $n$-butanol.

The rate of inhibition in the presence of substrate depends on the following factors: (1) the concentration of the inhibitor in the inhibition mixture and its $\rho$ value at this concentration; (2) the relative volumes of the inhibition and substrate solutions; (3) the degree to which uninhibited enzyme is complexed by substrate—complexing increases with increasing substrate concentration, but various factors place limits on the substrate concentration which can be used; and (4) the time taken to measure the velocity of the residual substrate reaction.

The first factor merely defines the problem since many of the better inhibitors are characterized by high $\rho$ values at the concentrations which must be used in order to evaluate the rate constants.

The second factor poses the question of the practical limits which can set on the volumes of the inhibition and substrate solutions. With inhibition reaction vessels (Fig. 2) the lowest volume commensurate with good mixing is about 0.4 ml. If the residual activity were measured by pH-stat, substrate volumes as high as 100 ml could be used conveniently. A dilution factor of 250-fold would result. Inhibition volumes of 0.02 ml have been used with substrate volumes of 15 ml by a "falling drop" method, permitting dilutions of 750-fold. The limiting factor to dilution was the enzyme concentration in the inhibition mixture. As the dilution increases, the initial concentration of enzyme must be increased in order to maintain a reasonable substrate velocity.

With the soluble choline esters the upper substrate concentration limit can be quite high, approaching 0.1 $M$, but optimal concentrations tend to range from 1 to 50 m$M$. The degree of enzyme complexing at the substrate concentration used is the critical factor. Since the cholinesterase substrate reaction does not follow Michaelis kinetics, $K_m$ values are difficult to estimate. Inhibition by organophosphates provides an alternative approach to determine $K_m$, since the rate of inhibition is proportional to the concentration of free enzyme. If it is assumed that the only effect which substrate has on inhibition is to reduce the enzyme concentration by complexing, then a complexing factor $\psi$ can be defined such that

$$\psi = e/e_0 = \rho_s/\rho \tag{12}$$

when $\psi$ is the fraction of free enzyme at any time during inhibition in the presence of substrate. The first-order rate constant in the presence of substrate is $\rho_s$. Evaluation of $\rho$ and $\rho_s$ will then give the degree of complexing directly. Equation (12) holds at the low inhibitor concentrations which result from dilution when $i \gg K_a$. It can then be shown [33] that

$$\rho_s = \frac{2.3 \log (v_0/v)}{t} = ik_i \frac{K_m}{(s + K_m)} \tag{13}$$

when $s = 0$, $\rho_s = \rho$ and Eq. (9) holds. Since $K_m$ is given by

$$K_m = se/(e_0 - e), \tag{14}$$

$$\rho/\rho_s = 1 + s/K_m = 1/\psi. \tag{15}$$

If the substrate reaction follows Michaelis kinetics, $K_m$ is constant, but if it does not, $K_m$ will vary. The plot of $1/\psi$ against $s$ for the hydrolysis of acetylcholine by acetylcholinesterase has been determined [36]. Values of $\rho_s$ are obtained from exactly the same kind of log $v$ against $t$ plots as were used to obtain $\rho$. The only difference is the way in which $v$ is measured, as described in Section IV,B,3.

This approach also provides an alternative method for determining $K_m$ through measurement of $(\rho/\rho_s)$.

The fourth factor tends to favor colorimetric over titrimetric methods of measuring the substrate velocity. Velocities cannot be reliably measured by pH-stat in less than 3 or 4 minutes, while colorimetric assays can be readily measured in 10 to 15 seconds. The disadvantage of colorimetric methods is the limited number of substrates and the relatively low limit on the concentrations which can be used. Colorimetric methods for these determinations have not been thoroughly explored, but it seems possible that they will become the method of choice.

### 4. Curved Plots as $i_0 \to e_0$

When the $i_0$ approaches $e_0$, $i$ does not remain constant over the course of inhibition. As a result, the log $v$ against $t$ plots curve, as shown in Fig. 1B. This case is not of critical importance to active-site-directed irreversible kinetics, since relatively high inhibitor concentrations are usually needed to determine the constants governing binding and rates of covalent bond formation ($K_a$ and $k_2$). However, Ooms (38) has used it to determine $k_i$ values. For present purposes, the assumption that $i_0 >> e_0$ normally holds. However, it is convenient to obtain at least one value of $\rho$ where $i << K_a$; and in these circumstances, $i_0$ might approach $e_0$. Second-order kinetics are also useful in designing experiments to determine the enzyme concentration. In addition, they bear on the problem of $I_{50}$ and its validity as a criterion of inhibitory power.

The rate of inhibition as $i_0 \to e_0$, assuming $i_0 << K_a$, is given by

$$-de/dt = k_i(e_0 - q)(i_0 - q) \qquad (16)$$

since $(i_0 - q) \not\cong i_0$ in these circumstances. The limited integration of Eq. (16) gives

$$k_i = \frac{2.3}{t(i_0 - e_0)} \log \frac{e_0(i_0 - q)}{i_0(e_0 - q)} \qquad (17)$$

To determine $k_i$, $e_0$ must be known, as well as $i_0$. A linear plot is obtained by plotting log $[(i_0 - q)/(e_0 - q)]$ against $t$ by a suitable rearrangement of Eq. (17). The curves shown in Fig. 1B suggest that $i_0$ should be at least $4e_0$ and preferably $10e_0$ when Eq. (8) is used to determine $k_i$.

The $I_{50}$ or $pI_{50}$ value is a much used and frequently questioned (28) criterion of inhibitory power. When $I_{50} >> e_0$, it is valid in this sense, since it is inversely proportional to $k_i$ at a given finite value of $t$.

$$I_{50} = \frac{2.3 \log 2}{tk_i} \qquad (18)$$

However, as $I_{50} \to e_0$, it reaches a limit equal to 0.5 $e_0$ and is then merely a measure of $e_0$ rather than of inhibitory power. The main problem with the $I_{50}$ is that there is no way of knowing from the experimental results which meaning it has. In addition, the precision associated with its use is poor and it cannot be used in a kinetic sense to investigate the mechanism of inhibition. These faults are also its greatest virtue, since one can always get an $I_{50}$, regardless of mechanism, enzyme concentration, and so on. A brief study of $I_{50}$ within the context of Eq. (17) suggests that $I_{50}$ will be inversely proportional to $k_i$ over a wide range of conditions. Still one wonders if the troubles that are avoided by its use compensate for the knowledge lost.

### 5. Curved Plots When Regeneration Is Significant

When the course of inhibition by a compound such as N-methyl phenyl carbamate is followed over a prolonged period, a plot such as that shown in Fig. 1C is obtained. The plot resolves into two regions which are approximately linear. In the first region $k_2$ predominates, since relatively little carbamylated enzyme has formed. As inhibition progresses, the concentration of free enzyme decreases, while that in the carbamylated form increases. After a time the rate at which the carbamylated enzyme breaks down to regenerate free enzyme equals the rate at which it is formed and a steady state (ss) is reached. As long as $i$ remains constant, this steady state will be reflected by the second linear region running parallel to the time axis. Eventually the curve will swing up since the inhibitor is being continuously depleted by this process. In effect, the inhibitor is a poor substrate, and the progress of the poor substrate reaction is followed with a better substrate. These plots have a characteristic shape and can be readily distinguished from most other curving plots.

### 6. Curved Plots Which Reflect Multiple Enzyme Systems

Recognition of this type of curving is relatively new (34). Previously the assumption was made, for kinetic purposes, that cholinesterases were homogeneous and existed in only one form. This assumption is implicit in all of the reaction schemes given to this point. Yet evidence has accumulated over a number of years which indicates that cholinesterases exist as a mixture of different forms (39), some of which are interconvertible (40). This is true of many other enzymes as well, some of which occur as isoenzymes, but whether the different forms of cholinesterase qualify as isoenzymes is not now known. The important fact, however, is that many enzymes, including cholinesterases, are not homogeneous but exist in systems of multiple forms. This may have important consequences insofar as the kinetics of their inhibition is concerned, since the different forms may react differently *(34)*.

Examples of such curving are shown in Fig. 1D and Fig. 4. When several different enzymes, or different forms of one enzyme, are inhibited irreversibly, the time course for the inhibition of one particular enzyme will be independent of the other. If inhibition of each enzyme follows first-order kinetics, $\rho$ will be given by Eq. (9). Since the different enzymes hydrolyze a common substrate and the substrate reactions occur independently, the velocity measured experimentally after inhibition for time $t$ will be the sum of the individual velocities ($\Sigma v$). In a system, for example, which contained three different species, $\Sigma v$ would be given by

$$\Sigma v = v^{\mathrm{I}} + v^{\mathrm{II}} + v^{\mathrm{III}} = v_0^{\mathrm{I}} e^{-\rho^{\mathrm{I}} t} + v_0^{\mathrm{II}} e^{-\rho^{\mathrm{II}} t} + v_0^{\mathrm{III}} e^{-\rho^{\mathrm{III}} t} \qquad (19)$$

where here $e$ is the base of the natural logarithms, and the individual enzymes are identified by the superscripts I, II, and III. Equation (19) indicates that the plot of log $\Sigma v$ against $t$ would curve providing the $\rho$ values of each enzyme differed and the $v_0$ values were of the same order. Curves such as the one shown in Fig. 1D have been interpreted through the use of Eq. (19).

The method of resolution is described by using, as an example, inhibition of a partially purified preparation of horse serum cholinesterase by $1 \times 10^{-5}$ $M$ tetram at 5°C, pH 7.0. The log $\Sigma v$ against $t$ plot is shown in Fig. 4 on three time scales as curves A, B, and C.

If several enzymes were irreversibly inhibited at different rates, after a time only one enzyme, the most slowly inhibited, would remain active. The log $\Sigma v$ against $t$ plot over this terminal portion of the curve should then be straight, assuming first-order inhibition. The terminal phase of the inhibition considered here is shown by curve C, Fig. 4. Between 10,600 and 61,200 seconds, when inhibition was 99.4% completed, the plot was linear, suggesting one enzyme.

This, the most slowly inhibited, is enzyme IV. The enzymes were numbered in order of decreasing rates of inhibition. The most rapidly inhibited was then enzyme I, the next enzyme II, and so on.

A straight line was fitted to the terminal points by regression analysis, which also gave the slope, $\rho^{\mathrm{IV}}/2.3 = 1.79 \times 10^{-5}$ seconds$^{-1}$, and intercept value, log $v_0^{\mathrm{IV}} = 1.441$.

The first point (10,600 seconds) was provisionally selected by inspection, using the criterion of linearity. This choice was later confirmed or

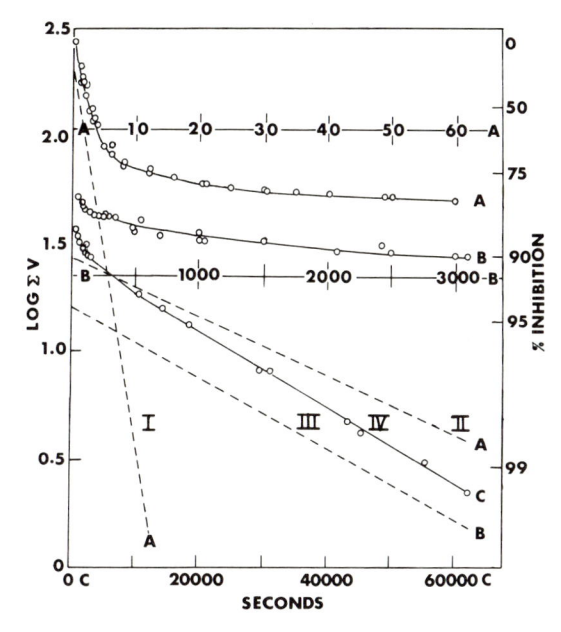

FIG. 4. Inhibition progress curve for the inhibition of partially purified horse serum cholinesterase by $1 \times 10^{-5}$ $M$ tetram at 5°C, pH 7.0. $\Sigma v$ is the sum of the velocities of each form. The broken lines are the first-order rate plots of the four forms of cholinesterase.

corrected by the lower time limit ($t_0$) of enzyme III preceding: $t_0$ defined the time at which the activity of a given enzyme became insignificant within the limits of resolution associated with measuring $v$. For enzyme III, $t_0 = 3590$ seconds, so that at 10,600 seconds no significant $v^{III}$ remained.

To calculate the slope and intercept of enzyme III, the $v^{IV}$ components of $\Sigma v$ values in the next time range, 104 to 3590 seconds, were calculated by substitution of $\rho^{IV}$ and $v_0^{IV}$ into Eq. (9). Then $v^{III} = \Sigma v - v^{IV}$, and a set of $v^{III}$ and $t$ values. As before, a provisional upper limit was selected by inspection of the $v^{III}$ against $t$ plot on the basis of linearity. This was later confirmed or corrected by the $t_0$ of isoenzyme II. The slope and intercept values were again calculated by regression analysis.

The slopes and intercept values of enzymes II and I were successively calculated by the same treatment. Thus the method involved obtaining provisional estimates of the slope and intercept values which were then used to define more closely the time ranges proper to the resolution of each enzyme. If necessary, terminal points were then either added or excluded; and the slopes and intercept values were again calculated by regression analysis to obtain a better estimate.

Each resolved curve typically consisted of at least 6 points and frequently more were used.

By this procedure, the log $\Sigma v$ against $t$ curve was resolved into four plots, each of which was sensibly linear to the limits of resolution commensurate with the precision attainable. They are shown by the broken lines in Fig. 4.

The inhibition progress curves considered so far have been determined by incubating enzyme and inhibitor and then adding substrate. In the next section, the effect of varying the inhibitor concentration on the first-order inhibition constants will be considered. Inhibition in the presence of substrate will be examined further within this context.

### B. $K_a$ and $k_2$: Binding and Rates of Covalent Bond Formation

At least three approaches can be used in deriving an equation from Scheme (I), which is rewritten below in a slightly different form.

$$\text{EH} + \text{AX} \underset{k_{-1}}{\overset{k_1}{\rightleftharpoons}} \text{EHAX} \xrightarrow{k_2} \text{EA} \quad \text{(VIII)}$$

with HX produced, and $k_i$ ($i \ll K_a$) regeneration.

The first approach, and the one that is usually used, assumes that EHAX is formed under equilibrium conditions, and that $k_3$ is negligible. For convenience this will be called the "initial phase" approach since regeneration is ignored. Equilibrium is approached when $k_{-1} \gg k_2$, but there appears to be no *a priori* reason for $k_{-1}$ to be greater than $k_2$. It is, however, a very useful assumption, since then $K_a = k_{-1}/k_1$, and is an equilibrium constant. As such, $K_a$ is a valid measure of binding and is of thermodynamic significance.

The second approach is the same as the first, but considers the reaction to involve the further regeneration step, as given in Scheme (II) *(9)*. The treatment utilizes the steady-state phase of inhibition and for convenience will be called the "steady-state" approach. The equation derived from Scheme (VIII) is then a special case of the one derived from Scheme (II), in which $k_3 = 0$.

The third approach is to derive an equation from Scheme (VIII) in which no assumptions are made concerning the relationship of $k_{-1}$ and $k_2$. $K_a$ then appears to have the meaning of a steady-state constant *(41)*.

## 2. ACTIVE-SITE-DIRECTED IRREVERSIBLE INHIBITION

### 1. BASIC KINETIC EQUATIONS: THE CASE OF ENZYME AND INHIBITOR REACTING ALONE, BEFORE ADDING SUBSTRATE— THE INITIAL PHASE APPROACH

When enzyme and inhibitor react alone, the reaction is described by Scheme (VIII). At the instant when substrate is added, the remaining free enzyme is complexed and the inhibition reaction reduces to the fate of the reversible complex existing at the moment of dilution

$$\text{EH} \xleftarrow{k_{-1}} \text{EHAX} \xrightarrow{k_2} \text{EA} \qquad \text{(IX)}$$
$$\downarrow$$
$$\text{HX}$$

then, EHAX can go either to EH or to EA. When the assumption is made that $k_{-1} \gg k_2$, it goes to EH. In measuring residual velocities, it is also assumed that the rate constants for the substrate reaction are considerably larger than those for inhibition. The conservation equation for enzyme from Scheme (VIII) is, $e_0 = (e + r + q)$ and it follows that the velocity of the substrate reaction will be proportional to $(e + r) = (e_0 - q)$. The rate of inhibition is then proportional to $(e + r)$ and is

$$- d(e + r) / dt = dq/dt = k_2 r. \qquad (20)$$

Assuming for the second time that $k_{-1} \gg k_2$ and that $i_0 \gg e_0$ so that $i$ remains constant, $K_a = (e_0 - r - q) i/r$, from which

$$r = \frac{(e_0 - q) i}{(i + K_a)}. \qquad (21)$$

Substituting (21) into (20) and arranging for integration,

$$\int \frac{dq}{(e_0 - q)} = \frac{k_2 i}{(i + K_a)} \int dt. \qquad (22)$$

Integrating between the limits $q = 0$ when $t = 0$ and $q = q$ when $t = t$, gives

$$\frac{\ln [e_0/(e_0 - q)]}{t} = \frac{k_2}{1 + (K_a/i)} = \rho. \qquad (23)$$

Remembering that $e_0 \propto v_0$ and $(e_0 - q) \propto v$

$$\rho = \frac{2.3 \log (v_0/v)}{t} = \frac{k_2}{(1 + (K_a/i)} \qquad (24)$$

Equation (24) has the same form as the differential Michaelis equation, Eq. (3). The velocity $v$ is analogous with $\rho$, $i$ is analogous with $s$, $K_a$ with $K_m$, and $k_2$ with $V_{max} = ke_0$. Consequently, Eq. (24) can be written in forms which are analogous with the linear Michaelis equations. The three principal linear equations are

$$\frac{1}{\rho} = \frac{K_a}{k_2} \cdot \frac{1}{i} + \frac{1}{k_2} \qquad (25)$$

$$\frac{i}{\rho} = \frac{i}{k_2} + \frac{K_a}{k_2} \qquad (26)$$

$$\rho = -\frac{\rho}{i} \cdot K_a + k_2 \qquad (27)$$

To determine $K_m$, $s$ values of the same order as $K_m$ must be used. Similarly $i$ values of the same order as $K_a$ are used to determine $K_a$. The arguments as to which form of the Michaelis equation should be used apply also to the various forms of Eq. (24).

To determine $K_a$ and $k_2$, a set of $\rho$ values are obtained over an appropriate range of inhibitor concentrations, as described in Section IV,A. A family of straight lines which intersect at a common point, log $v_0$, is obtained, as shown, for example, in Fig. 5A. If possible, the highest value of $i$ should approach $K_a$ (in the example, the highest DFP concentration was $2.24 \times 10^{-5}$ M and $K_a = 2.64 \times 10^{-5}$ M). The limiting value of $\rho$ is $k_2$, when $i \to \infty$, and is the broken line for the system illustrated (Fig. 5A). When $\rho = k_2$, all the free enzyme is in the form of the reversible complex.

When $i \ll K_a$, Eq. (24) approximates Eq. (11), which was derived from Scheme (IV). Scheme (IV) assumed a simple bimolecular reaction. From Eq. (11), $\rho = ik_i$, and from Eq. (24), when $i \ll K_a$, $\rho = ik_2/K_a$. It folows that

$$k_i = k_2/K_a. \qquad (28)$$

The overall rate of inhibition is then given by $k_i$. Since inhibitory power has typically been measured when $i \ll K_a$, $k_i$ has been a valid measure of inhibitory power, but it is only valid when $i \ll K_a$ and is not applicable as $i \to K_a$. The $\rho$ and $i$ values obtained from Fig. 5A were plotted according to Eq. (26) in Fig. 5B and according to Eq. (25) in Fig. 5C. Because $k_2$ values were of particular interest, the plot shown in Fig. 5B, in which the slope is $1/k_2$, has been preferred in a number of studies (6,34). The plot chosen will affect the range and concentrations

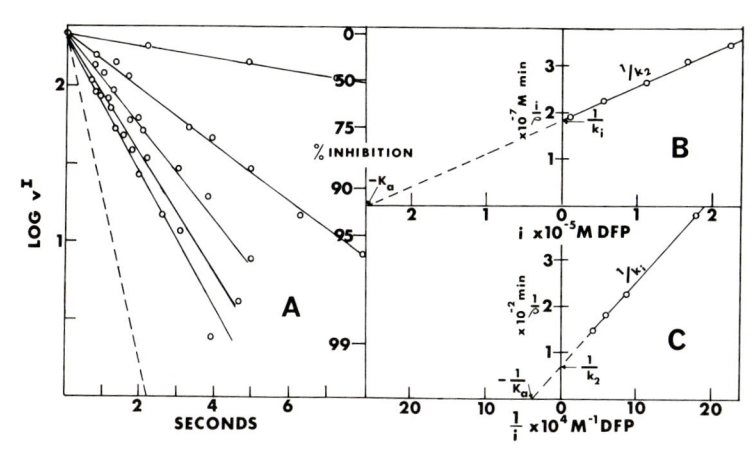

FIG. 5. (A) Resolved inhibition progress curves for the inhibition at 25°C, pH 7.0 of enzyme I in a partially purified preparation of horse serum cholinesterase by 1.12-, 5.60-, 11.2-, 16.8-, and 22.4-, all × 10⁻⁶ M DFP, reading from the top curve down. The broken line is the slope equivalent to $\rho$ where $i_0 \to \infty$. (B) Plot of the $\rho$ values obtained from Fig. 5A, according to Eq. (26). $K_a = 2.60 \pm 0.7 \times 10^{-5}$ M, $k_2 = 145 \pm 8$ minute⁻¹, $k_i = 5.5 \times 10^6$ $M^{-1}$ minute⁻¹. (C) Plot of $\rho$ values obtained from Fig. 5A according to Eq. (25).

of inhibitors employed. This plot (Fig. 5B) was also preferred because it makes the best use of the readily determined $\rho$ value when $i \ll K_a$; $i/\rho$ then approximates the $1/k_i$ intercept on the $i/\rho$ axis.

In determining $K_a$ and $k_2$ from plots such as those in Fig. 5B and C, the validity of the active-site-directed irreversible inhibition concept is also tested. A significant slope in the plot in Fig. 5B or significant intercept values in Fig. 5C are evidence of a reversible binding complex. The analogy with substrate reactions is exact in a fundamental sense. The concept of enzyme-catalyzed reactions involves formation of the enzyme–substrate complex. Similarly the active-site-directed irreversible inhibition concept involves the formation of a reversible enzyme–inhibitor complex, which places a limit on the rate of inhibition.

2. Kinetics When Regeneration Is Significant—The Steady-State Approach

In this treatment the time region in which the reaction between enzyme and inhibitor has reached a steady state is also utilized. At the steady state, enzyme is regenerated through the $k_3$-controlled regeneration reaction as fast as it is inhibited via Scheme (VIII). As a result, the inhibition progress curve levels out as shown in Fig. 1D. The progress curves are obtained experimentally as described in Section IV,A. Inhibitor and enzyme are incubated for a fixed time, after which substrate is added. The conditions and assumptions which were used in deriving Eq. (24) apply here: $i_0 \gg e_0$; $K_a = k_{-1}/k_1$; $v \propto (e + r) = (e_0 - q)$; and $e_0 = (e + r + q)$. The additional condition is the $k_3$-controlled step, as given in Scheme (II). The rate of inhibition is then

$$- d(e_0 - q)/dt = dq/dt = k_2 r - k_3 q. \qquad (29)$$

As before, $r = (e_0 - q) i / (i + K_a)$; substitution for $r$ in Eq. (29) and rearrangement for integration gives

$$\int \frac{dq}{e_0 - q \left[ 1 + \frac{k_3}{k_2}\left(1 + \frac{K_a}{i}\right)\right]} = \frac{k_2}{1 + \frac{K_a}{i}} \int dt. \qquad (30)$$

Integration between the limits $q = 0$ when $t = 0$ and $q = q$ when $t = t$, followed by rearrangement gives

$$\ln\left[\frac{(e_0 - q)}{e_0} - \frac{q}{e_0}\frac{k_3}{k_2}\left(1 + \frac{K_a}{i}\right)\right] = -t\left(\frac{k_2}{1 + \frac{K_a}{i}} + k_3\right). \qquad (31)$$

At the steady state, $dq/dt = 0$ and

$$k_2 r = k_3 q. \qquad (32)$$

Substituting for $r$ in (21) and rearranging gives

$$\left[\frac{(e_0 - q)}{q}\right]_{ss} = \frac{k_3}{k_2}\left(\frac{K_a}{i} + \frac{k_3}{k_2}\right) = \left[\frac{v}{(v_0 - v)}\right]_{ss} \qquad (33)$$

where the subscript ss indicates a steady state. Substituting (33) into (31)

$$\ln\left[\frac{(e_0 - q)}{e_0} - \frac{q}{e_0}\left(\frac{(e_0 - q)}{q}\right)_{ss}\right]$$
$$= y = -t\left\{\left[\frac{k_2}{1 + (K_a/i)}\right] + k_3\right\} \qquad (34)$$

Equations (33) and (34) have been used to evaluate $K_a$ and $k_2$ experimentally *(42)*. By plotting $y$ against $t$ at constant *(i)*, the slope $\{k_2/[1 + (K_a/i)]\} + k_3$ is obtained. Combining this slope value with Eq. (33) and remembering that $q = (e_0 - e)$, it can be shown that

$$k_3 = \left(\frac{e}{e_0}\right)_{ss} \frac{y}{t} = \left(\frac{v}{v_0}\right)_{ss} \frac{y}{t} \tag{35}$$

from which $k_3$ can be evaluated. The steady-state velocities, $v_{ss}$, are used with Eq. (33) by plotting $[v/(v_0 - v)]_{ss}$ against $1/i$. The slope of the straight line gives $(k_3 K_a/k_2)$, the intercept on the $y$ axis gives $k_3/k_2$, and the slope on the $1/i$ axis gives $-1/K_a$. Since the assumption that $k_{-1} \gg k_2$ has already been made and $k_2 > k_3$, it follows that $k_3 K_a/k_2 = K_{ss}$, the steady-state constant for the inhibition reaction. Since $k_3$ is known, $k_2$ is obtained from the intercept value, $k_3/k_2$. It would then appear that $k_2$, $k_3$, $K_a$, $K_m$, and $k_i$ ($= k_2/K_a$) can be obtained by this treatment.

For Eq. (33) to be used for evaluation of $K_a$ it is essential that $i$ values approaching $K_a$ be used. As $i \to K_a$, the intercept value $[v/(v_0 - v)]_{ss}$ approaches $k_3/k_2$. Consequently the application will be limited to systems for which $v_{ss}$ values in the range of $[(k_3/k_2)v_0]_{ss}$ can be measured with reasonable precision. The lower limits of resolution associated with the colorimetric and titrimetric methods by which substrate velocities are measured are normally in the order of 1% of $v_0$. Thus the $K_a$ and $k_2$ values of systems characterized by $k_3/k_2$ ratios of less than 0.01 could not then be determined reliably. The lower limits of $v_{ss}$ values which can be precisely measured bear the same relationship to the steady-state treatment as the shortest measurable times of incubation bear to the initial-phase approach. Unfortunately, the inhibition systems have sometimes been tailored to the limitations of the steady-state method rather than tailoring the method to the system. The result has been some unreasonably low $K_a$ and $k_2$ values. When $K_a$ and $k_2$ values of carbamates are to be determined, it would seem reasonable to take advantage of both the steady-state and initial-phase methods. As Metcalf *(43)* has pointed out, a disturbing number of inconsistent $K_a$ and $k_2$ values have been reported. It is time that the limitations of both methods were thoroughly understood and the results examined critically within the context of these limitations. It is not the basic data which are in question, but their interpretation. It is not a question of ethics, but of reason.

To illustrate the problem, the example of $N$-methylphenyl carbamate inhibition of bovine erythrocyte acetylcholinesterase will be considered briefly. In Fig. 1C, the $\rho$ value calculated from the initial phase of inhibition using $2 \times 10^{-4}$ $M$ $N$-methylphenyl carbamate was 0.056 minute$^{-1}$. From the equation, $\rho = ik_i$, $k_i = 2.8 \times 10^2$ $M^{-1}$ minute$^{-1}$. In Fig. 1C, $v_{ss} = 0.27$ $v_0$. From initial phase studies, $K_a$ was $2.37 \times 10^{-2}$ $M$ and $k_2$ was 6.82 minute$^{-1}$ *(44)*. Substituting these values into Eq. (31) and solving for $k_3$ gives $k_3 = 2.1 \times 10^{-2}$ minute$^{-1}$, which agrees with the $k_3$ reported by Wilson et al. *(45)*.

The ratio of $k_2/k_3$ for this system is then 325, which clearly indicates that obtaining $K_a$ for this compound by the steady-state method would have been difficult if not impossible. It may be noted too that $N$-methylphenyl carbamate is a poor inhibitor. Thus it appears that the effective use of the steady-state region to obtain $K_a$ values will in general be restricted to extremely poor inhibitors.

However, this method does give $K_{ss}$ as the slope. $K_{ss}$ is less than $K_a$ by the ratio $k_3/k_2$. In the example, $K_{ss}$ was $7.5 \times 10^{-5}$ $M$, while $K_a$ was $2.37 \times 10^{-2}$ $M$. There have been instances where $K_a$, the initial binding, has been confused with $K_{ss}$, the overall binding. As can be seen from this example, the error involved in confusing the two may be very large.

By combining constants obtained from the initial region with those from the steady-state region, $k_2$, $k_3$, $K_a$, $K_m$, and $k_i$ can be obtained. Of these, $k_2$ and $K_a$ can be most readily obtained from the initial region, while $K_{ss}$ and $k_3$ can be estimated from the steady-state region. The regeneration constant $k_3$ can also be determined from a regeneration curve.

In the absence of inhibitor, the rate of regeneration is proportional to the concentration of EA, thus

$$-dq/dt = k_3 q. \tag{36}$$

Integrating (36) between the limits $q = q_0$ when $t = 0$, and $q = q$ when $t = t$,

$$2.3 \log (q/q_0) = k_3 t = 2.3 \log (v/v_0') \tag{37}$$

where now $v_0'$ is the velocity when the regeneration timing begins and $v$ is the velocity measured after regenerating for time $t$. A straight line is obtained by plotting $\log v$ against $t$; the slope is $k_3/2.3$, from which $k_3$ is obtained.

3. KINETICS FOR INHIBITION IN THE PRESENCE OF SUBSTRATE

This approach has seen only occasional use *(33)*, but interest in it appears to be growing *(46)* and with good reason. It offers interesting pos-

## 2. ACTIVE-SITE-DIRECTED IRREVERSIBLE INHIBITION

sibilities for the rapid measurement of inhibition progress curves through the use of chromogenic substrates and time-based oscilloscopes or high-speed recorders. It also offers an unparalleled opportunity to explore the relationship between the interaction of the active-site-directed irreversible inhibitor and the substrate at the active site. The treatment proposed is based on the assumption that the inhibitors act in a purely competitive manner. With some substrates this appears to be true *(46)*. However, the range of substrates and inhibitors which were explored is extremely limited, as were the concentration ranges employed, so the full story has yet to be told—indeed it has hardly begun.

Kinetics based on simple bimolecular reaction between inhibitor and enzyme in the presence of substrate were described by Main and Dauterman *(33)*. When the concept of active-site-directed irreversible inhibition is considered, there are additional complications. The present derivation given here for the first time considers this case. The reaction schemes are

$$\text{EH} + \text{AX} \underset{}{\overset{K_a}{\rightleftharpoons}} \text{EHAX} \xrightarrow{k_2} \text{EA} + \text{HX}$$

$$\text{EH} + \text{CB} \underset{k_{-1}}{\overset{k_1}{\rightleftharpoons}} \text{EHCB} \xrightarrow{k_2'} \text{EC} + \text{HOH} \xrightarrow{k_3'} \text{EH} + \text{AOH}$$ 
$$\quad + \text{HB}$$

(X)

The substrate is CB and the assumptions and conditions are as follows: $e_0 \ll i_0$; $e_0 \ll s_0$; $i$ and $s$ remain constant over the course of inhibition; EHAX is formed under conditions approaching an equilibrium; $k_3 = 0$ for the inhibition reaction. The conservation equation for enzyme is

$$e_0 = (e + r + q + p),$$

where $p = (x_1 + x_2)$, and $x_1$ and $x_2$ are the concentrations of EHCB and EC, respectively.

Since velocities are measured continuously as inhibition procedes in the presence of substrate, EHAX does not revert to EH as $v$ *is* measured.

In the presence of substrate, therefore, $v \propto (e + p) = (e_0 - r - q)$, and we solve for $(e_0 - r - q)$. The rate of irreversible inhibition as before is,

$$dq/dt = k_2 r. \tag{38}$$

$K_m = [(e_0 - r - q - p) s/p]$ from which

$$p = \frac{(e_0 - r - q) s}{(s + K_m)} \tag{39}$$

$$K_a = \frac{(e_0 - r - q - p) i}{r}. \tag{40}$$

Substituting (39) into (40) and solving for $r$ gives,

$$r = \frac{(e_0 - r - q) i K_m}{(K_a K_m + s K_a)}. \tag{41}$$

Substituting $r$ in (41) into (38) and arranging for integration gives

$$\int \frac{dq}{(e_0 - q - r)} = \frac{k_2 i K_m}{(K_a K_m + s K_m)} \int dt \tag{42}$$

from (41)

$$r = \frac{(e_0 - q) i K_m}{(K_a K_m + s K_a + i K_m)} \tag{43}$$

and it follows that

$$\int \frac{dq}{(e_0 A - qA)} = \frac{k_2 i K_m}{(K_a K_m + s K_m)} \int dt \tag{44}$$

where

$$B = \frac{K_a (s + K_m)}{K_a (s + K_m) + i K_m} = \frac{(e_0 - r - q)}{(e_0 - q)}. \tag{45}$$

Integrating (44) between the limits $q = 0$ when $t = 0$ and $q = q$ when $t = t$ gives

$$\ln \left[ \frac{e_0 B}{(e_0 B - qB)} \right] = \frac{t k_2 i K_m}{K_a (s + K_m)} B. \tag{46}$$

Substituting the appropriate expressions for $A$ into both sides of (46) gives

$$\ln \left[ \frac{(e_0 - r)}{(e_0 - r - q)} \right] = \frac{t k_2 i K_m}{(s K_a + K_a K_m + i K_m)}. \tag{47}$$

## 2. ACTIVE-SITE-DIRECTED IRREVERSIBLE INHIBITION

Then, $v \propto (e_0 - r - q)$ and $v_0 \propto (e_0 - r)$ from which,

$$\frac{2.3 \log (v_0/v)}{t} = \rho = \frac{k_2}{1 + \dfrac{K_a}{i}\left(1 + \dfrac{s}{K_m}\right)}. \tag{48}$$

The linear form of Eq. (48) in which $1/k_2$ is the slope is

$$\frac{i}{\rho} = \frac{i}{k_2} + \frac{K_a}{k_2}\left(1 + \frac{s}{K_m}\right). \tag{49}$$

From Eq. (49) $k_2$ can be obtained directly, but in order to determine $K_a$, $K_m$ must be known.

Although $\rho$ is obtained from log $v$ against $t$ plots as described previously, the values of $v$ and $t$ used for the plots are not. They are obtained directly from what might be called "inhibited" substrate progress curves. An example is shown in Fig. 6A. The enzyme catalyzing the sub-

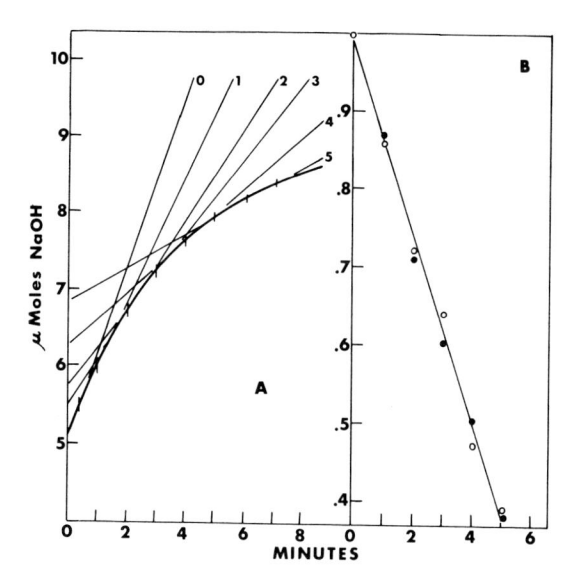

FIG. 6. Determination of first-order rate constants ($\rho$) from inhibited substrate progress curves. (A) The curve shown is a recorder trace from a radiometer pH-stat showing the hydrolysis of 2 mM dibutyl malate by rat liver carboxylesterase at 25°C, pH 7.6 in the presence of $1.07 \times 10^{-5}$ M dibutyl malaoxon. The tangents were drawn to the curve at the times indicated, following addition of inhibitor. (B) The plots of log $v$ against $t$ from the tangents (open circles) are compared with the plot obtained by the Guggenheim method. $\log[z_{(t+\tau)} - z_t]$ shown by closed circles, log $v$ shown by open circles, $\rho = 0.28$ minute$^{-1}$.

strate reaction is progressively removed by the action of the irreversible inhibitor present in the substrate and this causes the progress curve to bend. Conditions are arranged so that the progress curve in the absence of inhibitor is straight over the measured course of the reaction. This simply means that the substrate concentration remains constant over the period in question. Deviation from linearity when the inhibitor is added is then caused solely by inhibition.

The curve can be analyzed in two ways. The first involves taking tangents to the curves at various times *(33,47)*. The tangents are then the velocities $v$ of the substrate reactions at these times $t$. A plot of log $v$ against $t$ gives the desired inhibition progress curve.

The second approach employs the Guggenheim method and was suggested by Smissaert as reported in DeJong *(46)*. Equation (47) can be written

$$\ln (v/v_0) = -k_2 K t \tag{50}$$

where $K = [iK_m / (sK_a + K_a K_m + iK_m)]$. Written in the exponential form, Eq. (50) becomes

$$v/v_0 = \exp(-k_2 t K t). \tag{51}$$

The velocity of the substrate reaction is given by the rate at which product concentration $z$ changes with time, i.e.,

$$v = dz/dt \tag{52}$$

so that

$$dz/dt = v_0 \exp(k_2 K t). \tag{53}$$

Arranging (53) for integration gives

$$\int dz = v_0 \int \exp(-k_2 K t)\, dt. \tag{54}$$

Integrating (54) between the limits $z = 0$ when $t = 0$ and $z = z_t$ when $t = t$ gives

$$z_t = -\frac{v_0}{k_2 K} [\exp(-k_2 K t) - \exp(0)] = \frac{v_0}{k_2 K} [1 - \exp(-k_2 K t)] \tag{55}$$

then

$$z(t + \tau) = \frac{v_0}{k_2 K} - \frac{v_0}{k_2 K} \exp[-k_2 (t + \tau)] \tag{56}$$

where $\tau$ is any convenient, constant time and

$$z_t = \frac{v_0}{k_2 K} - \frac{v_0}{k_2 K} \exp(-k_2 K t). \tag{57}$$

Subtracting (57) from (56)

$$\{[z_{(t+\tau)} - z_t] = \frac{v_0}{k_2 K}[\exp(-k_2 K t)] - \exp[-k_2 K (t+\tau)]\} \tag{58}$$

and remembering that

$$\exp[-k_2 K (t+\tau)] = \exp(-k_2 K t) \cdot \exp(-k_2 K \tau),$$

then
$$[z_{(t+\tau)} - zt] = \exp(-k_2 K t)[1 - \exp(-k_2 K \tau)] \frac{v_0}{k_2 K} \tag{59}$$

in which $[1 - \exp(-kK\tau)] \dfrac{v_0}{k_2 K}$ is constant. Let it be $C$, then

$$[z_{(t+\tau)} - z_t] = \exp(-k_2 K t) C. \tag{60}$$

Writing (60) in the logarithmic form gives

$$\ln[z_{(t+\tau)} - z_t] = -k_2 K t + \ln C. \tag{61}$$

Substituting the expression for $K$ into (61) gives

$$\log[z_{(t+\tau)} - z_t] = \frac{-k_2 i K_m t}{(sK_a + K_a K_m + iK_m) 2.3} + \log C. \tag{62}$$

The plot of $\log[z_{(t+\tau)} - z_t]$ against $t$ will then give a straight line, the slope of which will be $\rho/2.3$. Perhaps the best way of explaining the use of Eq. (62) is to give an example. The inhibited progress curve in Fig. 6A was obtained by inhibiting the hydrolysis of 2 m$M$ dibutylmalate by rat liver carboxylase in the presence of $1.07 \times 10^{-5}$ $M$ dibutyl malaoxon. Figure 6A shows the trace of NaOH production against time obtained from the recorder of a pH-stat. The NaOH production was equivalent to the acid liberated.

The inhibition plot was obtained by taking tangents to the curve at various times as shown, and plotting the log of the tangents ($\equiv \log v$) against the appropriate times. The open circles in Fig. 6B are these points. The Guggenheim plot is shown by the filled circles and was obtained as shown in Table I.

Because inhibition is measured in the presence of substrate, EHAX remains. Consequently the log $v$ against $t$ plots at the various inhibitor con-

## TABLE I
### CALCULATION OF INHIBITED PROGRESS CURVE[a]

| $t$ (minutes) | $\tau$ (minutes) | $(t+\tau)$ (minutes) | $z_t$ ($\mu$ moles) | $z_{(t+\tau)}$ ($\mu$ moles) | $z_{(t+\tau)} - z_t$ ($\mu$ moles × 10) | $\log[z_{(t+\tau)} - z_t]$ |
|---|---|---|---|---|---|---|
| 0 | 1 | 1 | 5.0 | 6.0 | 10.0 | 1.0 |
| 1 | 1 | 2 | 6.0 | 6.74 | 7.4 | 0.87 |
| 2 | 1 | 3 | 6.74 | 7.25 | 5.1 | 0.71 |
| 3 | 1 | 4 | 7.25 | 7.65 | 4.1 | 0.60 |
| 4 | 1 | 5 | 7.65 | 7.97 | 3.2 | 0.51 |
| 5 | 1 | 6 | 7.97 | 8.20 | 2.3 | 0.36 |

[a] The Guggenheim method, Eq. (62), was applied to calculate the inhibited progress curve shown in Fig. 6A. The $\log[z_{(t+\tau)} - z_t]$ values are plotted in Fig. 6B, filled circles.

## 2. ACTIVE-SITE-DIRECTED IRREVERSIBLE INHIBITION

centrations will *not* extrapolate back to a common log $v_0$ at $t = 0$. Instead they will intersect at points progressively lower than $v_0{}^0$, where $v_0{}^0$ is $v$ at $i = 0$ and $t = 0$. If these log $v$ intercepts at $t = 0$ in the presence of inhibitor are called $v_0{}^i$, then it can be shown that

$$\frac{v_0{}^0}{(v_0{}^0 - v_0{}^i)} = 1 + \frac{K_a}{i}\left(1 + \frac{s}{K_m}\right). \tag{63}$$

This follows because at $t = 0$, $q = 0$ but $r = e_0 - (e + p) = (v_0{}^0 - v_0{}^i)$. As $i$ increases, $r$ increases and the difference $(v_0{}^0 - v_0{}^i)$ becomes greater. If $v_0{}^i$ is measured at various concentrations of both $s$ and $i$, Eq. (61) can be rewritten to take advantage of the Hunter and Downs *(48)* method of calculating $K_a$, since the system now is purely competitive and reversible. The equation is

$$\frac{i v_0{}^i}{(v_0{}^0 - v_0{}^i)} = s \frac{K_a}{K_m} + K_a. \tag{64}$$

The plot of $[iv_0{}^i/(v_0{}^0 - v_0{}^i)]$ against $s$ will be straight and will give an intercept of $K_a$ on the $y$ axis. If $s$ is kept constant and only $i$ is varied, then Eq. (63) can be used by plotting $[v_0{}^0/(v_0{}^0 - v_0{}^i)]$ against $1/i$. The intercept on the $1/i$ axis gives $1/[K_a(1 + K_m/s)]$ from which $K_a$ can be calculated if $K_m$ is known.

*The general derivation from Scheme (VIII)*—When no assumption is made regarding $k_{-1}$ and $k_2$, the rate of formation of EHAX is given by

$$dr/dt = k_1(e_0 - r - q)i - r(k_{-1} + k_2). \tag{65}$$

The formation of EA is

$$dq/dt = k_2 r. \tag{66}$$

The second derivative of $dq/dt$ is

$$d^2q/dt^2 = k_2\, dr/dt. \tag{67}$$

Equation (65) may be written

$$dr/dt = k_1(e_0 - q)i - r(k_1 i + k_{-1} + k_2). \tag{68}$$

Substituting $r$ and $dr/dt$ from (66) and (67), respectively, into (68) and rearranging,

$$d^2q/dt^2 + dq/dt\,(k_1 i + k_{-1} + k_2) - k_1 k_2(e_0 - q)i = 0. \tag{69}$$

The second derivative $d^2q/dt^2 \to 0$ when the initial phase of the reaction, in which EHAX is increasing from 0 is over. Then

$$dq/dt = \frac{k_1 k_2 (e_0 - q) i}{(k_1 i + k_{-1} + k_2)} = \frac{k_2 (e_0 - q) i}{i + [(k_{-1} + k_2)/k_1]} = \frac{k_2 (e_0 - q) i}{(i + K_a)} \tag{70}$$

from which it appears that $K_a = (k_{-1} + k_2)/k_1$ *(41)*. However the assumption that $d^2q/dt^2 = 0$ can be made only if the formation of EHAX has approached the steady state. With the present system, the only steady state which can be approached is an equilibrium, but for this to hold $k_{-1} > k_2$ and then $K_a = k_{-1}/k_1$. The solution to Eq. (69) has been derived *(49)* and is

$$\frac{(e_0 - q)}{e_0} = \left[\frac{A + (A^2 - 4B)^{1/2}}{2(A^2 - 4B)^{1/2}}\right] \exp\left[-\frac{t}{2}[A - (A^2 - 4B)^{1/2}]\right]$$
$$- \left[\frac{A - (A^2 - 4B)^{1/2}}{2(A^2 - 4B)^{1/2}}\right] \exp\left[-\frac{t}{2}[A + (A^2 - 4B)^{1/2}]\right] \tag{71}$$

where $A = (k_{-1} + k_2 + k_1 i)$ and $B = k_1 k_2 i$.

An attempt has been made to estimate how much greater $k_{-1}$ must be than $k_2$ for equations such as (24) and (49) to hold *(50)*, but it seems evident that more theoretical and experimental work is needed in order to gain a firm understanding of the problem.

**C. The Scope of the Present Treatment**

The basic kinetics and the main events leading to their development have been described. Emphasis has been given to organophosphate, carbamate, and organosulfonate inhibitors of cholinesterases and other hydrolytic enzymes. The reason is partly historical and partly because it was felt that the principal kinetic problems are associated with these reactions. The alkylating antimetabolites, while extremely interesting compounds, are not generally characterized by high rates of covalent bond formation, nor do they, to the same degree as the organophosphates and carbamates, mimic the mechanism of the substrate reaction. Consequently the kinetics applied to them emphasizes the "affinity" part of affinity labeling. Shaw *(49)* in a recent review, has given an excellent account of the active-site-directed reagents, by which the relative role of kinetics can be judged. In the present essay peripheral areas either have not been considered or have been mentioned only insofar as they were relevant to the central theme of this essay. These would include the phenomenon of aging (e.g., *51*), regenerating reagents (e.g., *29*), the kinetics of the transient state associated with the inhibition process (e.g., *50*), various methods of estimation of the active-site concentration (e.g., *19,52*), and perhaps, most relevant of all, structure-activity studies (e.g., *38,53*). The peripheral areas might also include alkylating reagents such as 1,1-dimethyl-2-phenylaziridinium *(54)* discussed by O'Brien *(55)* in the first volume of this serial publication. To deal with these topics in greater depth, and to explore their relationship with the kinetics of active-site-directed irreversible inhibition, is beyond the scope of this essay. Here I note only that the task remains.

There are other areas of more immediate concern which have also been ignored. They include the effect of pH *(56,57)*, temperature (e.g., *6*), and ionic strength. Suitable expressions dealing with each of these parameters have been or could readily be incorporated into the kinetics of active-site-directed irreversible inhibition. They would be based, in the first instance, on accepted theory. For example, the approach of Michaelis and Davidsohn to pH as developed by Dixon and Webb *(20)* and others, has been applied by Iverson *(57)*, but the results were difficult to interpret. Similarly, the effect of temperature can be considered within the context of the theory of absolute reaction rates proposed by Eyring *(58)*. Numerous studies have already been made of the effect of pH (e.g., *59*) and temperature (e.g., *38*) with these inhibitors, but not with the kinetics described here. The present kinetics evaluate an equilibrium constant $(K_a)$ and an elementary rate constant $(k_2)$ which would appear to make such studies a most inviting proposition. But there may be difficulties. One is related to the nature of the enzymes in question. As mentioned, cholinesterases appear to exist in multiple forms. These may be conformational isomers *(60)*, or they may be polymers *(40)*, or they may be both *(61)*. Both pH and temperature may well affect the distribution of the forms as well as the reaction rates. The two different effects must be sorted out before unequivocal effects on each can be ascertained.

Kinetic expressions which include the interaction of reversible and irreversible inhibitors present simultaneously in the reaction medium have also been considered in connection with the anionic site of acetylcholinesterase *(62)*. The treatment is analogous with that given for inhibition in the presence of substrate. A related area would consider systems in which two or more irreversible inhibitors were present. Such systems would give nonlinear $i/\rho$ against $i$ plots.

In general, it seems reasonable to suppose that Scheme (I), from which the basic kinetics have been derived, will frequently be too simple to describe many systems of interest. More complex systems would probably be reflected by $i/\rho$ against $i$ plots which are not linear, but curve significantly in a number of ways, depending on the complication. The analogy with substrate reactions is again appropriate, since there are a number of instances in which substrate reactions do not follow simple Michaelis kinetics.

The possibility that cholinesterase inhibition by haloxons *(35)* or by tetram *(34)* involves an allosteric site provides an example of how such complications might be handled within the context of the kinetics developed.

Inhibition involving an allosteric site would be described by the following reaction sequence

$$\begin{array}{ccccc}
& & K_{a1} & & k_2 \\
\text{E} & + & \text{PX} \rightleftharpoons \text{EPX} & \longrightarrow & \text{EP} \\
K_{a2} \updownarrow & & K'_{a2} \updownarrow & +\text{PX} & \\
& & K'_{a1} & & k'_2 \\
\text{PXE} & + & \text{PX} \rightleftharpoons \text{PXEPX} & \longrightarrow & \text{EP}
\end{array} \quad (\text{XI})$$

Binding to the allosteric site is controlled by $K_{a2}$ and $K'_{a2}$, while binding to the active site is governed by $K_{a1}$ and $K'_{a1}$. PXE signifies binding to the allosteric site. For this sequence the equation is

$$\rho = \left[ \frac{1}{(i^2 K_{a1} + i K_{a1} K_{a1}' + i K_{a1}' K_{a2} + K_{a1} K_{a1}' K_{a2})} \right]$$
$$\times \left[ i^2 k_2' K_{a1} + \frac{k_2 (i^2 K_{a1}' K_{a2} + i K_{a1} K_{a1}' K_{a2})}{(i + K_{a1})} \right]. \quad (72)$$

Despite its complexity, the right-hand side is constant at constant $i$, which means that the $\log v$ against $t$ plot from which $\rho$ is obtained will be straight.

In a system as complex as (XI), some of the reactions are almost certain to be insignificant relative to others. If the assumptions are made, for example, that

$k_2 \ll k_2'$ and $K_{a2} \gg K_{a2}'$ and $K_{a1} \gg K_{a1}'$, then Scheme (XI) reduces to

$$\text{E} + \text{PX} \underset{}{\overset{K_{a2}}{\rightleftharpoons}} \text{PXE} + \text{PX} \underset{}{\overset{K_{a1}'}{\rightleftharpoons}} \text{PXEPX} \overset{k_2'}{\longrightarrow} \text{EP} \rightarrow \quad (\text{XII})$$

and Eq. (72) reduces to

$$\frac{i}{\rho} = \frac{1}{k_2}\left( \frac{K_{a1}' K_{a2}}{i} + i \right) + \frac{K_{ai}'}{k_2'}. \quad (73)$$

## 2. ACTIVE-SITE-DIRECTED IRREVERSIBLE INHIBITION

Equation (73) is consistent with an $i/\rho$ against $i$ plot which swings up as $i \to 0$, as was observed for the reaction of tetram with horse serum cholinesterase *(34)*. According to this scheme, the allosteric site must be occupied before further phosphorylation can occur. The probability of such an assumption is, of course, open to question, but it does open an interesting line of study. Other assumptions, such as $K_{a1} = K_{a1}'$ and $K_{a2} = K_{a2}'$, will give an equation of the same form as (73), so that the validity of Scheme (XII) is not established.

This highlights an important feature of kinetic interpretations. They are by nature inferential and hence are not definitive. More than one set of premises (e.g., reaction schemes) and more than one interpretation can usually satisfy any given set of results. Thus the validity of $K_a$ as a measure of affinity and of $k_2$ as a measure of covalent bond formation are not definitively established by plots such as those shown in Fig. 5B or C. One should hasten to add that such plots certainly argue for their validity. But additional supporting evidence is needed insofar as organophosphates and carbamates are concerned, and it has come, for example, from studies with analogous substrate and inhibitor reaction series. One might expect that a similar series of substituents would result in parallel changes in the binding capacities on the one hand, and in parallel changes in rates of covalent bond formation and substrate velocities on the other. Such expectations have been realized experimentally *(32,44,54,62)*. The expectation too would be that the $K_a$ values of inhibitors, such as diethyl $p$-nitrophenylphosphate ($3.6 \times 10^{-4}$ $M$) and $N,N$-dimethyl-$p$-nitrophenyl carbamate ($3.2 \times 10^{-3}$ $M$), would be of the same order as the $K_m$ values of substrates such as $p$-nitrophenylacetate ($3.86 \times 10^{-3}$ $M$) in reaction with the same enzyme. That they are, as indicated by the values in parentheses *(44)*, lends further support to the validity of $K_a$. A growing body of evidence along these lines (e.g., 64–66) clearly indicates that the kinetics do, in fact, reflect the presence of a reversible-affinity binding complex.

Despite false starts and the inevitable contingent of questionable results, of both of which the author acknowledges his fair share, the validity of the kinetics of active-site-directed irreversible inhibition seems well established. Thus the first chapter in the story of active-site-directed irreversible inhibition kinetics can, with some satisfaction, be ended. But what of the future? The question of the allosteric binding site has been mentioned briefly. The multiple forms in which some enzymes appear to exist have been considered at greater length, but it is evident that the surface here has only been scratched. The area of pH-dependence and of temperature effects remain largely unexplored within this context, as does the question of conformational isomers *(60)*. Perhaps the most immediate problem, the upper limit of the rate of covalent bond formation, remains unanswered. The catalog is large, so in ending chapter one, the reader is advised that chapter two is already well begun. There seems no question that it will be as interesting, provocative, and frustrating as the first. One only hopes it will be as productive.

## REFERENCES

1. Baker, B. R. (1964). Factors in the design of active-site-directed irreversible inhibitors. *J. Pharm. Sci.* 53, 347–364.
2. Baker, B. R. (1959). The case for irreversible inhibitors as anticancer agents, an essay. *Cancer Chemother. Rep.*, pp. 1–10.
3. O'Brien, R. D. (1967). "Insecticides, Action and Metabolism." Academic Press, New York.
4. Baker, B. R. (1967). "Design of Active-Site-Directed Irreversible Inhibitors." Wiley, New York.
5. Main, A. R. (1964). Affinity and phosphorylation constants for the inhibition of esterases by organophosphates. *Science* 144, 992–993.
6. Main, A. R., and Iverson, F. (1966). Measurement of affinity and phosphorylation constants govering irreversible inhibition of cholinesterases by di-isopropyl phosphorofluoridate. *Biochem. J.* 100, 525–531.
7. Aldridge, W. N. (1954). Anticholinesterases. Inhibition of cholinesterase by organophosphorus compounds and reversal of this reaction: mechanisms involved. *Chem. Ind. (London)* pp. 473–476.
8. Aldridge, W. N., and Davison, A. N. (1953). The mechanism of inhibition of cholinesterases by organophosphorus compounds. *Biochem. J.* 55, 763–765.
9. Wilson, I. B., Hatch, M. A., and Ginsburg, S. (1960). Carbamylation of acetylcholinesterase. *J. Biol. Chem.* 235, 2312–2315.
10. Wilson, I. B. (1960). Acetylcholinesterase. In "The Enzymes" (P. D. Boyer, H. Lardy, and K. Myrbäck, eds.), 2nd ed., Vol. 4, pp. 501–520. Academic Press, New York.
11. Wilson, I. B., Bergmann, F., and Nachmansohn, D. (1950). Acetylcholinesterase. X. Mechanism of catalysis of acylation reactions. *J. Biol. Chem.* 186, 781–790.
12. Myers, D. K., and Kemp, A., Jr. (1954). Inhibition of esterases by the fluorides of organic acids. *Nature (London)* 173, 33–34.
13. Myers, D. K. (1956). Studies on cholinesterase. 10. Return of cholinesterase activity in the rat after inhibition by carbamoyl fluorides. *Biochem. J.* 62, 556–563.
14. Jansz, H. S., Brons, D., and Warringa, M. G. P. J. (1959). Chemical nature of the DFP-binding site of pseudocholinesterase. *Biochim. Biophys. Acta* 34, 573–575.
15. Gaddum, J. H. (1954). Anticholinesterase. The history of work on anticholinesterases. *Chem. Ind. (London)* pp. 266–268.
16. Easson, L. H., and Stedman, E. (1936–1937). The absolute activity of choline-esterase. *Proc. Roy. Soc. Ser. B* 121, 142–164.
17. Goldstein, A. (1944). The mechanism of enzyme-inhibitor-substrate reactions. Illustrated by the cholinesterase-physostigmine-acetylcholine system. *J. Gen. Physiol.* 27, 529–580.
18. Straus, O. H., and Goldstein, A. (1943). Zone behavior of enzymes. Illustrated by the effect of dissociation constant and dilution on the system cholinesterase–physostigmine. *J. Gen. Physiol.* 26, 559–585.

19. Myers, D. K. (1952). Studies on cholinesterase. 7. Determination of the molar concentration of pseudo-cholinesterase in serium. *Biochem. J.* **51**, 303–311.
20. Dixon, M., and Webb, E. C. (1964). "Enzymes," 2nd ed. Academic Press, New York.
21. Mazur, A., and Bodansky, O. (1946). The mechanism of *in vitro* and *in vivo* inhibition of cholinesterase activity by diisopropyl fluorophosphate. *J. Biol. Chem.* **163**, 261–276.
22. Holmstedt, B. (1951). Synthesis and pharmacology of dimethylamido-ethoxy-phosphoryl cyanide (Tabun) together with a description of some allied anticholinesterase compounds containing the N-P bond. *Acta Physiol. Scand.* **25**, Suppl. 90, 1–120.
23. Adrian, E. D., Feldberg, W., and Kilby, B. A. (1947). The cholinesterase inhibiting action of fluorophosphonates. *Brit. J. Pharmacol.* **2**, 56–58.
24. Mackworth, J. F., and Webb, E. C. (1948). The inhibition of serum cholinesterase by alkyl fluorophosphonates. *Biochem. J.* **42**, 91–95.
25. Boursnell, J. C., and Webb, E. C. (1949). Reaction of esterases with radioactive di-isopropyl fluorophosphonate. *Nature (London)* **164**, 875.
26. Aldridge, W. N. (1950). Some properties of specific cholinesterase with particular reference to the mechanism of inhibition by diethyl p-nitrophenyl thiophosphate (E 605) and analogues. *Biochem. J.* **46**, 451–460.
27. Aldridge, W. N. (1957). 3. Organo-phosphorus compounds and esterases. *Annu. Rep. Chem. Soc.* **54**, 294–305.
28. O'Brien, R. D. (1960). "Toxic Phosphorous Esters." Academic Press, New York.
29. Green, A. L., and Smith, H. J. (1958). The reactivation of cholinesterase inhibited with organophosphorus compounds. 1. Reactivation by 2-oxoaldoximes. *Biochem. J.* **68**, 28–31.
30. Main, A. R., and Braid, P. E. (1962). Hydrolysis of malathion by ali-esterases *in vitro* and *in vivo*. *Biochem. J.* **84**, 255–263.
31. Main, A. R., and Dauterman, W. C. (1967). Kinetics for the inhibition of carboxylesterase by malaoxon. *Can. J. Biochem.* **45**, 757–771.
32. Dauterman, W. C., and Main, A. R. (1966). Relationship between acute toxicity and *in vitro* inhibition and hydrolysis of a series of carboalkoxy homologs of malathion. *Toxicol. Appl. Pharmacol.* **9**, 408–418.
33. Main, A. R., and Dauterman, W. C. (1963). Determination of the bimolecular rate constant for the reaction between organophosphorus inhibitors and esterases in the presence of substrate. *Nature (London)* **198**, 1–5.
34. Main, A. R. (1969). Kinetic evidence of multiple reversible cholinesterases based on inhibition by organophosphates. *J. Biol. Chem.* **244**, 829–840.
35. Aldridge, W. N., and Reiner, E. (1969). Acetylcholinesterase. Two types of inhibition by an organophosphorous compound: one the formation of phosphorylated enzyme and the other analogous to inhibition by substrate. *Biochem. J.* **115**, 147–162.
36. Main, A. R. (1967). Evaluation of phosphorylation and carbamylation rate constants. *In* "Structure and Reactions of DFP-Sensitive Enzymes" (E. Heilbronn, ed.), p. 129. Swedish Res. Inst. Nat. Defence, Stockholm.
37. Ellman, G. L., Courtney, D. K., Andres, V., Jr., and Featherstone, R. M. (1961). A new and rapid colorimetric determination of acetylcholinesterase activity. *Biochem. Pharmacol.* **1**, 88–95.
38. Ooms, A. J. J. (1961). De reactiviteit van organische fosforverbindingen ten opzichte van een aantal esterasen. Ph.D. Thesis, Univ. of Leiden, Netherlands.

39. Svensmark, O. (1965). Molecular properties of cholinesterases. *Acta Physiol. Scand.* **64**, Suppl. 245, 9–74.
40. La Motta, R. V., McComb, R. B., and Noll, C. R., Jr. (1968). Multiple forms of serum cholinesterase. *Arch. Biochem. Biophys.* **124**, 299–305.
41. Gold, A. M., and Fahrney, D. (1964). Sulfonyl fluorides as inhibitors of esterases. II. Formation and reactions of phenylmethanesulfonyl $\alpha$-chymotrypsin. *Biochemistry* **3**, 783–791.
42. Hellenbrand, K. (1967). Inhibition of housefly acetylcholinesterase by carbamates. *J. Agr. Food Chem.* **15**, 825–829.
43. Metcalf, R. L. (1971). Structure-activity relationships for insecticidal carbamates. *Bull. W. H. O.* **44**, 43–78.
44. Hastings, F. L., Main, A. R., and Iverson, F. (1970). Carbamylation and affinity constants of some carbamate inhibitors of acetylcholinesterase and their relation to analogous substrate constants. *J. Agr. Food Chem.* **18**, 497–502.
45. Wilson, I. B., Harrison, M. A., and Ginsburg, S. (1961). Carbamyl derivatives of acetylcholinesterase. *J. Biol. Chem.* **236**, 1498–1500.
46. DeJong, L. P. A. (1970). Inhibition of acetylcholinesterase and butyrylcholinesterase by organophosphorus compounds in the presence of substrates. Chemisch Laboratorium, National Defence Research Organization, TNO, Rijswijk, Netherlands, Report 1970-22: 26 pp.
47. Main, A. R., and Dauterman, W. C. (1967). Kinetics for the inhibition of carboxylesterase by malaoxon. *Can. J. Biochem.* **45**, 757–771.
48. Hunter, A., and Downs, C. E. (1945). The inhibition of arginase by amino acids. *J. Biol. Chem.* **157**, 427–445.
49. Shaw, E. (1970). Modification of active-site-directed reagents. *In* "The Enzymes," 3rd ed. (P. D. Boyer, ed.), Vol. I, pp. 91–146. Academic Press, New York.
50. Main, A. R. (1969). Kinetics of cholinesterase inhibition by organophosphate and carbamate insecticides. *Can. Med. Ass. J.* **100**, 161–167.
51. Oosterbaan, R. A., Warringa, M. G. P. J., Janz, F. B., and Cohen, J. A. (1958). The reaction of pseudocholinesterase with diisopropyl phosphorofluoridate. *Proc. Int. Congr. Biochem., 4th, Vienna, Abstr.* 4–12, 38.
52. Wilson, I. B., and Harrison, M. A. (1961). Turnover number of acetylcholinesterase. *J. Biol. Chem.* **236**, 2292–2295.
53. Main, A. R., and Hastings, F. L. (1966). A comparison of acylation, phosphorylation, and binding in related substrates and inhibitors of serum cholinesterase. *Biochem. J.* **101**, 584–590.
54. Purdie, J. E., and McIvor, R. A. (1966). Modification of the esteratic activity of acetylcholinesterase by alkylation with 1, 1-dimethyl-2-phenylaziridinium ion. *Biochim. Biophys. Acta* **128**, 590–593.
55. O'Brien, R. D. (1969). Poisons as tools in studying the nervous systems. *Essays Toxicol.* **1**, 1–59.
56. Hartley, B. S. (1956). The site of action of inhibitors of $\alpha$ chymotrypsin. *Biochem. J.* **64**, 27P.
57. Iverson, F. (1968). Comparison of carbamylation and binding constants of charged and non-charged carbamates in reaction with eel and erythrocyte acetylcholinesterase. Ph.D. Thesis, Dept. of Biochemistry, North Carolina State Univ., Raleigh, North Carolina.
58. Eyring, H. (1935). The activated complex in chemical reactions. *J. Chem. Phys.* **3**, 107–115.

59. Davies, D. R., and Green, A. L. (1956). The kinetics of reactivation, by oximes, of cholinesterase inhibited by organophosphorus compounds. *Biochem. J.* **63**, 529–535.
60. Wilson, I. B. (1967). Conformation changes in acetylcholinesterase. *Ann. N. Y. Acad. Sci.* **144**, Art. 2, 664–674.
61. Main, A. R., Tarkan, E., Aull, J. L., and Soucie, W. G. (1972). Purification of horse serum cholinesterase by preparative polyacrylamide gel electrophoresis. *J. Biol. Chem.* **247**, 566–571.
62. Iverson, F., and Main, A. R. (1969). Effect of charge on the carbamylation and binding constants of eel acetylcholinesterase in reaction with neostigmine and related carbamates. *Biochemistry* **8**, 1889–1895.
63. Iverson, F. (1971). The influence of tetraethylammonium ion on the reaction between acetylcholinesterase and selected irreversible inhibitors. *J. Mol. Pharmacol.* **7**, 129–135.
64. Braid, P. E., and Nix, M. (1969). The kinetic constants for the inhibition of acetylcholinesterase by phosdrin, sumioxon, DDVP, and phosphamidon. *Can. J. Biochem.* **47**, 1–6.
65. Chiu, Y. C., Main, A. R., and Dauterman, W. C. (1969). Affinity and phosphorylation constants of a series of O, O-dialkyl malaoxons and paraoxons with acetylcholinesterase. *Biochem. Pharmacol.* **18**, 2171–2177.
66. Main, A. R., and Hastings, F. L. (1966). Carbamylation and binding constants for the inhibition of acetylcholinesterase by physostigmine (eserine). *Science* **154**, 400–402.

Chapter 3

# Recondite Toxicity of Trace Elements*

*HENRY A. SCHROEDER*

|       |                                                                         |     |
|-------|-------------------------------------------------------------------------|-----|
| I.    | Introduction                                                            | 108 |
| II.   | Specific Considerations                                                 | 112 |
|       | A. "Metal-free" Environment                                             | 112 |
|       | B. Low Trace Element Diet                                               | 113 |
| III.  | General Conclusions                                                     | 115 |
| IV.   | Recondite Toxicity in Terms of Growth                                   | 115 |
| V.    | Effects on Body Weights of Aged Animals                                 | 124 |
| VI.   | Effects of Trace Elements on Survival and Longevity                     | 124 |
| VII.  | Effects on Tumors                                                       | 126 |
| VIII. | Longevity and Median Life-Span                                          | 129 |
|       | A. Correlation of Effects on Growth and Longevity in Rats and Mice      | 129 |
|       | B. Longevity as Affected by the Environment Alone                       | 129 |
|       | C. Some Long-Lived and Less-Long-Lived Rats and Mice                    | 131 |
|       | D. Life-Span of Rats and Mice in Our Laboratory                         | 132 |
| IX.   | Other Manifestations of Recondite Toxicity                              | 132 |
|       | A. Amyloidosis                                                          | 132 |
|       | B. Blanched Teeth                                                       | 133 |
|       | C. Fatty Changes in Liver and Kidney                                    | 133 |
|       | D. Response to Epidemic Infection (Pneumonia)                           | 136 |
|       | E. Arteriolar Disease of the Kidneys                                    | 137 |
|       | F. Urinary Abnormalities                                                | 138 |
|       | G. Serum Constituents, Glucose                                          | 139 |
|       | H. Serum Constituents, Cholesterol                                      | 143 |
|       | I. Serum Constituents, Uric Acid                                        | 148 |

\* Supported by grants from the National Institutes of Health (grant-in-aid ES 00699-13A1), CIBA Pharmaceutical Company, and Cooper Laboratories, Inc.

107

J. Effects of the Metals in the Basic Water on Serum Glucose and
Cholesterol of Rats ............................................. 148
X. Recondite Toxicity of Trace Elements as Expressed by Effects on
Reproduction of Rats and Mice ................................. 151
XI. Some Clues to Mechanisms of Toxicity ............................. 156
  A. Cellular Toxicity ................................................ 158
  B. Oral Toxicity ................................................... 159
  C. Accumulation with Age during Constant Oral Exposure ............ 162
  D. Accumulation from Respiratory Exposures ....................... 163
  E. Prediction of Toxicity of an Element ............................ 163
  F. Interactions of Trace Elements ................................. 164
  G. Other Mechanisms of Toxicity ................................. 171
XII. Production of Chronic Diseases Simulating Human Disorders ......... 174
  A. Cadmium Hypertension ......................................... 174
  B. Overt Cadmium Toxicity ....................................... 177
  C. Atherosclerosis in Rats ........................................ 177
  D. Aortic Lipids and Plaques ..................................... 179
  E. Human Atherosclerosis ......................................... 181
XIII. Recondite Toxicity of Other Metals or Elements in Man ............. 186
XIV. Innate Toxicity from Water ......................................... 188
  Other Diseases Caused by Recondite Toxicity ..................... 192
XV. Summary and Conclusions .......................................... 193
  References ....................................................... 194

## I. INTRODUCTION

The overt toxicities of the metals and other elements are well known (Browning, 1969). Most of them have been studied in terms of effects from parenteral injection of salts or complexes, or by giving large doses by mouth to experimental animals. When a soluble substance is injected, it is usually distributed throughout the body via the blood stream, and, until deposited in organ depots or excreted, it exerts its effects on every cell. When doses are large enough, the animal dies. This form of cellular toxicity, although governed in part by the efficiency of excretory mechanisms, is in many respects similar to the direct application of the substance to living cells. It would be even more similar if the experimental animal were nephrectomized and hepatectomized.

There is an area of toxicity of a substance given to mammals in low doses for life, by mouth. This area we can consider as recondite toxicity. It is in many respects similar to the experiments man has unwittingly performed on himself by exposure to environmental contaminants, usually of industrial origin. Exposures are often subthreshold, in that they exert their effects subtly, and may in some cases mimic certain chronic diseases. No one can predict what these effects will be.

Table I shows the extent of the problem. Potential human exposures in terms of annual industrial consumption of elements in the United States (when divided into essential, relatively inert, and toxic elements) reveal large disparities in the consumption of lead, antimony, cadmium, mercury, tin, and arsenic compared to the abundances of these elements in the earth's crust, and a probable increase in human body burdens above natural or background levels in land and sea. For the essential elements and most others, there is no such increase in the body of man.

This essay is concerned principally with recondite toxicity of trace elements. Major criteria for evaluating recondite toxicity include rate of growth, survival in terms of median life-span, longevity in terms of mean age of the last surviving 10% of animals, the incidences of spontaneous tumors and malignant tumors, excessive loss of weight of old animals, susceptibility to infections, and gross and microscopic pathology. Minor criteria include elevation of blood pressure, abnormalities in serum constituents (glucose, cholesterol, uric acid), and urinary constituents (proteinuria, glycosuria, ketonuria), as well as deposition of lipids in the aorta. Such changes can be correlated with accumulation of the element in organs and tissues.

No discussion of trace elements can avoid consideration of the essential trace elements chromium, manganese, iron, cobalt, copper, zinc, selenium, molybdenum, and fluorine. Deficiency of one, whether from dietary deficiency or conditioning by an elemental antimetabolite, may produce signs of "toxicity" indistinguishable from recondite toxicity of another element. These essential trace elements therefore will be considered along with the abnormal elements we have studied.

Rats, mice, and hamsters are the only mammals of conveniently small size and practically short life-span to study in this way. Larger animals take up too much space, live too long for multiple experiments to be performed, and are too expensive to maintain in numbers large enough for statistical evaluation, although they have advantages for short-term studies. Hamsters have not been well studied in chronic experiments.

In order to study trace elements by this approach, the following are necessary:

    a. An environment—a laboratory—as free of contamination with airborne, water-borne, food-borne, and people-borne trace elements as possible. No metals or paint should be in it.

    b. A low trace element diet, made from bulk foods on the spot.

    c. Deionized water, hot and cold.

    d. Filtered, electrostatically precipitated air under positive pressure.

    e. A closed environment, allowing only technicians with stocking feet or slippers, and no visitors.

    f. A laboratory for analysis of tissues for trace elements.

## TABLE I

Approximate Annual United States Industrial Consumption of Metals and Nonmetals (1968), Their Amounts in the Human Body, and Their Abundances on the Earth's Crust and in Seawater[a]

| Metal | Industrial consumption (thousands of tons) | Amounts in reference man (mg) | Igneous rocks, earth's crust (ppm) | Seawater (ppb) | Human disease from excess |
|---|---|---|---|---|---|
| *Essential for Life or Health* | | | | | |
| Iron | 109,000 | 4,200 | 56,300 | 10 | Hemochromatosis (genetic) |
| Calcium | 86,273 | 1,000,000 | 41,500 | 400,000 | |
| Sodium | 15,091 | 100,000 | 28,600 | 10,500,000 | |
| Potassium | 3,230 | 140,000 | 20,900 | 380,000 | |
| Manganese | 1,050 | 12 | 1,000 | 2 | Manganism |
| Zinc | 1,278 | 2,300 | 70 | 10 | |
| Copper | 1,400 | 72 | 55 | 3 | Hepatolenticular degeneration (genetic) |
| Chromium | 459 | 1.5 | 100 | 0.5 | Cancer (Cr VI) |
| Fluorine[b] | 587 | 2,600 | 700 | 1,300 | Fluorosis |
| Nickel[c] | 170 | 10 | 75 | 5.4 | Nickel-carbonyl cancer |
| Magnesium | 89 | 19,000 | 23,300 | 1,350,000 | |
| Molybdenum | 25 | 9 | 1.5 | 10 | |
| Cobalt | 6 | 1.5 | 25 | 0.27 | |
| Strontium[d] | 6 | 320 | 375 | 8100 | |
| Vanadium | 5 | 18 | 135 | 2 | |
| Iodine | — | 11 | 0.5 | 60 | |
| Selenium | 0.5 | 13 | 0.05 | 0.09 | Cancer, rats |
| *Toxic to Living Things* | | | | | |
| Lead | 816 | 121 (9–480) | 10 | 0.03 | Plumbism |
| Antimony | 19 | 8 | 0.2 | 0.33 | Heart disease |
| Beryllium | 0.3 | 0.04 | 2.8 | 0.0006 | Berylliosis |
| Cadmium | 7 | 50 | 0.2 | 0.11 | Hypertension, emphysema |
| Mercury | 3 | 13 | 0.1 | 0.03 | Poisoning |

## Slightly Toxic to Some Life Processes

| | | | |
|---|---|---|---|
| Tin | 59 | 6 | 2 | 3 |
| Arsenic | 22 | *18* | 1.8 | 3 | Cancer |
| Tungsten | 7 | + | 1.5 | 0.1 |
| Germanium | 11 | + | 5.4 | 0.07 |
| Uranium | 2.7 | 0.09 | 2.7 | 3 | Kidney disease, animals |
| Bismuth | 1 | 0.2 | 0.2 | 0.017 |
| Tellurium | 0.1 | 8 | 0.001 | — |
| Palladium | 0.02 | + | 0.01 | — |
| Rhodium | 0.002 | + | 0.001 | — |

## Probably Inert in Living Things

| | | | |
|---|---|---|---|
| Aluminum | 3,534 | 61 | 82,300 | 10 |
| Barium | 700 | 22 | 425 | 30 | Baritosis |
| Titanium | 413 | 9 | 5,700 | 1 |
| Zirconium | 61 | 420 | 165 | 0.022 |
| Lithium | 2.6 | 2 | 20 | 180 |
| Silver | 0.03 | 0.8 | 0.1 | 0.3 | Argyria |
| Niobium | 2 | 110 | 20 | 0.01 |
| Boron[e] | 70 | 14 | 10 | 4,600 |

---

[a] Numbers in italics are considered to be larger than normal for uncontaminated man. Data from references *1–3*.
[b] Nonmetal, essential for healthy bones and teeth.
[c] Essential for birds, possibly essential for mammals.
[d] Possibly essential.
[e] Essential for plants.

g. Unfailing patience.

Experiments with life-term studies in rats usually last 42 months and occasionally 48 months. One lasted 5 years. With mice, they last 2–3 years.

The experience on which this essay is based comprises 30 trace elements given to mice for life, with 3 repeat experiments and 7 sets of controls, involving a total of 4320 mice, plus 18 trace elements given to rats for life, with 5 sets of controls, involving 2600 rats. Animals were equally divided as to sex.

## II. SPECIFIC CONSIDERATIONS

### A. "Metal-free" Environment

A hilltop in Southern Vermont was chosen for the laboratory *(4,5)*. Winds are generally northwesterly over the Green Mountains, a situation which largely avoids fallout of contaminants from the Albany–Troy–Schenectady industrial complex, as well as the centers in upper New York State. The laboratory, a 40- by 20-foot building, was built entirely of wood on a concrete slab. All building materials were analyzed for cadmium and lead as indicator contaminants before use, and choices were made of those with lowest concentrations *(6)*.

The laboratory was later expanded by the addition of a second building 40 by 20 feet, making a work area of 80 by 20 feet divided into two rooms. The interior of the first building was lined with Sheetrock and that of the second with plywood; both were coated with six coats of tough plastic varnish (Fabulon) used for bowling alley floors. Nail heads were countersunk and the holes filled with plastic wood of a low-lead type. Door bars and handles were made of wood. All windows were sealed airtight.

The laboratory is entered through a 25- by 26-foot converted garage which has been rebuilt as a work space for autopsies, calculations, paper work, and storage for grain and bedding. It is kept clean. Animals are not brought into this area.

Animal racks were built of wood with nylon casters and covered with six coats of the varnish. Animal cages were acrylic plastic (Keystone Plastics) with stainless steel covers and feeding troughs. Water bottles were polyethylene, with rubber corks and stainless steel drinking tubes. Bedding was made of wood shavings from a local sawmill. The only metal objects inside the animal quarters were two gas heaters which vented outdoors.

Inside at the entrance to the laboratory was a small isolation room protected by a plastic screen door, for incoming animals. Another room, divided by a wood partition, contained a soapstone sink, deionizing and water-softening equipment, 2-gallon polyethylene bottles for drinking water solutions, a wooden table for mixing food, a hot plate, and a low work shelf for weighing, for taking blood samples, and for measuring blood pressure. Chairs and stools were wooden.

Water came from two covered forest springs through black polyethylene pipe. Because cadmium and lead are used as plasticizers, the pipes gave up traces of these elements to water *(6)*. The soft spring water, of about 18 ppm hardness, is therefore softened to protect the deionizer, and then deionized in bulk (Culligan). From there it enters a short copper pipe to two glass-lined heaters to provide hot water for washing cages. As it takes up copper from the pipes, it is again deionized in a laboratory apparatus to be used for drinking water (Barnstead). The treated water is kept at a resistance of 5 M $\Omega$.

At the other end of the laboratory is an electrostatic precipitator enclosed in a wooden box and blowing air through a wooden conduit, the size of which is controlled by a simple slotted board. A positive pressure of 1.5–2.0 cm of water is maintained in the building. The air enters the precipitator box through a hole in the building to which is attached a 150-foot length of aluminum pipe, 3 feet in diameter. At the other end of the pipe is a screened wooden box placed on a trestle deep in the forest, in a damp area where ferns grow. The dust from the precipitator is analyzed at yearly intervals for lead and cadmium. The precipitator is so sensitive that it crackled at one time when a bulldozer was digging a swimming pond for a summer camp a half mile away. "Leadfree" gasoline is used in personal motor vehicles, and no refuse is burned on the place. It takes 2 weeks for lead to be detected in fallen snow *(7)*.

Because the laboratory is situated one mile up a steep hill via a dirt road through a forest, and, except for the author's house, is a mile away from human habitation, and because of the listed precautions, we believe that we have provided an environment as free of industrial metallic contaminants as possible and practical in today's civilized world. Frequent monitoring of dust and snow has strengthened this belief.

## B. Low Trace Element Diet

After many analyses of ingredients, a diet low in trace elements and economical enough for large-scale use was evolved. It consists of wholeseed Balboa rye from New York State ground locally into flour, 60%; bulk dried skim milk, 30%; corn oil, 9%; iodized sodium chloride, 1%;

TABLE II

CONCENTRATIONS OF TRACE ELEMENTS OCCURRING NATURALLY IN MOUSE AND RAT STARCH DIET (WET WEIGHT), AND ADDED TO DRINKING WATER

| Essential elements | Contained in food ($\mu$g/gm) | Given in water ($\mu$g/ml) | Nonessential elements | Contained in food ($\mu$g/gm) | Given in water ($\mu$g/ml) |
|---|---|---|---|---|---|
| Chromium | 0.14[a] | 5 | Scandium | 0.2[b] | 5 |
| Manganese | 12.7[a] | 10 | Titanium | 0.06[c] | 5 |
| Iron | 100+ | — | Vanadium | 3.24[c] | 5 |
| Cobalt | 0.4[a] | 1 | Nickel | 0.44[a] | 5 |
| Copper | 1.36[a] | 5 | Gallium | <0.25[d] | 5 |
| Zinc | 22.3[a] | 50 | Germanium | 0.32[c] | 5 |
| Molybdenum | 0.25[c] | 1 | Arsenic | 0.05[c] | 5 |
| Selenium | 0.05[e] | 3 | Yttrium | 0.3[b] | 5 |
| | | | Zirconium | 2.66[c] | 5 |
| | | | Niobium | 1.62[c] | 5 |
| | | | Rhodium | <1.0[d] | 5 |
| | | | Palladium | <0.25[d] | 5 |
| | | | Cadmium | 0.07[a] | 10 |
| | | | Indium | <0.05[a] | 5 |
| | | | Tin | 0.28[c] | 5 |
| | | | Antimony | N.D.[f] | 5 |
| | | | Tellurium | 0.16[a] | 2 |
| | | | Lead | 0.20[a] | 25 |

[a] Analysis by atomic absorption spectrophotometry.
[b] Neutron-activation analysis.
[c] Colorimetry.
[d] Emission spectrography.
[e] Photofluorimetry.
[f] N.D. = Not detected.

iron as ferrous sulfate, 100 mg/kg diet; and added vitamins *(4)*. The flour and milk powder are mixed with a wooden spoon in a stainless steel cauldron 10 kg at a time. Deionized water is warmed and the water-soluble vitamins and iron dissolved in it in a Pyrex beaker. Fat-soluble vitamins are dissolved in the corn oil. About 1 liter of water is used for each batch. A thick dough is made by hand (polyethylene gloves are used), rolled with a wooden rolling pin, and cut into strips with a stainless steel spatula. Animals are fed twice a week. The annual cost of the diet is about $1.00 per animal.

Because the diet is low or marginal in several trace metals (Table II), they are given in luxus amounts in the drinking water at the following concentrations (ppm): zinc (acetate), 50; manganese (acetate), 10; cuprous (acetate), 5; chromic (acetate), 5; cobaltus (chloride), 1; molybdenum as (sodium) molybdate, 1. These concentrations approximate those in a standard commercial chow. The salts are dissolved in 1- or 2-

liter polyethylene bottles in concentrated form, so that 25 ml added to 8 l of doubly deionized water makes up the final concentrations for the animals. In this way, the intake of trace elements can be measured by measuring water consumed.

A diet of torula yeast, 30%; sucrose, 50%; commercial lard, 15%; salt mixture without trace elements, 4%; and vitamin mixture, 1% was also given to rats. It was marginal or deficient in all essential trace metals but zinc. Selenium to a concentration of 0.2 ppm was added as sodium selenite, and $\alpha$-tocopherol at 100 mg/kg of diet was necessary. The trace metals were provided in drinking water.

## III. GENERAL CONCLUSIONS

Although it is not usual to give conclusions at this point in an essay, several general findings have been revealed which the reader should keep in mind in respect to recondite toxicity by the oral route.

1. Doses of a trace element tolerable for growth may not be tolerable for prolonged survival or longevity.
2. Doses of a trace element tolerable for longevity may not be tolerable for normal reproduction. Experiments on reproduction are the most sensitive for detecting recondite toxicity.
3. Some chronic diseases of man can be mimicked by life exposures of rats to certain trace elements.
4. Recondite toxicity to ordinary doses of essential trace metals is virtually nil. Mammalian homeostatic mechanisms are usually excellent and no accumulation with age can be detected.
5. Elements showing greatest toxicity to mammals are those which occur in nature—seawater and the earth's crust—in lowest concentrations. Conversely, elements which occur naturally in high concentrations have low orders of toxicity.
6. Elements on the right side of the periodic table are regularly more toxic than those on the left side, except when the latter occur in nature in very low concentrations. Orders of toxicity also increase vertically downward in periodic groups.
7. In most cases female animals are more tolerant to toxic elements than are males.

## IV. RECONDITE TOXICITY IN TERMS OF GROWTH

*Rats.* The rats used in these experiments came from Long-Evans [BLU: (LE)] strain random-bred pregnant females, delivered from the supplier. Litters were weaned at 21–23 days of age, and weanlings were divided as litter mates into controls and 3 or 4 metal groups. They were divided as to sex and placed 4 to a cage. They remained in the same cage all their lives. Each group comprised about 52 males and 52 females, a number large enough for statistical evaluation. The controls received the basic water, whereas each experimental group received the same water plus the element to be tested until they died.

The dose of each element was chosen on the basis of known cellular and oral toxicity, and it was deliberately small in order to show any recondite toxicity. With two exceptions, selenite and methyl mercury, the concentrations used were tolerated. Early mortality of rats after weaning almost never occurred in this closed environment; when it did, it was a significant sign of overt toxicity.

At the time these experiments were begun, only six trace metals were recognized as essential for mammals. Since then, two metals and two nonmetals have been shown to have required biological activities. One

TABLE III

EFFECTS OF TRACE ELEMENTS ON GROWTH OF RATS, BY ATOMIC NUMBER, SIGNIFICANT DIFFERENCES FROM CONTROLS IN MEAN WEIGHTS AT VARIOUS INTERVALS, $p < 0.05$–$0.005$

| Age (days) | Beryllium (gm) | Chromium III (gm) | Nickel (gm) | Selenium (IV) (gm) | Molybdenum (gm) |
|---|---|---|---|---|---|
| *Males* | | | | | |
| 30 | — | +24 | — | −22 | −26 |
| 60 | −24 | +24 | +25 | −73 | −13 |
| 90 | −36 | +40 | +24 | −34 | — |
| 120 | −34 | +24 | +47 | −45 | — |
| 150 | — | +25 | +34 | −34 | — |
| 180 | −34 | +30 | — | −49 | −34 |
| *Females* | | | | | |
| 30 | — | +16 | — | −28 | −14 |
| 60 | — | +12 | — | −60 | — |
| 90 | — | +16 | +18 | −67 | — |
| 120 | — | +12 | +16 | −62 | — |
| 150 | — | +11 | — | −53 | — |
| 180 | — | — | — | −48 | — |
| Intake (ppm) | | | | | |
| Diet | <0.1 | 0.14 | 0.44 | 0.05 | 0.25 |
| Water | 10 | 5 | 5 | 3 | 50 |

Note: There was no significant effect from vanadium, germanium, arsenic, or aluminum, and inconstant effects of selenate at 30 days only. There were about 52 rats of each sex in each group. Data in Tables III and IV from references 4–6, 8–11, 18, and personal observations.

## TABLE IV

Effects of Trace Elements on Growth of Rats, by Atomic Number, Significant Differences from Controls in Mean Weights at Various Intervals, $p < 0.05$–$0.005$

| Age (days) | Zirconium (gm) | Niobium (gm) | Cadmium (gm) | Antimony (gm) | Barium (gm) |
|---|---|---|---|---|---|
| *Males* | | | | | |
| 30 | +16 | +20 | — | +27 | — |
| 60 | — | — | — | +18 | — |
| 90 | — | +40 | −27 | — | — |
| 120 | — | +51 | −40 | — | — |
| 150 | +36 | +43 | −32 | — | — |
| 180 | +27 | +28 | −29 | — | — |
| *Females* | | | | | |
| 30 | +17 | +25 | — | +18 | — |
| 60 | — | — | — | — | — |
| 90 | — | — | — | — | — |
| 120 | — | — | — | — | +19 |
| 150 | +11 | — | −21 | — | +17 |
| 180 | — | — | −17 | — | −40 |
| Intake (ppm) | | | | | |
| Diet | 2.66 | 1.62 | 0.02 | <0.1 | ? |
| Water | 5 | 5 | 10 | 5 | 10 |

Note: There was no effect of tellurite on growth. There was an increase of 23gm in tungsten-fed males at 180 days, otherwise no effect. Weights of males and females fed tin were 15 and 22gm larger than their controls at 30 days only and weights of males fed lead were 16 and 18gm lighter at 30 to 60 days. There were about 52 rats of each sex in each group.

manifestation of essentiality for life or optimal function is enhancement of growth in the presence of low dietary intakes. Table III shows examples. Chromium (III) feeding produced regular enhancement of growth *(8)* and can be considered a growth factor. It is now included among the essential trace elements. Increased growth was also associated with the feeding of nickel at four ages in males and two in females, of niobium at five intervals in males and one in females *(9)*, and of zirconium at five intervals *(9)*. Effects in females were less than in males, except in the case of barium (Table IV).

Enhancement of growth by itself cannot be considered a toxic manifestation, but may suggest essentiality.

Suppression of growth was found with selenite, which was overtly toxic in terms of survival *(10)*. Selenate given at the same rate (selenium, 3 ppm) was not. Lead in males suppressed early growth *(9)* as did molybdenum and beryllium in males. Cadmium suppressed later growth.

## TABLE V

Effects of Trace Elements on Growth of Mice, Significant Differences from Controls in Mean Weight at Various Intervals, $p < 0.05$–$0.005$. Elements According to Atomic Number

| Age (days) | Beryllium (gm) | Fluorine (gm) | Scandium (gm) | Titanium (gm) | Vanadium (gm) | Chromium (III) (gm) | Chromium (VI) (gm) |
|---|---|---|---|---|---|---|---|
| *Males* | | | | | | | |
| 30  | +2.7 | —   | —    | +2.2 | +2.4 | —    | −3.6 |
| 60  | —    | —   | −3.6 | +2.1 | +3.6 | —    | —    |
| 90  | —    | +2.2 | −4.6 | —   | +2.3 | +3.2 | −2.9 |
| 120 | —    | —   | −2.9 | —   | —    | +5.0 | −2.9 |
| 150 | —    | —   | —    | —   | +2.2 | +5.0 | −2.7 |
| 180 | —    | —   | —    | —   | +3.4 | +6.4 | —    |
| *Females* | | | | | | | |
| 30  | —    | —   | −2.3 | —   | −3.0 | —    | −2.8 |
| 60  | —    | —   | −4.6 | +3.1 | —    | —    | —    |
| 90  | +2.4 | —   | −1.8 | —   | —    | +2.0 | —    |
| 120 | −3.2 | +4.2 | —    | —   | —    | +3.6 | −2.6 |
| 150 | —    | —   | —    | —   | —    | +3.8 | −2.3 |
| 180 | −3.0 | +4.8 | −2.6 | —   | —    | +4.0 | —    |
| Amounts in water (ppm) | 5 | 10 | 5 | 5 | 5 | 5 | 5 |
| Diet (ppm) | Tr | 1? | 0.2 | 0.06 | 3.24 | 0.14 | 0.14 |

Note: There was no significant effect from nickel or aluminum. There were 54 or more mice of each sex in each group.

No effects on growth of rats were observed from vanadium *(9)*, germanium *(11)*, arsenic *(11)*, aluminum, and tellurite *(10)*. Inconstant effects appeared with selenate *(11)*, tin *(11)*, antimony *(9)*, and tungsten, usually at the earliest age a week after weaning. At this interval, effects are probably of little significance.

The metals in the basic water without chromium did not improve growth, when growth was compared to that of a group given plain water. When chromium was added to the basic water, typical effects on growth appeared.

The diet contained more than 1 ppm vanadium, zirconium, and niobium (Table II). Addition of 5 ppm vanadium to the water may not have influenced growth because of adequate intake of this element from the diet. Vanadium has been shown to be a growth factor for rats, and is probably an essential element *(12)*.

Therefore, of 18 elements tested in rats, marked suppression of growth was found in only one case, that of selenite, and sporadic suppression in

TABLE VI

EFFECTS OF TRACE ELEMENTS ON GROWTH OF MICE, SIGNIFICANT DIFFERENCES FROM CONTROLS IN MEAN WEIGHT AT VARIOUS INTERVALS, $p < 0.05$–$0.005$. ELEMENTS ACCORDING TO ATOMIC NUMBER

| Age (days) | Gallium (gm) | Selenium (IV) (gm) | Yttrium (gm) | Niobium (gm) | Rhodium (gm) | Palladium (gm) |
|---|---|---|---|---|---|---|
| *Males* | | | | | | |
| 30 | −4.3 | − | −7.6 | − | −7.0 | −2.5 |
| 60 | −5.0 | − | − | − | −4.0 | −5.2 |
| 90 | −5.3 | +3.1 | −3.1 | −2.7 | −4.0 | −4.1 |
| 120 | −3.3 | +5.0 | −6.3 | − | −2.0 | −2.9 |
| 150 | −3.6 | +7.3 | −7.6 | − | − | −3.6 |
| 180 | − | +7.9 | −2.3 | − | − | −3.6 |
| *Females* | | | | | | |
| 30 | − | −2.2 | −5.0 | − | −4.5 | − |
| 60 | − | −2.8 | −1.2 | − | − | − |
| 90 | − | −3.1 | − | − | −2.8 | −3.7 |
| 120 | − | −3.3 | −5.3 | − | − | − |
| 150 | − | − | −5.1 | −4.7 | − | − |
| 180 | − | − | −5.6 | −3.1 | − | − |
| Amounts in water (ppm) | 5 | 3 | 5 | 5 | 5 | 5 |
| Diet (ppm) | <0.25 | 0.05 | 0.03 | 1.62 | <1.0 | <0.025 |

Note: There was no significant effect from germanium, arsenic, hexavalent selenium, fluorine, and inconstant effects of zirconium in 90-day-old males (loss) and in 60-day-old females (gain). There were 54 or more mice in each group. Data in Tables V–VII from references *10, 13–17,* and personal observations.

four: lead, cadmium, beryllium, and molybdenum. Enhancement of growth occurred with chromium, nickel, and niobium, and sporadic enhancement with zirconium, barium, and antimony.

*Mice.* Random-bred pregnant mice of the Charles River CD strain were brought to term in our laboratory, and the young were weaned at 19–21 days of age. Litter mates were divided among several groups, six to a cage, and treated exactly as were the rats.

Of the 18 elements given to rats, significant growth enhancement occurred with chromium *(4)*, vanadium in males, and selenite in males *(13)* (Tables V–VII). An additional 12 elements were given to mice for life. Growth was increased somewhat by titanium *(4)* and markedly increased by 1 ppm methyl mercury. Suppression of growth occurred from 5 ppm methyl mercury, scandium, hexavalent chromium, gallium (in

TABLE VII

EFFECTS OF TRACE ELEMENTS ON GROWTH OF MICE, SIGNIFICANT DIFFERENCES FROM CONTROLS IN MEAN WEIGHT AT VARIOUS INTERVALS ($p < 0.05$–$0.005$). ELEMENTS ACCORDING TO ATOMIC NUMBER

| Age (days) | Indium (gm) | Antimony (gm) | Tellurium (VI) (gm) | MeHg[a] (gm) | MeHg[b] (gm) | Mercury[c] (gm) |
|---|---|---|---|---|---|---|
| *Males* | | | | | | |
| 30 | −3.3 | − | −1.4 | − | +0.9 | − |
| 60 | −3.6 | − | − | −3.0 | +2.8 | − |
| 90 | −4.6 | −2.2 | −2.1 | −5.5 | +2.7 | − |
| 120 | − | − | − | −5.4 | +2.7 | − |
| 150 | − | −2.8 | − | −5.7 | +2.6 | − |
| 180 | − | − | − | −5.2 | +4.3 | − |
| *Females* | | | | | | |
| 30 | −3.4 | − | − | −1.7 | +5.1 | − |
| 60 | −3.1 | − | − | −3.9 | +5.3 | +2.5 |
| 90 | −5.6 | − | − | −5.1 | +4.0 | − |
| 120 | − | − | − | −6.8 | +2.2 | − |
| 150 | − | −4.7 | − | −7.1 | +3.7 | − |
| 180 | − | −3.1 | − | −8.3 | +3.9 | − |
| Amount in water (ppm) | 5 | 5 | 2 | 5–1 | 1 | 5 |
| Diet (ppm) | <0.05 | <0.01 | 0.16 | Tr | Tr | Tr |

[a] Series begun on methyl mercury, 5 ppm Hg, mercury changed after 60 days to 1 ppm.
[b] Series begun on methyl mercury, 1ppm Hg mercury.
[c] Series begun on mercuric chloride, 5 ppm Hg mercury.
Note: There was no significant effect from tetravalent telliurium, lead, barium, or cadmium. There were 54 or more mice of each sex in each group.

## TABLE VIII
### MEDIAN LIFE-SPANS AND MEAN LONGEVITIES (±SEM) OF RATS FED TRACE ELEMENTS FOR LIFE

| Element | ppm | Males 50% dead (days) | Males Longevity (days) | $p^a$ | $p^b$ | Females 50% dead (days) | Females Longevity (days) | $p^a$ | $p^b$ |
|---|---|---|---|---|---|---|---|---|---|
| 0 | 0 | 978 | 1141±13.2 | — | — | 945 | 1245±36.0 | — | — |
| Chromium (III) | 5 | 922 | 1249±33.2 | — | <0.01 | 950 | 1288±13.9 | — | — |
| Cadmium | 5 | 822 | 1221±20.2 | <0.005 | — | 805 | 1146±19.4 | <0.005 | <0.005 |
| Lead | 25 | 729 | 1123±24.2 | <0.0005 | — | 727 | 1162±33.5 | <0.0005 | <0.005 |
| 0 + Chromium | 1 | 872 | 1160±27.8 | — | — | 912 | 1304±36.0 | — | — |
| Zirconium | 5 | 881 | 1127±23.0 | — | — | 947 | 1247±17.4 | — | — |
| Niobium | 5 | 892 | 1045±4.1 | — | <0.001 | 998 | 1247±21.3 | — | — |
| Antimony | 5 | 766 | 999±7.8 | — | <0.001 | 805 | 1092±30.0 | <0.025 | <0.001 |
| Lead | 25 | 883 | 1071±66.0 | — | — | — | — | — | — |
| Vanadium | 5 | 860 | 1147±35.5 | — | — | 961 | 1269±34.5 | — | — |
| 0 + Chromium | 1 | 872 | 1160±27.8 | — | — | 912 | 1304±36.0 | — | — |
| Arsenic | 5 | 825 | 1220±96.0 | — | — | 912 | 1249±24.9 | — | — |
| Germanium | 5 | 738 | 1177±58.8 | <0.005 | — | 833 | 1231±25.6 | — | — |
| Tin | 5 | 876 | 1134±22.8 | — | — | 830 | 1160±27.5 | — | <0.005 |
| 0 + Chromium | 5 | 853 | 1118±17.3 | — | — | 872 | 1177±28.4 | — | — |
| Selenium (IV) | 3 | 58 | — | <0.0001 | — | 348 | — | <0.0001 | — |
| Selenium (VI) | 3 | 962 | 1117±17.8 | — | — | 1014 | 1314±130.1 | — | — |
| Tellurium (IV) | 2 | 844 | 1163±17.0 | — | — | 908 | 1117±19.1 | — | — |
| 0 + Chromium | 5 | 834 | 1190±23.4 | — | — | 890 | 1190±28.2 | — | — |
| Nickel | 5 | 837 | 1122±10.7 | — | <0.025 | 924 | 1217±7.4 | — | — |
| Molybdenum | 50 | 916 | 1128±12.0 | — | <0.05 | 930 | 1270±26.4 | — | — |
| Cadmium | 10 | 870 | 1106±25.8 | — | <0.025 | 1012 | 1218±20.0 | — | <0.01 |

$^a p$ is the significance of the difference from control values by chi-square analysis.
$^b p$ is the significance of the difference from control values by Student's $t$.
Note: 0 signifies controls, 0 + Chromium shows concentration of chromium in control and treated groups' water, from 1–5 ppm.

TABLE IX

Medium Life-Spans and Mean Longevities (± SEM) of Mice Fed Trace Elements for Life

| Elements | ppm | Males 50% dead (days) | $p^a$ | Males Longevity (days) | $p^b$ | Females 50% dead (days) | $p^a$ | Females Longevity (days) | $p^b$ |
|---|---|---|---|---|---|---|---|---|---|
| 0 | 0 | 496 | — | 957±48.4 | — | 565 | — | 966±29.0 | — |
| Chromium | 5 | 587 | <0.001 | 831±49.6 | <0.05 | 625 | — | 940±45.0 | — |
| Lead | 25 | 464 | <0.025 | 865±27.3 | <0.025 | 670 | <0.05 | 888±23.2 | <0.01 |
| Cadmium | 5 | 454 | <0.01 | 814±18.0 | <0.005 | 624 | — | 904±18.1 | — |
| Nickel | 5 | 427 | <0.01 | 896±47.3 | — | 703 | — | 929±43.7 | — |
| Titanium | 5 | 570 | — | 760±14.2 | <0.005 | 629 | — | 884±38.3 | <0.05 |
| 0 | 0 | 510 | — | 802±50.2 | — | 570 | — | 735±29.0 | — |
| Vanadium | 5 | 500 | — | 779±37.6 | — | 590 | — | 805±93.0 | — |
| Tin | 5 | 548 | — | 896±35.9 | — | 554 | — | 761±14.1 | — |
| 0 + Chromium | 1 | 570 | — | 831±49.6 | — | 624 | — | 910±45.0$^c$ | <0.005 |
| Arsenic | 5 | 496 | — | 694±7.4 | <0.025 | 548 | — | 789±22.4 | <0.025 |
| Germanium | 5 | 478 | <0.01 | 712±29.2 | <0.05 | 589 | — | 829±35.9 | — |
| 0 + Chromium | 1 | 546 | — | 806±34.3 | — | 618 | — | 855±29.3 | — |
| Zirconium | 5 | 543 | — | 760±17.4 | — | 558 | — | 901±21.0 | — |
| Niobium | 5 | 563 | — | 910±21.1 | <0.025 | 560 | — | 803±23.1 | — |
| Antimony | 5 | 582 | — | 786±32.7 | — | 576 | — | 843±47.8 | — |
| Fluorine | 10 | 599 | — | 830±28.3 | — | 630 | — | 838±14.5 | — |
| 0 + Chromium | 5 | 419 | — | 696±19.2 | — | 511 | — | 817±18.8 | — |
| Scandium | 5 | 453 | — | 686±13.1 | — | 484 | — | 783±27.8 | — |
| Gallium | 5 | 516 | — | 663±24.0 | — | 534 | — | 730±31.0 | <0.025 |
| Rhodium | 5 | 509 | <0.0005 | 708±16.5 | — | 531 | — | 818±25.4 | — |
| Palladium | 5 | 554 | <0.0005 | 815±27.1 | <0.005 | 572 | <0.025 | 851±26.8 | — |
| Indium | 5 | 487 | — | 678±28.8 | — | 504 | — | 785±23.8 | — |

| Group | N | | | | | | | |
|---|---|---|---|---|---|---|---|---|
| 0 +Chromium | 5 | 505 | — | 631±7.6 | — | 623 | — | 821±16.1 | — |
| Chromium (VI) | 5 | 493 | — | 721±55.7 | — | 570 | — | 830±36.8 | — |
| Yttrium | 5 | 494 | — | 710±30.4 | <0.025 | 574 | — | 908±36.0 | <0.05 |
| 0 +Chromium | 5 | 568 | — | 763±14.4 | — | 547 | — | 790±19.7 | — |
| Titanium | 5 | 536 | — | 791±31.5 | — | 545 | — | 760±17.5 | — |
| Nickel | 5 | 528 | — | 831±49.6 | — | 577 | — | 864±11.4 | <0.005 |
| Vanadium | 5 | 569 | — | 880±36.0 | <0.005 | 615 | — | 878±30.8 | <0.025 |
| Lead | 25 | 542 | — | 748±11.4 | — | 632 | — | 804±18.9 | — |
| 0 +Chromium | 1 | 419 | — | 673±19.8 | — | 511 | — | 798±15.2 | — |
| Selenium (IV) | 3 | 530 | — | 702±26.7 | — | 536 | — | 746±4.4 | <0.005 |
| Tellurium IV | 2 | 468 | — | 663±19.8 | — | 568 | — | 725±17.7 | <0.005 |
| 0 +Chromium | 5 | 505 | — | 621±7.6 | — | 623 | — | 819±2.8 | — |
| Selenium VI | 3 | 528 | — | 672±13.0 | <0.005 | 633 | — | 782±19.2 | <0.05 |
| Tellurium VI | 2 | 551 | — | 662±5.4 | <0.001 | 583 | — | 812±17.9 | — |

[a] $p$ is significance of difference from controls by chi-square analysis.
[b] $p$ is significance of difference from controls by Student's $t$.
[c] $p$ Differs from previous no-chromium controls.

males), yttrium, rhodium, palladium, indium *(14)*, and occasionally from antimony and niobium *(15)* as well as selenite (in females) *(13)*. No consistent effects on growth from beryllium, fluorine *(15)*, aluminum, nickel, germanium, arsenic *(16)*, cadmium, tellurite, lead *(4)*, hexavalent selenium, or zirconium were observed.

In our total experience with both rats and mice, chromium (III) was the only trace element consistently active in increasing growth in both species. Germanium, arsenic, tin, tellurite, and selenate were apparently inert in both species. No element depressed growth in both species, although in mice chromium (VI), scandium, gallium, yttrium, rhodium, palladium, indium, tellurite, and 5 ppm (but not 1 ppm) methyl mercury showed toxicity in this respect.

## V. EFFECTS ON BODY WEIGHTS OF AGED ANIMALS

*Rats.* One of the subtle toxic effects of some trace elements is to decrease the body weight of aging animals. The weights of rats at 30 and 36 months, or at death, as compared to controls, showed that significant weight losses of 10% or more occurred in rats fed lead, tin, and selenite, but in no others.

*Mice.* A similar comparison of mice at death showed significant loss of weight in those given gallium, scandium, lead, and yttrium, but in no others. Therefore, lead appears to be active in this respect in both species.

## VI. EFFECTS OF TRACE ELEMENTS ON SURVIVAL AND LONGEVITY

*Rats.* Median life spans and mean ages of the last surviving 10% to die are given in Table VIII. Toxicity in one or both of these terms was shown by cadmium, lead *(6)*, antimony, nickel (in males only) *(9)*, by niobium *(9)*, germanium, and molybdenum (in males) *(11)*, and by tin (in females) *(11)*, compared to controls. Selenite was overtly toxic.

Longevity of males was increased by chromium (III) *(6)*, and of females by molybdenum.

*Mice.* Table IX shows median life spans and longevities of mice given 22 trace elements. Toxicity in one or both of these terms was demonstrated by lead, titanium, and arsenic in both sexes; cadmium, nickel, and germanium in males; and gallium, selenium, and tellurite in females *(14–17)*.

Longevity of females was increased by 1 ppm chromium. Longevity of males was increased by 5 ppm chromium but not by 1 ppm. Median life span and/or longevity was increased by yttrium and palladium in both sexes; by nickel and vanadium in females; and by niobium, selenate, and tellurate in males.

When the parameters were compared in rats and mice, only three elements were constantly toxic: cadmium, lead, and selenite. Only chromium (III) consistently enhanced life-span or longevity. Toxicity in males of both species was caused by germanium. Three metals were toxic to rats but not to mice: niobium, tin, and antimony. Four were toxic to mice but not to rats: nickel, arsenic, selenate (females), and tellurite (females). Vanadium and zirconium were nontoxic to either species. Survival

TABLE X

EFFECTS OF CHROMIUM ON THE TOXICITY OF LEAD AND CADMIUM IN RATS. DIFFERENCES IN SURVIVAL TIMES FROM CONTROLS IN DAYS

| Metal in water | No. rats dead $<$3 mos. | 50% Dead | 75% Dead | 90% Dead | Last survivor | Longevity |
|---|---|---|---|---|---|---|
| *Males* | | | | | | |
| No chromium Lead (25 ppm) | 10[a] | −249[a] | −113[a] | −14 | +12 | −18 |
| Chromium (1 ppm) Lead (25 ppm) | 0 | +11 | −43 | −106 | +30 | +11 |
| Difference | | +260 | +70 | −92 | +18 | +29 |
| *Females* | | | | | | |
| No chromium Lead (25 ppm) | 10[a] | −218[a] | −111[a] | −87 | −73 | −83[b] |
| *Males* | | | | | | |
| No chromium Cadmium (5 ppm) | 12[a] | −156[a] | −20 | +51 | +82 | +80 |
| Chromium (5 ppm) Cadmium (10 ppm) | 0 | −2 | +32 | +77 | −77 | −54 |
| Difference | | +154 | +52 | +26 | −159 | −134 |
| *Females* | | | | | | |
| No chromium Cadmium (5 ppm) | 8 | −140[a] | −134[a] | −138 | −187 | −92[b] |
| Chromium (5 ppm) Cadmium (10 ppm) | 0 | +178 | +133 | +120 | +18 | +28 |
| Difference | | +318 | +267 | +258 | +205 | +120 |

[a] Differs from control group, $p$ <0.005–0.0005 by chi-square analysis.
[b] Differs from control group, $p$ <0.005 by Student's $t$.
Note: the series on lead in females was not repeated. Mortality data were corrected by excluding early deaths. There were 52 rats in each group.

of male rats at various intervals was considerably less than that of controls when lead without chromium was given in drinking water; when chromium at 1 ppm was added, survival was more comparable to that of controls. The difference at the median life-span amounted to 260 days. Early mortality of nearly 20% of animals occurred in the group not given chromium; there were no deaths before three months of age in the chromium-fed group (Table X).

Chromium appeared to have a similar effect on cadmium toxicity—in the absence of chromium it was manifest by a decrease in median life-span of 156 and 140 days in males and females, respectively, compared to controls, and a sizeable early mortality. The addition of chromium at 5 ppm resulted in survivals comparable to or exceeding that of controls, and no early mortality. Differences in the median life-spans between the chromium-deficient and chromium-fed groups were 154 days in males and 318 days in females.

Similar effects were found in mice, especially on longevity. Mice given 25 ppm lead in drinking water had longevities (corrected for those of controls) which were 77 days greater in males and 92 days greater in females when chromium (5 ppm) was added then when it was not. Similar experiments on cadmium were not done. Therefore, animals with marginal intakes of chromium appeared to have increased susceptibilities to the recondite toxicities of lead and cadmium.

## VII. EFFECTS ON TUMORS

The habit of exposing rats to a possible carcinogen for only 2 years, or about the median life-span, does not reproduce the human experiment. It will pick up strong carcinogens having early effects, will detect weaker carcinogens given in larger doses, and can demonstrate a relationship of dose of a known carcinogen to time of appearance of the first tumor. When small doses are given, however, it will not demonstrate late carcinogenicity unless the experiments are carried on for the lives of the animals.

Because the incidence of tumors in mice, rats, and man increases with age, experiments on late carcinogenicity must be interpreted carefully, and it is essential that life-spans of the controls and treated animals be reasonably similar in order to exclude the effect of age on spontaneous tumors. When half the animals of a control and a treated group, however, are dead at approximately the same age, and when most of the treated animals subsequently have tumors with few in the control group, we consider that the substance to which they were exposed showed recondite carcinogenicity. Such findings cannot be discounted any more than can the high incidence of cancer in human beings older than 70 years, which is about our median life-span.

Therefore, we have examined animals fed trace elements for tumors and malignant tumors, throughout their lives. In Table XI are the results on microscopie sections of mice, with the sexes grouped together. There were no significant differences between the degrees of increased inci-

TABLE XI
Tumors in Mice Given Various Trace Elements for Life, Both Sexes

| Element fed | No. mice examined | Tumors No. | % | $p^a$ | Malignant tumors No. | % | $p^a$ |
|---|---|---|---|---|---|---|---|
| Control-1 | 104 | 33 | 31.1 | — | 22 | 21.1 | — |
| Cadmium | 87 | 11 | 12.7 | <0.01 | 7 | 8.2 | <0.05 |
| Lead | 68 | 12 | 17.7 | — | 8 | 11.8 | — |
| Nickel | 74 | 10 | 13.5 | <0.025 | 9 | 12.2 | — |
| Titanium | 72 | 11 | 15.2 | <0.05 | 8 | 11.4 | — |
| Chromium | 68 | 15 | 22.1 | — | 10 | 14.7 | — |
| Control-2 | 170 | 55 | 30.8 | — | 15 | 8.8 | — |
| Arsenic | 103 | 11 | 10.7 | <0.0005 | 6 | 5.8 | — |
| Germanium | 131 | 25 | 19.0 | <0.025 | 7 | 5.3 | — |
| Tin | 86 | 22 | 25.5 | — | 6 | 7.0 | — |
| Vanadium | 47 | 15 | 32.0 | — | 9 | 19.1 | — |
| Control-3 | 71 | 24 | 33.8 | — | 8 | 11.3 | — |
| Zirconium | 72 | 15 | 20.8 | — | 5 | 6.9 | — |
| Niobium | 79 | 18 | 22.8 | — | 5 | 6.3 | — |
| Antimony | 76 | 18 | 23.7 | — | 6 | 7.6 | — |
| Fluorine | 72 | 22 | 30.6 | — | 5 | 6.9 | — |
| Control-4 | 119 | 23 | 19.3 | — | 10 | 8.4 | — |
| Selenite | 47 | 9 | 19.1 | — | 9 | 19.1 | — |
| Tellurite | 50 | 7 | 14.0 | — | 7 | 14.0 | — |
| Control-4 | 80 | 13 | 16.3 | — | 11 | 13.8 | — |
| Scandium | 73 | 19 | 26.0 | — | 17 | 23.3 | — |
| Gallium | 66 | 16 | 24.2 | — | 16 | 24.2 | — |
| Rhodium | 59 | 17 | 28.8 | — | 17 | 28.8 | <0.05 |
| Palladium | 65 | 19 | 29.2 | — | 18 | 27.7 | <0.05 |
| Indium | 54 | 7 | 12.9 | — | 6 | 11.1 | — |
| Control-5 | 41 | 11 | 24.4 | — | 6 | 14.6 | — |
| Chromium (VI) | 29 | 8 | 27.6 | — | 8 | 27.6 | — |
| Yttrium | 33 | 11 | 33.3 | — | 11 | 33.3 | — |
| Selenate | 41 | 9 | 22.0 | — | 9 | 22.0 | — |
| Tellurate | 40 | 11 | 27.5 | — | 7 | 17.5 | — |

[a] $p$ is the significance of the difference from controls by chi-square analysis.

dence in males and females, although females in general had more tumors, at a ratio of about 1.1 : 1. Incidences were suppressed somewhat by cadmium, nickel, arsenic, germanium, and titanium.

Only 2 of the 24 metals [rhodium and palladium (14)] showed mild carcinogenicity. However, there were many multiple, presumably malignant, tumors in mice not sectioned for microscopic analysis because of postmortem autolysis. Addition of these tumors would make the incidences significantly elevated in mice fed chromium (VI) ($p < 0.005$), selenate, and yttrium ($p < 0.025$).

In Table XII are the incidences of tumors and malignant tumors in rats given various trace elements for life. Only selenate was carcinogenic, with a high incidence of late cancers. Five eighths had tumors, of which two thirds were malignant (18). These results confirm those of others (19,20). Almost every rat fed selenate and living over 30 months of age had a malignant tumor, whereas there were few in the controls or in rats

TABLE XII

TUMORS IN RATS GIVEN 14 TRACE ELEMENTS FOR LIFE

| Element | No. rats examined[a] | No. tumors | % Tumors | p | No. Malignant tumors | % Malignant tumors | p |
|---|---|---|---|---|---|---|---|
| Control-1 | 34 | 10 | 29.4 | — | 2 | 5.9 | — |
| Cadmium | 47 | 22 | 46.8 | — | 7 | 14.8 | — |
| Chromium | 56 | 28 | 50.0 | — | 7 | 12.5 | — |
| Lead | 32 | 7 | 21.9 | — | 2 | 6.3 | — |
| Control-2 | 82 | 31 | 37.8 | — | 9 | 11.0 | — |
| Arsenic | 91 | 25 | 27.4 | — | 3 | 3.3 | — |
| Germanium | 98 | 25 | 25.5 | — | 2 | 2.0 | <0.05 |
| Tin | 94 | 29 | 30.8 | — | 5 | 5.3 | — |
| Control-3 | 65 | 20 | 30.8 | — | 11 | 16.9 | — |
| Selenate | 48 | 30[b] | 62.5 | <0.001 | 20 | 41.7 | <0.01 |
| Tellurite | 44 | 16[c] | 36.4 | — | 8 | 18.2 | — |
| Zirconium | 64 | 26 | 40.6 | — | 14 | 21.9 | — |
| Niobium | 78 | 30 | 38.5 | — | 17 | 21.8 | — |
| Antimony | 60 | 15 | 25.0 | — | 8 | 13.3 | — |
| Vanadium | 39 | 6 | 15.4 | — | 2 | 5.1 | — |
| Lead | 29 | 6 | 20.7 | — | 4 | 13.8 | — |
| Nickel | 43 | 13 | 30.2 | — | 5 | 11.6 | — |

[a] Examined and sections made.

[b] There were 13 additional tumors not sectioned, of which 7 were multiple and presumably malignant. Inclusion of these would increase the significance of the difference from controls to $p < 0.0005$.

[c] There were 13 additional tumors not sectioned, of which 1 was multiple.

fed tellurite. More females than males had tumors, at a ratio of 2.2 : 1. Germanium slightly suppressed malignant tumors.

A study such as this is difficult to make, because animals dying of old age autolyze rapidly. In spite of surveying the colony daily, nearly half of dead animals in some groups were unsuitable for sectioning. In fact, animals have been found unsuitable a few hours after death. We have not heard of this phenomenon, but it occurs in aged rats and mice.

## VIII. LONGEVITY AND MEDIAN LIFE-SPAN

### A. Correlation of Effects on Growth and Longevity in Rats and Mice

In order to compare effects of these trace elements in both species of animals of both sexes, an attempt was made to ascertain whether growth and/or longevity were enhanced or depressed, and whether each bore a relationship to the other (Tables III–IX). For each metal, there were eight groups determined by sex, species, and parameter (i.e., male and female rats, and mice studied in regard to growth and longevity). In seven of the eight groups no effects were observed from vanadium and tin, and in six none from germanium, arsenic, selenate, zirconium, and tellurite. In seven, both parameters were increased by chromium. They were depressed in four by lead and antimony, and in five by selenite. Therefore, chromium stands out as active in enhancement; selenite, lead, and antimony as active in depression; and vanadium and tin as largely inactive.

In rats, both growth and longevity were decreased by selenite and lead, and in males, by molybdenum. In mice no element depressed both functions. Therefore, the adverse effects of an element on growth are seldom manifested by similar effects on longevity.

### B. Longevity as Affected by the Environment Alone

We have long suspected that our "metal-free" environment increased the life-spans of rats and mice, as compared to those animals in the contaminated environment of the usual animal quarters in institutes and medical schools. We have had no experience with life-term studies conducted in dirty quarters, but mortality of young rats has been found sizeable. In all survival curves reported on rats, there is a dip at young ages amounting to about 10% of all animals.

## TABLE XIII
### Median Life-Spans of Male Rats in Other Laboratories and in Our "Metal-Free" Laboratory

| Laboratory and breed | Median life-span (days) | Age of last survivor (days) | Reference or condition |
|---|---|---|---|
| *Other laboratories* | | | |
| Sprague-Dawley | 696 | — | (22) |
| Sprague-Dawley | 750 | 1200 | (23) |
| Sprague-Dawley | 705 | 1170 | (24) |
| Wistar | 750 | — | (25) |
| Holtzman | 670 | — | (26) |
| Mean | 714 ± 15.6 | 1185 ± 14.3 | |
| Sprague-Dawley food restricted | 870 | 1300 | (21) |
| *Our laboratory* | | | |
| Long-Evans, Control-1 | 978 | 1185 | No Chromium |
| Long Evans, Control-2 | 872 | 1232 | Chromium, 1 ppm |
| Long-Evans, Control-3 | 853 | 1160 | Chromium, 1 ppm |
| Long-Evans, Control-4 | 834 | 1264 | Chromium, 5 ppm |
| Long-Evans, Chromium | 922 | 1320 | Chromium, 5 ppm |
| Mean | 892 ± 27.0[a] | 1232 ± 27.8[b] | |

[a] Differs from previous groups by Student's $t$, $p < 0.001$.
[b] Not significant.

We first noted that, in our laboratory, no weanlings died until 15 to 18 months of age, and the survival curves were flat. Another phenomenon was not realized until 4 years later, when our first experiments were complete. Median life-spans were considerably longer than those reported in the literature (Table XIII). Although the Long-Evans rat may have an inherently longer life than other strains of rats, two facts strongly suggest that there is a real environmental difference. McCay et al. *(21)* restricted food for life and prolonged life-span to that of our rats, but in the Sprague-Dawley strain. The ages of the last survivors of two series did not differ from those of our rats. The conclusion can be drawn that rats in a dirty environment breathe, or more likely eat, something which shortens life-span but allows a few resistant animals to survive. We believe that this substance is lead or cadmium or both, for commercial diets have contained much lead and cadmium, both of which decrease life-span, and the other subtly toxic metals (antimony, tin, and niobium) are found only in small quantities in foods.

TABLE XIV

Some Long- and Short-Lived Animals. Age of Last Survivor

|  | Rats | | Mice | |
| --- | --- | --- | --- | --- |
| Element | Male (days) | Female (days) | Male (days) | Female (days) |
| Controls | 1232±27.0 | 1322±27.8 | 895±64.5 | 942±44.6 |
| + 2 S.D. | 1356 | 1447 | 1024 | 1031 |
| − 2 S.D. | 1108 | 1198 | 766 | 853 |
| | | *Long-lived* | | |
| Selenate | — | 1830 | — | — |
| Arsenite | 1596 | — | — | — |
| Tellurite | — | — | — | 1232 |
| Selenite | — | — | 1161 | — |
| Vanadium | — | — | — | 1084 |
| Nickel | — | — | — | 1042 |
| | | *Short-lived* | | |
| Antimony | 1030 | 1195 | — | — |
| Niobium | 1061 | — | — | — |
| Tellurite | — | 1179 | — | — |
| Selenate | — | — | — | 849 |
| Arsenite | — | — | 706 | 849 |
| Gallium | — | — | 741 | 853 |
| Rhodium | — | — | 748 | — |
| Indium | — | — | 766 | — |

Note: Values shown are those exceeding the means of 5 control rat and 6 control mouse groups by ± 2 S.D. Significance, $p < 0.05$.

## C. Some Long-Lived and Less-Long-Lived Rats and Mice

Whereas the age of the last survivor of a group of animals may be influenced by extraneous factors, in a laboratory such as ours with adequate pure food and "tender loving care" such factors are minimal. We have had a few extraordinarily long-lived animals. In Table XIV are shown the ages of those last survivors which exceed by 2 standard deviations (S.D.) the mean ages of five control rat and six control mouse groups, comprising 520 and 648 animals, respectively. According to this criterion, long-lived rats received selenate and arsenite; short-lived rats were given antimony, niobium, and tellurite, each of which showed some form of recondite toxicity in rats.

This parameter differed in mice. Long-lived animals were fed tellurite, selenite, vanadium, and nickel, whereas short-lived ones were taking selenate and arsenite. In addition, gallium, rhodium, and indium had depressed growth (Tables VI and VII) and their groups contained short-lived survivors. Therefore, the two species differed in respect to the influences of these elements on the age of the last survivor.

### D. Life-Span of Rats and Mice in Our Laboratory

The median life-spans of rats in five control series under the conditions of our "metalfree" laboratory were (days): males, $892 \pm 27.0$; females, $914 \pm 16.1$. The median life-spans of mice in six control series were: males, $501 \pm 27.9$; females, $575 \pm 24.6$. The mean ages of the last survivors of the same groups are shown in Table XIV. Therefore, an experiment begun on weanling rats can be expected to last more than 43 months and rarely may last 60 months. An experiment begun on weanling mice can be expected to last 30 months or more, and rarely may last nearly 41 months.

The greatest age achieved by a male rat (fed arsenite) was 52.1 months and that achieved by a female rat (fed selenate) was 60.1 months. The oldest control male rat lived 43.4 months and the oldest control female lived 46 months. These ages can be considered the total life-spans of rats in a controlled environment. The oldest male control mouse lived 33 months, and the oldest female control lived 34.7 months. The oldest male mouse (fed selenite) was 38.2 months of age and the oldest female (fed tellurite) was 40.5 months. These ages can be considered the total life-spans of mice under the conditions of the experiment.

Whereas increase in total life-span occurs only when an element is nontoxic, and decrease occurs when an element is subtly toxic, the parameter of life span must be considered with others to support either thesis and cannot be used alone. Prolonged total life span in a single animal fed a trace element may be a bizarre, isolated phenomenon, not applying to animals of another sex or another species, and must not be attributed to any special quality of the element. This lack of uniformity of effect is partly illustrated in Table XIV, and would be more obvious if all of the data, omitted for clarity of presentation, were exhibited.

### IX. OTHER MANIFESTATIONS OF RECONDITE TOXICITY

#### A. Amyloidosis

By careful observations, one can sometimes discover changes in the frequency of some normal process, or a new manifestation, associated

TABLE XV
AMYLOIDOSIS AND BLANCHING OF THE INCISOR TEETH IN MICE FED VARIOUS TRACE ELEMENTS FOR LIFE

| Element | Amyloidosis (%) | $p^a$ | White teeth | $p$ |
|---|---|---|---|---|
| Control | 30.6 | — | 13.3 | — |
| Scandium | 32.4 | — | 0 | <0.0001 |
| Gallium | 35.6 | — | 0 | <0.0001 |
| Chromium (VI) | 36.5 | — | 36.8 | <0.0001 |
| Yttrium | 34.6 | — | 21.1 | — |
| Rhodium | 52.8 | <0.025 | 15.4 | — |
| Palladium | 57.8 | <0.01 | 19.0 | — |
| Indium | 33.4 | — | 5.8 | — |
| Control | 29.8 | — | 12.4 | — |
| Selenium | 58.3 | <0.001 | 16.6 | — |
| Tellurium | 40.3 | — | 13.0 | — |

$^a$ $p$ is significance of difference from controls by chi-square analysis.

with the feeding of a trace element. One example is amyloidosis in mice. This condition is a normal development in aged mice, but may be enhanced by some trace elements (Table XV). Rhodium, palladium, and selenium appeared to favor amyloidosis; six other elements did not.

## B. Blanched Teeth

Blanching of the incisor teeth occurs regularly in most aged rats and mice, regardless of element fed. It was suppressed, however, in mice fed scandium and gallium, and increased in those fed chromium (VI).

## C. Fatty Changes in Liver and Kidney

Fatty degeneration of the liver has been found to some degree in most groups of mice (Table XVI). The incidence was increased in those fed niobium and decreased in the tin-fed group. This pathological lesion was also found in rats, where it was increased by germanium, tin, and selenite, but decreased in the group fed chromium (Table XVII).

Fatty infiltration and vacuolization of the proximal convoluted tubules of the kidney also was found in 11–32% of rats; it was enhanced somewhat by tin.

From these data, it appears that some recondite toxicity tolerable for life-span is caused by feeding germanium and tin to rats—both belonging to the same periodic group as lead—and by feeding niobium to mice. There was a species difference in the response to tin.

TABLE XVI

FATTY DEGENERATION OF THE LIVER IN MICE FED TRACE ELEMENTS

|           | No. mice | 1 + | 2 + and 3 + | Total | %    | $p^a$  |
|-----------|----------|-----|-------------|-------|------|--------|
| Control   | 99       | 4   | 18          | 22    | 22.2 | —      |
| Zirconium | 60       | 8   | 14          | 22    | 36.7 | —      |
| Niobium   | 68       | 8   | 20          | 28    | 41.2 | <0.02  |
| Antimony  | 67       | 2   | 9           | 11    | 16.4 | —      |
| Fluorine  | 56       | 4   | 9           | 13    | 23.2 | —      |
| Arsenic   | 55       | 2   | 5           | 7     | 12.7 | —      |
| Germanium | 75       | 1   | 13          | 14    | 18.7 | —      |
| Tin       | 24       | 1   | 0           | 1     | 4.2  | <0.05  |
| Vanadium  | 19       | 2   | 1           | 3     | 15.8 | —      |

[a] $p$ is significance of difference from controls by chi-square analysis.

TABLE XVII

PATHOLOGICAL LESIONS IN LIVERS AND KIDNEYS OF RATS FED VARIOUS TRACE ELEMENTS

| Element   | No. rats | No. | %    | $p^a$   | No. | %    | $p^a$   |
|-----------|----------|-----|------|---------|-----|------|---------|
| Liver     |          | Fatty degeneration |||  Cellular degeneration and necrosis |||
| Control   | 88       | 33  | 37.5 | —       | 21  | 23.9 | —       |
| Arsenic   | 83       | 42  | 50.6 | —       | 19  | 22.8 | —       |
| Germanium | 86       | 54  | 62.8 | <0.005  | 12  | 14.0 | —       |
| Tin       | 80       | 54  | 67.5 | <0.001  | 14  | 17.5 | —       |
| Chromium  | 28       | 5   | 17.9 | <0.05   | 12  | 42.9 | —       |
| Cadmium   | 24       | 8   | 33.3 | —       | 9   | 37.5 | —       |
| Selenite  | 34       | 34  | 100.0| <0.001  | 26  | 76.6 | <0.001  |
| Kidney    |          | Vacuolar tubular changes ||| Pyelonephritis[b] |||
| Control   | 88       | 16  | 18.2 | —       | 33  | 41.6 | —       |
| Arsenic   | 77       | 23  | 29.8 | —       | 31  | 43.1 | —       |
| Germanium | 84       | 22  | 26.2 | —       | 19  | 29.7 | —       |
| Tin       | 81       | 26  | 32.1 | <0.05   | 17  | 32.1 | —       |
| Chromium  | 27       | 3   | 11.1 | —       | 21  | 80.7 | <0.001  |
| Cadmium   | 35       | 4   | 11.4 | —       | 16  | 48.5 | —       |

[a] $p$ is significance of difference from controls by chi-square analysis.
[b] Based on slightly smaller numbers of rats (25).

Note: Chromium-fed rats lived longer than others, which may account for pyelonephritis.

## TABLE XVIII
RESPONSE OF RATS TO THREE EPIDEMICS OF PNEUMONIA IN THE LABORATORY, AS AFFECTED BY THE TRACE ELEMENT FED, AND INFECTIOUS DEATHS IN MICE

| Element | Chromium in water (ppm) | No. rats in group | No. surviving before epidemic | No. dead in epidemic | Mortality (%) | $p^a$ | Age (months) |
|---|---|---|---|---|---|---|---|
| *Epidemic 1, 1963* | | | | | | | |
| | | | *Males* | | | | |
| Control | 0 | 52 | 44 | 12 | 27.3 | — | 27 |
| Chromium | 5 | 54 | 45 | 12 | 26.7 | — | |
| Cadmium | 0 | 69 | 34 | 8 | 23.6 | — | |
| Lead | 0 | 62 | 25 | 9 | 36.0 | — | |
| Total | | 237 | 148 | 41 | 27.7 | — | |
| | | | *Females* | | | | |
| Control | 0 | 52 | 39 | 10 | 25.6 | — | 27 |
| Chromium | 5 | 54 | 51 | 4 | 7.8 | <0.05 | |
| Cadmium | 0 | 58 | 25 | 8 | 32.0 | — | |
| Lead | 0 | 60 | 36 | 5 | 13.9 | — | |
| Total | | 224 | 151 | 27 | 17.9 | — | |
| *Epidemic 2, 1968* | | | | | | | |
| | | | *Males* | | | | |
| Control | 1 | 52 | 55 | 19 | 34.6 | — | 28 |
| Zirconium | 1 | 56 | 35 | 5 | 14.3 | — | |
| Niobium | 1 | 52 | 32 | 12 | 37.5 | — | |
| Antimony | 1 | 51 | 20 | 9 | 45.0 | — | |
| Vanadium | 1 | 52 | 30 | 17 | 56.6 | <0.025 | |
| Lead | 1 | 52 | 28 | 22 | 78.5 | <0.0005 | |
| Total | | 315 | 200 | 84 | 42.0 | | |
| Control | 5 | 55 | 52 | 19 | 36.5 | — | 21 |
| Selenate | 5 | 49 | 44 | 22 | 48.9 | — | |
| Tellurite | 5 | 52 | 52 | 19 | 36.8 | — | |
| Total | | 156 | 148 | 60 | 40.6 | | |
| | | | *Females* | | | | |
| Control | 1 | 54 | 31 | 12 | 38.7 | — | 28 |
| Zirconium | 1 | 58 | 45 | 4 | 8.9 | <0.01 | |
| Niobium | 1 | 56 | 39 | 6 | 15.4 | — | |
| Antimony | 1 | 59 | 39 | 3 | 7.7 | <0.01 | |
| Vanadium | 1 | 61 | 49 | 17 | 34.7 | — | |
| Total | | 288 | 203 | 42 | 20.7 | — | |
| Control | 5 | 50 | 44 | 12 | 27.3 | — | 21 |
| Selenate | 5 | 55 | 54 | 8 | 14.8 | — | |
| Tellurite | 5 | 53 | 53 | 13 | 24.4 | — | |
| Total | | 158 | 151 | 33 | 21.8 | | |

*(continued)*

TABLE XVIII (continued)

| Element | Chromium in water (ppm) | No. rats in group | No. surviving before epidemic | No. dead in epidemic | Mortality (%) | $p^a$ | Age (months) |
|---|---|---|---|---|---|---|---|
| *Epidemic 3, 1971* | | | | | | | |
| | | | *Males* | | | | |
| Control | 5 | 52 | 48 | 19 | 39.6 | — | 20 |
| Aluminum | 5 | 54 | 46 | 11 | 23.9 | — | |
| Barium | 5 | 52 | 40 | 12 | 30.0 | — | |
| Beryllium | 5 | 52 | 50 | 20 | 40.0 | — | |
| Tungsten | 5 | 37 | 31 | 13 | 42.0 | — | |
| Total | | 247 | 215 | 75 | 34.9 | — | |
| | | | *Females* | | | | |
| Control | 5 | 52 | 48 | 11 | 22.9 | — | 20 |
| Aluminum | 5 | 52 | 49 | 13 | 26.5 | — | |
| Barium | 5 | 52 | 46 | 6 | 13.0 | — | |
| Beryllium | 5 | 52 | 48 | 9 | 18.8 | — | |
| Tungsten | 5 | 35 | 30 | 10 | 33.3 | — | |
| Total | | 243 | 221 | 49 | 22.2 | — | |
| *Mice, spontaneous infections* | | | | | | | |
| | | | *Males* | | | | |
| Control | 0 | 44 | — | 5 | 11.3 | — | |
| Chromium | 5 | 39 | — | 11 | 28.2 | — | |
| Cadmium | 0 | 48 | — | 4 | 8.3 | — | |
| Nickel | 0 | 41 | — | 9 | 22.0 | — | |
| Titanium | 0 | 40 | — | 5 | 12.5 | — | |
| Lead | 0 | 39 | — | 15 | 38.4 | <0.01 | |
| Total | | 251 | | 49 | 19.5 | | |
| | | | *Females* | | | | |
| Control | 0 | 60 | — | 11 | 18.3 | — | |
| Chromium | 5 | 29 | — | 11 | 38.2 | <0.05 | |
| Cadmium | 0 | 39 | — | 6 | 15.4 | — | |
| Nickel | 0 | 33 | — | 12 | 36.4 | — | |
| Titanium | 0 | 32 | — | 9 | 28.1 | — | |
| Lead | 0 | 29 | — | 10 | 34.5 | — | |
| Total | | 222 | — | 59 | 26.6 | — | |

[a] $p$ is significance of difference from appropriate controls by chi-square analysis.
Note: Mice show number examined and number of dead of infections.

## D. Response to Epidemic Infection (Pneumonia)

Three epidemics of pneumonia appeared in our closed environment, subsequent to bringing new pregnant rats into the laboratory in 1963,

## TABLE XIX
### Renal Vascular Lesions in Rats Fed Various Trace Elements[a]

| Element and No. | Glomerular capillaries |   |    |     | Arterioles |   |    |     | Small arteries |   |    |     |
|---|---|---|---|---|---|---|---|---|---|---|---|---|
|   | 0 | + | ++ | +++ | 0 | + | ++ | +++ | 0 | + | ++ | +++ |
| Controls (79) | 69 | 4 | 6 | 0 | 78 | 1 | 0 | 0 | 79 | 0 | 0 | 0 |
| Chromium (26) | 19 | 1 | 6 | 0 | 26 | 0 | 0 | 0 | 26 | 0 | 0 | 0 |
| Germanium (64) | 59 | 1 | 4 | 0 | 63 | 1 | 0 | 0 | 64 | 0 | 0 | 0 |
| Arsenic (72) | 70 | 1 | 1 | 0 | 72 | 0 | 0 | 0 | 72 | 0 | 0 | 0 |
| Tin (53) | 51 | 0 | 2 | 0 | 53 | 0 | 0 | 0 | 53 | 0 | 0 | 0 |
| Lead (22) | 21 | 1 | 0 | 0 | 20 | 1 | 1 | 0 | 20 | 0 | 1 | 1 |
| Total | 289 | 8 | 19 | 0 | 240 | 3 | 1 | 0 | 243 | 0 | 1 | 1 |
| Cadmium (33) | 4 | 14 | 11 | 4 | 6 | 11 | 10 | 6 | 8 | 8 | 9 | 8 |
| With lesions (%) |   |   |   |   |   |   |   |   |   |   |   |   |
| Controls (79) |   | 12.7 |   |   |   | 1.3 |   |   |   | 0.0 |   |   |
| Other (237) |   | 7.2 |   |   |   | 1.3 |   |   |   | 0.8 |   |   |
| Cadmium (33) |   | 88.0 ($p < 0.0001$)[b] |   |   |   | 81.7 ($p < 0.0001$) |   |   |   | 75.8 ($p < 0.0001$) |   |   |

[a] Data from reference 25.
[b] $p$ is significance of difference from controls.

1968, and 1971. The mortality differed somewhat in the various groups, although it spread to all groups and all animal racks. In most instances, more male than female rats died (Table XVIII). The metals increasing mortality associated with infection were lead and vanadium in males, especially lead. Metals apparently protecting against mortality associated with infection were chromium, zirconium, and antimony in females. Male mice given lead died of spontaneous (not epidemic) infections in a higher incidence than those fed other metals. More females than males died of infections. Lead appears to increase susceptibility to infections in male mice and rats.

### E. Arteriolar Disease of the Kidneys

Seldom were arteriolar changes found in the kidneys of rats, except in proximity to pyelonephritis. There was one marked exception—cadmium feeding (27). Over 81% of kidneys of rats fed cadmium showed arteriolar thickening and muscular hypertrophy characteristic of chronic hypertension (Table XIX). Likewise, 88% of these kidneys had thickening of the glomerular capillaries characteristic of hypertension, and nearly 76% had hypertrophy and narrowing of the small arteries. These changes are associated with chronic elevation of the blood pressure. Kidneys of mice fed cadmium also showed similar lesions (17).

## F. Urinary Abnormalities

In Table XX are shown the percentages of rats in the various groups showing glycosuria and proteinuria by paper-strip, semiquantitative analysis. Zirconium, niobium, arsenic, and lead appeared to promote glycosuria, and cadmium promoted severe proteinuria. Germanium also tended to have this effect.

TABLE XX

Urinary Abnormalities and Blanching of Incisor Teeth in Rats Given Various Trace Elements

| Element | Glycosuria (%) | $p^a$ | Proteinuria 2+ to 4+ (%) | $p^b$ | Blanching of incisors (%) |
|---|---|---|---|---|---|
| Control, chromium (1 ppm) | 20.8 | — | 27.3 | — | 15.8 |
| Arsenic | 45.0 | <0.05 | 20.0 | — | 27.3 |
| Tin | 27.2 | — | 36.4 | — | 20.0 |
| Germanium | 15.0 | — | 45.0 | <0.05 | 14.9 |
| Control, chromium (5 ppm) | 25.0 | — | 54.2 | — | 12.5 |
| Selenate | 51.8 | — | 58.5 | — | 20.0 |
| Tellurate | 37.3 | — | 41.7 | — | 18.7 |
| Control, chromium (1 ppm) | 23.0 | — | 29.3 | — | 15.8 |
| Zirconium | 52.0 | <0.01 | 62.5 | <0.05 | 7.1 |
| Niobium | 71.0 | <0.0001 | 37.5 | — | 5.1 |
| Antimony | 43.0 | — | 75.0 | <0.01 | 5.2 |
| Lead | 63.0 | <0.005 | 91.6 | <0.001 | 20.9 |
| Vanadium | 12.0 | — | 50.0 | — | 12.8 |
| Control, no chromium | 54.6 | — | 30.4 | — | 3.5 |
| Chromium | 10.3 | <0.0005 | 35.2 | — | 13.6$^b$ |
| Cadmium | 66.7 | — | 100.0 | <0.005 | 5.2 |
| Lead | 100.0 | <0.0005 | 78.0 | <0.01 | 2.1 |
| Vitamin E Deficient | 80.0 | | | | |
| Deficient + chromium (2 ppm) | 5.5 | <0.0005 | | | |
| Supplemented | 83.3 | | | | |
| Supplemented + chromium (2 ppm) | 93.8 | | | | |

$^a$ $p$ is the difference in incidence from the controls by chi-square analyses.
$^b$ Differs from controls $p$ <0.05.
Note: Urinary constituents were measured semiquantitatively with paper strips (Combistix, Ames Co., Elkart, Indiana); blanching of teeth was measured by inspection of dead animals.

Glycosuria was frequent in chromium-deficient rats, and was largely prevented by chromium. In vitamin-E-deficient young rats, chromium virtually abolished the glycosuria which was present in 80% of chromium-deficient, E-deficient rats. However, in vitamin-E-supplemented young rats on the torula diet, chromium did not affect glycosuria significantly.

In Table XX are also shown the incidences of blanched incisors. As chromium promoted longevity, it was not unexpected that this change, a function of age, appeared.

## G. Serum Constituents, Glucose

Serum true glucose levels in rats fasted 18 hours after being fed various trace elements are shown in Table XXI. Elements depressing serum glucose in both sexes were chromium, barium, and molybdenum; depressing glucose in males were arsenic, beryllium, and lead; those depressing glucose in females were nickel, aluminum, and tungsten. Elements apparently raising serum glucose levels were tellurite and tungsten (in both sexes); selenate and molybdenum (50 ppm) without chromium (in males); and vanadium, germanium, zirconium, cadmium, tin, and selenite (in females).

There was an inverse relationship between the amount of chromium fed to rats and fasting serum glucose levels (Table XXI). Means of means of groups fed no chromium at various ages differed significantly from those given 1 ppm and 5 ppm in both sexes. Total decline in glucose produced by chromium in water was: males, 21.4%; females, 26.3%. The effect appeared within 2 to 3 weeks of supplementation. Therefore, chromium is a hypoglycemic agent, and deficiency of it is hyperglycemic, causing a disease simulating mild diabetes mellitus (8).

A rough glucose tolerance test was evaluated by comparing fasting with nonfasting serum glucose levels (Table XXII). Male rats fed lead had nonfasting glucose levels averaging 65 mg/100 ml of serum above their fasting levels. A normal response was a rise of about 25 mg/100 ml shown in controls, in the male zirconium, niobium, nickel, and tellurite groups, and in the female vanadium, selenate, selenite, and chromium groups. A bizarre response characterized by a fall in nonfasting levels occurred in the antimony group, in the male selenate, and in the female tellurite groups. This fall is unexplained, but probably is a manifestation of recondite toxicity affecting carbohydrate metabolism.

Therefore, it appears that carbohydrate metabolism is regularized by chromium; that arsenic, nickel, molybdenum and lead also affect it; and that it is depressed by selenate, tellurite, germanium, zirconium, cad-

## TABLE XXI
### Fasting Serum Glucose Levels in Rats Fed 17 Trace Elements, Starch Diet

| Element | Chromium (ppm) | Age (days) | Males (mg/100 ml + SEM) | $p^a$ | Females (mg/100 ml ± SEM) | $p^a$ |
|---|---|---|---|---|---|---|
| *Control* | | | | | | |
| Series I | 0 | 115 | 115±5.0 | — | 129±3.6 | — |
| | | 125 | 120±4.5 | — | 112±3.2 | — |
| | | 204 | 138±6.8 | — | 138±4.8 | — |
| | | 250 | 137±6.6 | — | 111±3.8 | — |
| | | 425 | 112±3.7 | — | 138±4.4 | — |
| | | 738 | 134±5.1 | — | 102±4.5 | — |
| Mean | | | 126±4.7 | | 122±6.3 | |
| Series II | 1 | 136 | 102±9.2 | — | — | — |
| | | 509 | 110±2.8 | — | 97±8.8 | — |
| | | 642 | 117±1.7 | — | 96±6.5 | — |
| | | 718 | 107±3.6 | — | 80±8.2 | — |
| | | 752 | 117±3.5 | — | 114±5.8 | — |
| Mean | | | 111±2.9[b] | <0.025 | 97±6.9[b] | <0.025 |
| Series III | 5 | 90 | 114±3.3 | — | 95±5.4 | — |
| | | 414 | 101±5.5 | — | 90±2.1 | — |
| | | 537 | 95±4.7 | — | 89±3.7 | — |
| | | 750 | 83±2.9 | — | 85±4.6 | — |
| Mean | | | 98±6.5[b] | <0.005 | 90±2.1[b] | <0.001 |
| Females | 12 | 480 | — | — | 75±3.0 | — |
| | | 912 | — | — | 87±3.8 | — |
| Mean | | | | | 81±6.0[b] | <0.001 |
| Vanadium | 1 | 697 | 108±8.9 | — | 96±2.5 | <0.025 |
| Nickel | 5 | 414 | 95±2.2 | — | 78±4.2 | <0.05 |
| Germanium | 1 | 557 | 108±4.7 | — | 100±3.6 | <0.01 |
| Arsenic | 1 | 780 | 79±4.4 | <0.001 | 78±5.8 | — |
| Selenate | 5 | 487 | 106±2.3 | — | 98±4.5 | — |
| | | 801 | 101±4.1 | <0.005 | 76±4.9 | — |
| Zirconium | 1 | 156 | 107±4.4 | — | 112±5.1 | — |
| | | 921 | 106±9.9 | — | 111±5.6 | <0.005 |
| Niobium | 1 | 166 | 108±6.1 | — | — | — |
| | | 889 | 112±5.7 | — | 94±5.3 | — |
| Molybdenum (50 ppm) | 0 | 480 | 128±4.0 | <0.001 | 90±2.3 | — |
| Molybdenum (10ppm) | 5 | 315 | 78±5.1 | <0.005 | 63±1.7 | <0.001 |
| Cadmium | 1 | 102 | — | — | 137±3.0 | <0.001 |
| | | 487 | 104±5.0 | — | 99±4.9 | — |
| | | 509 | 110±2.8 | — | — | — |
| | | 697 | 102±4.8 | — | 104±3.8 | <0.001 |
| Tin | 1 | 520 | 101±4.2 | — | 120±4.8 | <0.001 |
| Antimony | | 148 | 94±3.9 | — | 108±2.8 | — |
| | | 852 | 115±6.8 | — | 86±5.0 | — |

*(continued)*

TABLE XXI (continued)

| Element | Chromium (ppm) | Age (days) | Males (mg/100 ml + SEM) | $p^a$ | Females (mg/100 ml ± SEM) | $p^a$ |
|---|---|---|---|---|---|---|
| Tellurite | 5 | 482 | 102±3.4 | — | 100±2.8 | <0.005 |
|  |  | 793 | 97±4.1 | <0.025 | 82±5.7 | — |
| Lead | 1 | 737 | 82±3.6 | <0.01 | — | — |
| Selenite | 5 | — | — | — | 100±3.4 | <0.025 |
| Aluminum | 5 | 97 | 116±2.1 | — | 98±2.4 | — |
|  |  | 425 | 107±3.2 | — | 73±5.3 | <0.01 |
| Barium | 5 | 98 | 122±3.1 | — | 77±6.8 | <0.05 |
|  |  | 532 | 53±9.2 | <0.005 | 90±3.0 | — |
| Tungsten | 5 | 116 | 149±1.7 | <0.001 | 132±3.1 | <0.001 |
|  |  | 180 | 74±4.2 | — | 90±4.8 | — |
|  |  | 525 | 97±2.7 | — | 45±5.0 | <0.001 |
| Beryllium | 5 | 475 | 73±5.0 | <0.001 | 83±4.7 | — |
| Litter mates |  |  |  |  |  |  |
| Control | 0 | 128 | 125±4.1 |  |  |  |
| Chromium (2 weeks) | 1 | 128 | 107±4.7 | <0.005 |  |  |
| Chromium (3 weeks) | 1 | 136 | 102±9.2 | <0.01 |  |  |

[a] $p$ is the significance of the difference between value shown and comparable control.
[b] Differs from no-chromium group in mean of means.
Note: There were 12 rats in each group.

TABLE XXII

CHANGE IN SERUM GLUCOSE LEVELS OF RATS FROM FASTING TO NONFASTING STATE, AS RELATED TO TRACE ELEMENTS

| Element | Days | Males difference (mg/100 ml) | $p^a$ | Females difference (mg/100 ml) | $p^a$ |
|---|---|---|---|---|---|
| Control, chromium (1 ppm) | 718 | +27 | <0.005 | +34 | <0.001 |
| Zirconium | 921 | +27 | <0.01 | +9 | — |
| Niobium | 889 | +25 | <0.05 | +13 | <0.05 |
| Antimony | 852 | −24 | <0.025 | −4 | — |
| Lead | 737 | +65 | <0.001 | — | — |
| Vanadium | 697 | +13 | — | +20 | <0.005 |
| Control, chromium (5 ppm) | 406 | +6 | — | +24 | <0.001 |
| Nickel | 414 | +20 | <0.01 | +8 | — |
| Selenate | 487 | −9 | — | +24 | <0.005 |
| Selenite | 466 | — | — | +28 | <0.001 |
| Tellurite | 482 | +22 | <0.001 | −13 | <0.025 |
| Mean of those rising |  | +26 |  | +20 |  |

[a] $p$ is the significance of the difference of the means fasting and nonfasting.

## TABLE XXIII
### Fasting Serum Cholesterol Levels in Rats Fed 17 Trace Elements, Starch Diet

| Element | Chromium (ppm) | Age (days) | Males mg/100 ml | $p^a$ | Females mg/100 ml | $p^a$ |
|---|---|---|---|---|---|---|
| Control |  |  |  |  |  |  |
| Series I | 0 | 115 | 114±5.0 | — | 110±2.7 | — |
|  |  | 228 | 123±10.1 | — | 91±6.1 | <0.005 |
|  |  | 360 | 102±4.5 | — | — | — |
|  |  | 510 | 108±4.4 | — | 80±7.3 | — |
|  |  | 761 | 123±8.2 | — | 95±11.2 | — |
| Mean |  |  | 114±4.1 |  | 94±6.2 |  |
| Series II | 1 | 405 | 111±8.7 | — | 72±5.3 | — |
|  |  | 657 | 76±2.9 | <0.001 | 120±9.3 | <0.001 |
|  |  | 668 | 78±2.1 | — | 116±6.1 | — |
|  |  | 718 | 92±5.3 | <0.025 | 109±4.0 | — |
| Mean |  |  | 89±8.1 | <0.01[b] | 104±11.0 |  |
| Series III | 5 | 90 | 84±1.9 | — | 74±4.0 | — |
|  |  | 129 | 46±1.7 | <0.001 | 60±3.4 | <0.005 |
|  |  | 402 | 86±3.2 | <0.001 | 94±3.7 | <0.001 |
|  |  | 476 | 88±2.4 | — | 85±5.8 | — |
|  |  | 716 | 67±5.1 | <0.005 | 77±5.2 | — |
|  |  | 810 | 100±7.3 | <0.001 | 85±5.8 | — |
| Mean |  |  | 78±7.8 | <0.001[b,c] | 79±4.8 | <0.001[b,c] |
| Females | 12 | 480 | — | — | 62±2.7 | — |
|  |  | 912 | — | — | 86±3.4 | <0.001 |
| Mean |  |  |  |  | 74±12.1 |  |
| Vanadium | 1 | 697 | 92±5.1 | <0.005 | 68±9.2 | — |
| Nickel | 5 | 342 | 75±2.6 | <0.005 | 75±3.8 | — |
|  |  | 663 | 49±4.8 | <0.001 | 80±4.7 | — |
| Germanium | 1 | 557 | 63±3.2 | <0.001 | 108±5.9 | <0.001 |
| Arsenic | 1 | 770 | 91±10.5 | — | 110±7.4 | <0.001 |
|  |  | 804 | 91±10.1 | — | — | — |
| Selenate | 5 | 445 | 110±6.1 | <0.005 | 90±5.0 | <0.005 |
|  |  | 821 | 85±4.5 | <0.01 | 74±5.4 | — |
| Selenite | 5 | 466 | — | — | 90±3.5 | <0.005 |
| Zirconium | 1 | 270 | 69±3.8 | — | 76±1.8 | — |
|  |  | 921 | 90±5.6 | <0.01 | 101±9.0 | — |
| Niobium | 1 | 166 | 69±3.4 | — | 81±3.7 | — |
|  |  | 655 | 70±2.9 | — | — | — |
|  |  | 889 | 76±2.7 | <0.01 | 79±4.8 | <0.001 |
| Molybdenum (10 ppm) | 5 | 151 | 79±4.2 | — | 77±2.4 | — |
|  |  | 315 | 76±5.8 | — | 83±5.4 | — |
| Molybdenum (50 ppm) | 0 | 135 | 51±2.2 | — | 57±1.5 | — |
|  |  | 477 | 76±4.6 | <0.025 | 74±5.4 | <0.005 |
|  |  | 813 | 76±3.5 | <0.005 | 97±4.2 | <0.05 |
| Aluminum | 5 | 97 | 73±3.5 | <0.025 | 68±2.8 | — |
|  |  | 425 | 62±3.4 | <0.001 | 82±4.3 | — |

*(continued)*

3. RECONDITE TOXICITY OF TRACE ELEMENTS 143

TABLE XXIII (continued)

| Element | Chromium (ppm) | Age (days) | Males mg/100 ml | $p^a$ | Females mg/100 ml | $p^a$ |
|---|---|---|---|---|---|---|
| Barium | 5 | 98 | 77±2.5 | — | 78±4.1 | — |
|  |  | 532 | 90±4.6 | — | 99±4.3 | <0.001 |
| Tungsten | 5 | 117 | 94±3.2 | <0.01 | 86±3.7 | <0.025 |
|  |  | 180 | 96±4.1 | — | 106±6.0 | <0.005 |
|  |  | 525 | 73±2.6 | <0.001 | 87±4.5 | — |
| Beryllium | 5 | 475 | 90±5.0 | — | 105±5.3 | <0.001 |
| Cadmium | 1 | 231 | 74±4.2 | — | 64±2.4 | — |
|  |  | 510 | 68±2.8 | — | 87±9.8 | — |
|  |  | 576 | 107±6.1 | <0.005 | 88±2.8 | <0.05 |
|  |  | 719 | 89±8.7 | — | 113±9.0 | <0.01 |
|  |  | 750 | 99±5.2 | — | 97±4.2 | — |
|  |  | 917 | 111±12.4 | <0.001 | 85±5.9 | — |
| Tin | 1 | 520 | 83±3.4 | — | 105±3.5 | <0.001 |
| Antimony | 1 | 125 | 77±2.4 | — | 86±4.4 | — |
|  |  | 852 | 98±4.9 | <0.005 | 97±5.6 | <0.01 |
| Tellurite | 5 | 405 | 111±3.0 | <0.005 | 110±9.9 | <0.001 |
|  |  | 793 | 84±4.5 | — | 83±5.4 | — |
| Lead | 1 | 300 | 72±4.7 | — | — | — |
|  |  | 510 | 79±6.5 | — | 103±7.1 | — |
|  |  | 695 | 87±6.7 | — | — | — |
|  |  | 750 | 74±10.0 | — | 104±8.5 | — |

[a] $p$ is significance of difference of man from that of comparable control group, by Student's $t$.
[b] Mean of all means in group. $p$ is significance of differences from preceding mean of means.
[c] Differs from all preceding mean of means, i.e., 1 ppm and no-chromium groups.
Note: There were 12 rats in each group. Regular starch diet. Mean ± SEM.

mium, and tin in one or both sexes. Chromium is more active on this function in females than in males.

Molybdenum (50 ppm) in deionized water resulted in hyperglycemia in males to a level consistent with chromium deficiency. Molybdenum (10 ppm) plus chromium, however, acted synergistically, causing lower glucose levels than in their controls, which received 1 ppm molybdenum. Molybdenum therefore may act somewhat like chromium on carbohydrate metabolism, but not when it is given alone.

## H. Serum Constituents, Cholesterol

Fasting serum cholesterol levels in the various groups are shown in Table XXIII. A metal which lowered cholesterol levels was chromium (III). There was an inverse relationship between the means of mean levels and the amount of chromium fed to rats. Therefore, chromium affects cholesterol metabolism and presumably is as essential for this function as it is for carbohydrate metabolism. Chromium was more active in males than in females.

When the feeding of an element elevates cholesterol levels we can assume that the element is exerting toxicity on lipid metabolism, i.e., depressing it. Such an effect was shown in rats of both sexes by selenate, tungsten, cadmium, antimony, and tellurite; in males by no other metal; and in females by germanium, arsenic, tin, selenite, barium, and beryllium.

It is noteworthy that in most cases serum cholesterol levels of males and females were remarkably similar at the same ages, and that changes with time were in the same direction. Marked differences in levels of the two sexes (>20 mg/100 ml serum) were found in the groups given vanadium, germanium, cadmium, tin, and lead.

When the feeding of an element depresses serum cholesterol levels, the effect is either physiological, as in the case of chromium, or possibly toxic to hepatic lipid metabolism. It is likely that such toxic effects were exerted by germanium and niobium in males, but by no element in females. On the other hand, because vanadium is an essential trace metal for rats, and nickel may be, effects of these two may be synergistic or antagonistic with chromium on lipid metabolism. Vanadium increases cholesterol and fatty acid synthesis in rats (28). Molybdenum, an essential trace metal in the same periodic group as chromium, also appears to affect cholesterol metabolism. In Table XXIII are shown the data: molyb-

TABLE XXIV

Essential Trace Metals in Torula Yeast Diets Containing Various Sugars, Compared to Regular Starch Diet

| Metal | White sugar diet ($\mu$g/gm) | Brown sugar diet ($\mu$g/gm) | Raw sugar diet ($\mu$g/gm) | Regular starch diet ($\mu$g/gm) |
|---|---|---|---|---|
| Chromium | 0.08[a] | 0.16 | 0.14[a] | 0.14[a] |
| Manganese | 3.05 | 4.35 | 1.55[a] | 12.7 |
| Cobalt | 0.08 | 0.23 | <0.03 | 0.41 |
| Copper | 1.95[a] | 4.58 | 1.18[a] | 1.36[a] |
| Zinc | 28.6 | 27.7 | 17.1[a] | 22.3[a] |
| Molybdenum | 0.09[a] | 0.04[a] | 0.04[a] | 0.25 |
| Nickel[b] | 0.08 | 0.30 | 0.13 | 0.4 |
| Strontium[b] | 5.43 | 14.45 | 7.15 | 5.23 |
| Ash of sugar (%)[c] | 0.16 | 2.24 | 1.28 | — |

[a] Probably marginal or deficient.
[b] Possibly essential.
[c] As the diet contained 4% salt mixture, the ash weights were not too different.

denum (10 ppm) plus chromium (5 ppm) in the basic water resulted in low normal cholesterol levels in both sexes; molybdenum (50 ppm) in deionized water resulted in lower levels in 5-month-old rats and normal levels in older rats; the basic water without chromium resulted in high levels. The addition of chromium (5 ppm) to the basic water caused levels similar to those produced by molybdenum alone.

Thus, molybdenum acts like chromium on lipid metabolism, but not as strongly.

Further confirmation of the effect of chromium on cholesterol and glucose metabolism is afforded by experiments on feeding rats the torula yeast–lard–sugar diet, using white, brown, and raw sugar. The essential trace elements in this diet are given in Table XXIV. Several of the elements are present in marginal or deficient amounts, for which the basic water compensates.

In Table XXV are shown the effects on fasting serum cholesterol and glucose levels of chromium in the three sugars. Natural chromium occurs as a complex which is readily absorbed from the gastrointestinal tract; chromic acetate is absorbed poorly, to the extent of only 2–3%. Thus, of the 5 ppm of chromium in water given to rats, only 0.1 ppm could be expected to be absorbed.

Serum cholesterol levels rose with age in rats fed refined white sugar, but were lower and rose to a lesser extent in those fed brown or raw sugar, or in those fed white sugar and given chromium in their water. The effects were striking *(29)*.

The action of chromium supplements on fasting serum glucose was opposite to that expected from the experiments with the regular starch diet. Levels rose progressively with age, whereas without chromium the rise was either less or a fall occurred. Brown and raw sugars slowed the rise and, at two younger ages, effectively prevented it. Therefore, inorganic chromium alone was not sufficient to effect normal carbohydrate metabolism, although something in brown sugar, but not in raw sugar, was active. One can only speculate on what this active substance might be. From Table XXI it may be seen that arsenic, nickel, and lead are hypoglycemic to some extent, and traces of all of them are found in brown sugar.

These rats were deficient in vitamin E, and deficient rats do not respond to chromium in respect to growth *(30)*—nor did these rats. Furthermore, young rats on this diet apparently elevate serum glucose in response to chromium regardless of whether they are deficient in vitamin E (Table XXIII), which is similar to the response found in rats fed white sugar plus chromium. Growth was affected favorably in vitamin-E-deficient rats in response to chromium *(8)*, as were glycosuria and mortality.

TABLE XXV

EFFECT OF CHROMIUM SUPPLEMENTS AND CHROMIUM IN 3 SUGARS ON FASTING SERUM CHOLESTEROL AND GLUCOSE LEVELS OF RATS FED A TORULA YEAST–SUGAR–LARD DIET (±SEM)

| Age (months) | White (mg/100 ml) | $p^a$ | Type of sugar White + Cr (mg/100 ml) | $p^a$ | Brown (mg/100 ml) | $p^b$ | Raw (mg/100 ml) |
|---|---|---|---|---|---|---|---|
| *Cholesterol* | | | *Males* | | | | |
| 5 | 74±2.7 | N.S. | 68±3.1 | N.S. | 62±4.7 | <0.025 | — |
| 11 | 104±6.8$^c$ | <0.001 | 57±3.5 | N.S. | 55±3.3 | <0.001 | — |
| 22–23 | 109±4.1 | <0.001 | 85±5.5$^c$ | N.S. | 83±3.4$^c$ | <0.001 | — |
| 4 | 60±3.2 | <0.05 | — | — | — | — | 53±1.7 |
| 16 | 87±3.1$^c$ | <0.001 | — | — | — | — | 62±3.5$^d$ |
| | | | *Females* | | | | |
| 5 | — | — | — | — | 69±3.1 | <0.001 | — |
| 11 | 110±11.4 | <0.001 | 59±4.4 | N.S. | 77±2.2$^c$ | <0.001 | — |
| 22–23 | 123±14.3 | <0.001 | 81±8.3$^c$ | N.S. | — | — | — |
| 4 | 60±1.5 | <0.001 | — | — | — | — | 44±1.7 |
| 16 | 96±2.3$^c$ | <0.001 | — | — | — | — | 76±2.3$^c$ |
| *Glucose* | | | *Males* | | | | |
| 5 | 107±4.5 | <0.05 | 97±2.9 | <0.001 | 86±1.7 | <0.001 | — |
| 11 | 104±4.0 | N.S. | 109±3.7$^f$ | <0.001 | 86±3.8 | <0.001 | — |
| 22–23 | 109±3.1 | <0.001 | 141±5.6$^c$ | <0.001 | 105±7.5$^f$ | N.S. | — |
| 4 | 122±3.8 | <0.05 | — | — | — | — | 110±4.9 |
| 16 | 105±5.5$^c$ | N.S. | — | — | — | — | 105±5.5 |

3. RECONDITE TOXICITY OF TRACE ELEMENTS

|  | Females |  |  |  | Males |  |  |
|---|---|---|---|---|---|---|---|
| 5 | — |  | — |  | 98±3.0 |  | — |
| 11 | 118±3.4 | <0.001 | 83±4.6 | — | 85±4.1[f] | <0.001 | — |
| 22–23 | 107±7.6 | <0.005 | 134±4.6[c] | N.S. | 126±3.7[c] | <0.001 | — |
| 4 | 132±3.8 | <0.01 | — | — | — |  | 119±5.1 |
| 16 | 88±8.1[c] | N.S. | — | — | — |  | 94±3.3[c] |
| *Vitamin E deficiency* |  |  |  |  |  |  |  |
| 4 |  |  |  |  |  |  |  |
| Deficient | 84±13.9 |  |  |  |  |  |  |
| Deficient + Chromium | 109±4.0 | <0.02 |  |  |  |  |  |
| E-supplemented | 73±4.5 |  |  |  |  |  |  |
| E + Chromium | 96±3.8 | <0.001 |  |  |  |  |  |
| Chromium in diet and water | 0.08 ppm |  | 5.08 ppm |  | 0.16 ppm |  | 0.14 ppm |

[a] Significance of difference between contiguous mean values, by Student's *t*. N.S. Not significant.
[b] Significance of difference between brown and white sugar groups.
[c] Value differs from that of preceding age, $p < 0.001$.
[d] $p < 0.025$.
[e] $p < 0.005$.
[f] $p < 0.01$.

Note: There were two experiments done at different times. The first series was measured at 5, 11 and 22–23 months of age, the second at 4 and 16 months. The experiments with Vitamin E were also done at a different time.

TABLE XXVI

LIFE-SPANS AND LONGEVITIES OF RATS FED THE TORULA YEAST–SUGAR–LARD DIET

| Sugar in diet | Males 50% Dead (days) | Males Longevity (days) | Females 50% Dead (days) | Females Longevity (days) |
|---|---|---|---|---|
| Brown | 800 | 924±22.8 | 782 | 921±14.2 |
| White-A | 740 | 864±9.5[b] | 667 | 823±11.2[b] |
| Raw | 680 | 849±13.6 | 698 | 870±27.4 |
| White+chromium | 601[a] | 732±12.5[b,d] | 636[a] | 917±31.7[d] |
| White-B | 592 | 801±8.3[c] | 630 | 759±21.4[c] |

[a] Significance of difference from brown sugar group by chi-square analysis, $p < 0.005$.
[b] Significance of difference from brown sugar group by student's $t$, $p < 0.005$.
[c] Differs from raw sugar group. $p < 0.005$.
[d] Differs from white sugar group. $p < 0.005$.

Therefore, there is something missing in the torula–white sugar diet which is present in the torula–brown sugar diet and which allows chromium to exert its hypoglycemic action. That substance also affected longevity (Table XXVI). Rats fed brown or raw sugar lived longer than rats fed white sugar.

### I. Serum Constituents, Uric Acid

Fasting serum uric acid measured on 104 groups of rats fed various trace elements showed values ranging regularly from 2.0 to 4.0 mg/100 ml. Levels were suppressed in rats fed tellurite and tungsten, and were elevated in rats fed selenate. Mean levels in control males were 3.1 ± 0.11 mg/100 ml and levels in females were 2.6 ± 0.26 mg/100 ml; the means plus 3 S.D.s. were (mg/100 ml): males, 2.3 to 3.8; females, 1.7 to 4.5. In tungsten-fed males and females, respectively, they were 2.2 and 1.9 mg/100 ml. In tellurite-fed animals they were 2.0 and 1.0 mg/100 ml. High values were found in selenate-fed males (4.0 mg), and in females (4.2 mg/100 ml), and also in nickel- and vanadium-fed males (4.2 mg). Tungsten is an antimetabolite for molybdenum, a constituent of xanthine oxidase.

### J. Effects of the Metals in the Basic Water on Serum Glucose and Cholesterol of Rats

In order to evaluate glycolytic and cholesterolytic effects of the essential trace metals in the basic water, three groups of rats were given water,

TABLE XXVII

Fasting Serum Glucose Levels of Rats Partly Deficient in a Trace Metal Given a Torula Yeast–Sucrose–Lard Diet

| Metal fed in water | Age (days) | Males (mg/100 ml) Mean[b] | Change | $p^a$ | Females (mg/100 ml) Mean[b] | Change | $p^a$ |
|---|---|---|---|---|---|---|---|
| Zinc, manganese, copper, molybdenum | 128 | 122±3.8 | — | — | 132±3.8 | — | — |
|  | 457 | 105±5.5[f] | −17 | <0.001 | 88±8.1[c] | −44 | <0.001 |
| Zinc, manganese, copper | 122 | 83±4.2 | — | — | 95±6.0 | — | — |
|  | 491 | 110±4.5[c] | +27 | — | 84±5.1 | −11 | — |
|  | 564 | 97±3.8[d] | −13 | — | 81±3.4 | −3 | — |
| Zinc-deficient | 108 | 104±2.1 | — | — | 101±3.3 | — | — |
|  | 352 | 113±3.8[e] | +9 | <0.001 | 118±4.2[c] | +17 | <0.001 |
|  | 473 | 89±3.0[c] | −24 | <0.05 | 63±3.3[c] | −55 | <0.001 |
| Manganese-deficient | 188 | 122±3.3 | — | <0.001 | 89±2.7 | — | — |
|  | 484 | 100±5.0[f] | −22 | — | 74±3.0[c] | −15 | <0.001 |
|  | 576 | 82±7.1[d] | −18 | <0.05 | 66±2.5[c] | −8 | <0.025 |
| Copper-deficient | 111 | 93±7.2 | — | — | 109±2.1 | — | — |
|  | 406 | 91±6.4 | −2 | <0.025 | 83±3.4[c] | −26 | — |
|  | 518 | 80±4.1 | −11 | <0.005 | 85±2.8 | +2 | — |

[a] Significance of difference from value of zinc, manganese, and copper group at comparable age.
[b] Mean ± SEM.
[c] Differs from value at younger age, $p < 0.001$.
[d] $p < 0.025$.
[e] $p < 0.05$.
[f] $p < 0.01$.

Note: There were 12 rats in each group. One metal was omitted from the water.

## TABLE XXVIII

Fasting Serum Cholesterol Levels in Rats Partly Deficient in a Trace Element and Fed a Torula Yeast–Sucrose–Lard Diet

| Metal given | Age | Males mg/100 ml[a] | Rise | p[b] | Females mg/100 ml[a] | Rise | p[b] |
|---|---|---|---|---|---|---|---|
| Zinc, manganese, copper, molybdenum | 128 | 60±3.2 | — | | 60±1.5 | — | |
|  | 457 | 87±3.1[c] | 27 | <0.001 | 96±2.3[d] | 36 | <0.005 |
| Zinc, manganese, copper | 154 | 90±8.1 | — | | 75±3.0 | — | <0.001 |
|  | 453 | 115±7.7[e] | 25 | — | 118±5.8[c] | 43 | — |
|  | 564 | 118±11.2 | 3 | — | 104±3.1[e] | −14 | — |
| Zinc-deficient | 108 | 69±4.2 | — | <0.025 | 66±3.2 | — | <0.025 |
|  | 352 | 93±4.2[c] | 24 | <0.001 | 88±4.9[c] | 22 | <0.001 |
|  | 473 | 75±2.6[c] | −18 | <0.001 | 114±3.8[c] | 26 | <0.025 |
| Manganese-deficient | 188 | 70±2.7 | — | <0.01 | 53±2.0 | — | <0.001 |
|  | 484 | 83±6.5[f] | 13 | <0.001 | 63±2.4[d] | 10 | <0.001 |
|  | 596 | 71±3.8 | −12 | <0.001 | 82±4.5[c] | 19 | <0.001 |
| Copper-deficient | 111 | 91±2.6 | — | — | 79±2.8 | — | — |
|  | 406 | 92±6.9 | 1 | <0.025 | 88±3.7[f] | 9 | <0.001 |
|  | 518 | 103±3.5 | 11 | — | 79±3.2[f] | −9 | <0.001 |

[a] ± SEM.
[b] p is the significance of the difference from the zinc, manganese, and copper group at comparable ages.
[c] Differs from younger age values. p <0.001.
[d] p <0.005.
[e] p <0.025.
[f] p <0.05.

Note: There were 12 rats in each group. One metal was omitted from the water. Means ± SEM.

omitting zinc, manganese, or copper. Data on glucose are shown in Table XXVII. These rats were deficient in both chromium and molybdenum. At the greatest ages, male rats deficient in zinc, manganese, or copper had lower glucose levels than did rats given all three metals; females deficient in zinc and manganese had lower levels. At the other ages, differences were inconstant. Manganese- and copper-deficient rats, however, lowered their glucose levels with age, whereas zinc-deficient rats did not. This decline with age also occurred in the group given molybdenum.

Cholesterol levels of these same rats are given in Table XXVIII. Levels for all of the deficient rats, and those of the rats given molybdenum, were lower than were those fed zinc, manganese, and copper. Furthermore, significant rises with age, expected in rats deficient in chromium (Table XXIII), occurred in those given the three metals or the three metals and molybdenum. Considering rises from the youngest to the oldest rats, they were significant in zinc-deficient females and manganese-deficient females, but not in copper-deficient females, and they were significant in copper-deficient males but not in the other two groups. The data are confusing, but suggest that copper affects cholesterol metabolism in males by preventing a rise with age, that copper may also affect it in females, but that zinc is more concerned with it in that sex.

## X. RECONDITE TOXICITY OF TRACE ELEMENTS AS EXPRESSED BY EFFECTS ON REPRODUCTION OF RATS AND MICE

We have discovered that exposure of breeding animals to trace elements is a considerably more sensitive way of detecting recondite toxicity than is exposure for life. Doses tolerable for growth and survival often show severe effects on fertility and viability of offspring *(31)*.

By confining five pair of weanling rats or mice, each pair to a cage, one can expect 50 or so offspring at the first mating, and perhaps 200 by the last—each pair breeds about four times. A pair from each litter is then confined, and after breeding, a pair from each subsequent litter, providing three generations. Control mice so bred produced 687 offspring, whereas rats produced 348. Delayed pregnancies, failures to breed, unusual sex ratios of offspring, decreased sizes of litters, dead offspring, and runts were used as indices of toxicity.

In Table XXIX are shown the effects of selenate (3 ppm), arsenite (5 ppm), lead (25 ppm), molybdate (10 ppm), and cadmium (10 ppm) (doses in terms of elemental concentration) in drinking water of mice exposed for three generations. In addition, mice were given mercury (5 ppm) and methyl mercury (1 ppm).

## TABLE XXIX

Effects of Trace Elements in Drinking Water on Fertility and Viability of Offspring of Breeding Mice for Three Generations

| Generation and element | No. litters | Ave. litter size | ♂:♀ ratio | Runts | Dead litters | Young deaths | Failure to breed | No. mice |
|---|---|---|---|---|---|---|---|---|
| Control |  |  |  |  |  |  |  |  |
| $F_1$ | 19 | 11.0 | 0.94 | 0 | 0 | 0 | 0 | 209 |
| $F_2$ | 23 | 10.3 | 1.03 | 2 | 0 | 6 | 0 | 248 |
| $F_3$ | 22 | 10.5 | 1.00 | 0 | 0 | 1 | 0 | 230 |
| Mean and Total | 21.3 | 10.6 | 0.99 | 2 | 0 | 7 | 0 | 687 |
| Cadmium (5 ppm) |  |  |  |  |  |  |  |  |
| $F_1$ | 14 | 13.1 | 1.05 | 25[b] | 0 | 39[b] | 0 | 184 |
| $F_2$ | 11 | 9.2 | 0.78 | 9[a] | 2 | 48[b] | 3 | 101 |
| $F_3$ | — | — | — | — | — | — | — | — |
| Mean and Total | 12.5 | 11.1 | 0.91 | 34[b] | 2 | 87[b] | 3 | 285 |
| Lead (25 ppm) |  |  |  |  |  |  |  |  |
| $F_1$ | 8 | 12.0 | 1.05 | 69[b] | 2 | 9[b] | 0 | 72 |
| $F_2$ | 2 | 11.5 | 0.92 | 0 | 0 | 0 | 1 | 23 |
| $F_3$ | — | — | — | — | — | — | — | — |
| Mean and Total | 5 | 11.7 | 0.99 | 69[b] | 2 | 9[a] | 1 | 95 |

| | | | | | | | |
|---|---|---|---|---|---|---|---|
| **Selenium (3 ppm)** | | | | | | | |
| $F_1$ | 16 | 12.3 | 1.50 | 36[a] | 1 | 13[a] | 2 | 197 |
| $F_2$ | 17 | 10.0 | 1.44 | 41[b] | 0 | 10 | 2 | 169 |
| $F_3$ | 3 | 7.6 | 1.30 | 16[b] | 0 | 0 | 3 | 23 |
| Mean and Total | 12 | 10.0 | 1.41 | 93[b] | 1 | 23[b] | 7 | 389 |
| **Arsenic (5 ppm)** | | | | | | | |
| $F_1$ | 19 | 8.2 | 0.93 | 0 | 0 | 1 | 0 | 147 |
| $F_2$ | 25 | 9.6 | 1.30 | 0 | 0 | 0 | 1 | 290 |
| $F_3$ | 7 | 8.1 | 1.71 | 0 | 0 | 0 | 0 | 57 |
| Mean and Total | 17 | 8.6 | 1.31 | 0 | 0 | 8 | 1 | 494 |
| **Molybdenum (10 ppm)** | | | | | | | |
| $F_1$ | 21 | 11.3 | 1.05 | 0 | 0 | 15[c] | 0 | 238 |
| $F_2$ | 26 | 10.3 | 1.32 | 2 | 5 | 7 | 1 | 242 |
| $F_3$ | 14 | 8.8 | 0.90 | 11 | 4[d] | 34[b] | 3 | 123 |
| Mean and Total | 20.3 | 10.1 | 1.09 | 13 | 9 | 56[b] | 4 | 603 |

[a] Differs from controls by chi-square analysis, $p < 0.0005$.
[b] $p < 0.0001$.
[c] $p < 0.001$.
[d] $p < 0.05$.

Note: Maternal deaths occurred in the 6 groups as follows: control 1, cadmium 2, lead 0, selenium 1, arsenic 0, molybdenum 5. Delayed pregnancies occurred in the cadmium and lead groups.

## TABLE XXX

Effects of Nickel, Titanium and Lead on the Fertility and Viability of Offspring of Breeding Rats Given the Metals in Drinking Water

| Generation and element | No. litter | Ave. size litter | ♂:♀ ratio | Runts | Dead litters | Young deaths | Failure to breed | No. rats |
|---|---|---|---|---|---|---|---|---|
| **Control** | | | | | | | | |
| $F_1$ | 10 | 11.4 | 1.14 | 0 | 0 | 0 | 0 | 114 |
| $F_2$ | 10 | 11.3 | 1.10 | 1 | 0 | 0 | 0 | 113 |
| $F_3$ | 11 | 11.0 | 1.06 | 0 | 0 | 1 | 0 | 121 |
| Mean and Total | 10.3 | 11.2 | 1.10 | 1 | 0 | 1 | 0 | 348 |
| **Lead** | | | | | | | | |
| $F_1$ | 19 | 9.1 | 0.68 | $40^b$ | 2 | $12^b$ | 1 | 173 |
| $F_2$ | 32 | 10.3 | 1.16 | $26^b$ | 1 | $35^b$ | 3 | 311 |
| $F_3$ | 6 | 8.0 | 0.91 | 4 | 1 | 2 | 1 | 22 |
| Mean and Total | 19 | 9.1 | 0.92 | $70^b$ | 4 | $49^b$ | $5^c$ | 506 |
| **Nickel** | | | | | | | | |
| $F_1$ | 11 | 11.0 | 1.20 | $37^b$ | 0 | $11^a$ | 0 | 121 |
| $F_2$ | 15 | 10.5 | 1.18 | 8 | 0 | $16^b$ | 2 | 157 |
| $F_3$ | 10 | 8.1 | 0.44 | 5 | 0 | $17^b$ | 0 | 81 |
| Mean and Total | 12 | 9.5 | 0.87 | $50^b$ | 0 | $44^b$ | 2 | 359 |
| **Titanium** | | | | | | | | |
| $F_1$ | 11 | 9.4 | 1.43 | $23^b$ | 0 | 1 | 0 | 103 |
| $F_2$ | 16 | 10.9 | 0.99 | $14^d$ | 0 | 25 | 4 | 174 |
| $F_3$ | 2 | 8.0 | 0.60 | $6^d$ | 0 | 0 | 0 | 16 |
| Mean and Total | 9.7 | 9.4 | 1.01 | $43^b$ | 0 | $25^b$ | 4 | 293 |

[a] Differs from controls by chi-square analysis, $p < 0.005$.
[b] $p < 0.0001$.
[c] $p < 0.025$.
[d] $p < 0.01$.

Note: Delayed pregnancies occurred in the $F_1$ lead generation. Maternal deaths were as follows: nickel 1, titanium 1, lead 2.

Methyl mercury was extremely toxic to fertility and viability. Cadmium, selenium, and molybdenum decreased fertility. Viability of offspring was decreased by cadmium, lead, selenium, and molybdenum. There were many runts in the selenium, lead, and cadmium groups. The strains of mice given lead and cadmium virtually died out in the second generation, terminating the experiment. There were more males than females born to mice given selenium and arsenic. Litter size was reduced by arsenic.

In Table XXX are the effects on rats of nickel (5 ppm), titanium (5 ppm), and lead (25 ppm) in water. Again, lead was very toxic. Fertility was reduced by lead and titanium, and the latter especially reduced the number of litters in the $F_3$ generation. Viability of offspring was reduced

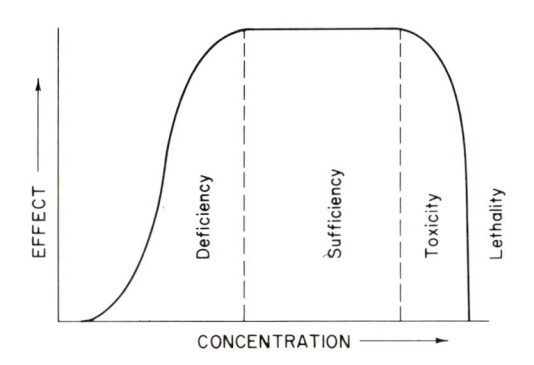

FIG. 1. Schematic illustration of Bertrand's law of optimal nutritive concentration of an essential trace element. When there is no element present there is no growth or function. The first part of the curve indicates a state of deficiency which becomes less as the concentration increases. The plateau indicates a state of sufficiency of the element when function is at its highest level. The width of this plateau varies with different elements and living things, but in mammals is wide, as the animal can get rid of excesses which it does not need. When high concentrations exceed the ability of the animal to repel or excrete excesses, the element becomes toxic, and is lethal at the point where the curve descends perpendicularly. This curve applies to all living things and may be quite narrow in the case of plants and especially marine organisms. It is important to note that growth is not necessarily a sign of optimal function when the element is somewhat deficient. For example, bacteria may grow well when an element is partially deficient, but may not produce compounds which ordinarily would be produced in the presence of sufficient element (Weinberg's principle).

by all three metals, especially by lead, and there were many runts, which could not breed.

These experiments indicate that the breeding animal may be very sensitive to abnormal trace metals in doses tolerable for growth and survival. Essential metals apparently are not teratogenic *(32)*, but abnormal ones, when injected into hamsters, produced characteristic congenital abnormalities specific for the metal *(32a,33)* in the cases of cadmium, arsenic, lead, and indium *(33a)*.

It is clear that toxicity of all of the common abnormal trace metals should be ascertained in this manner. Of those tested, the order of toxicity was mercury > cadmium > lead > selenium > molybdenum > titanium > nickel > arsenic.

## XI. SOME CLUES TO MECHANISMS OF TOXICITY

Here we can review briefly the possible mechanisms by which an element exerts recondite toxicity. Of course, all elements—in fact, all substances—are toxic in large enough amounts; in fact, water has the lowest ratio of normal to toxic doses of almost any substance in mammals. A

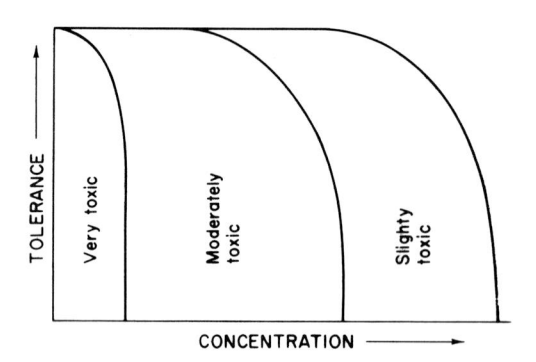

FIG. 2. Schematic illustration of effects of toxic trace elements which have no biological function. A certain concentration is tolerable but slight excesses may show increasing toxicity and eventual lethality. The first curve on the left, for example, can represent cadmium, beryllium, or mercury for which there are definite but very small tolerances. The middle curve can represent lead, for which there is more tolerance. The curve on the right can represent nickel, germanium, or tin, for which tolerance in the mammal may be evident only by a shortening of life span. For toxic elements there are differing thresholds at which effects appear; this phenomenon is common to all living things. In actual fact, all soluble elements can be toxic in large amounts.

man can drink 3 to 4 liters a day and excrete it, but if he drinks 9 to 12 liters his kidneys may fail, his cells become hydropic, and he may die.

There are sharply divided differences in the orders of toxicity of the essential and nonessential elements when given orally to mammals. The essential metals have low orders of toxicity. They are controlled by efficient homeostatic mechanisms, which repel or excrete excesses and conserve in the face of deficiencies, and so prevent accumulation. For every element, however, homeostasis may break down under excesses. Figure 1 illustrates the Law of Optimal Nutritive Concentration sometimes attributed to Gabriel Bertrand. The biological effect of an essential trace element increases in proportion to concentration until a plateau is reached. There homeostasis operates fully. Weinberg (34) showed that this plateau of concentration was necessary for full function of an organism, although most of its activity, growth, and reproduction could proceed with marginal amounts of the element (Weinberg's Principle). Increasing concentrations lead to toxicity and death as homeostatic mechanisms are exceeded. This Law, and probably this Principle, apply to all living things.

Many of the nonessential elements accumulate in mammals. Those which do are those low in abundance in sea water and on the earth's

TABLE XXXI

Acute Cellular Toxicities of Trace Elements in Experimental Animals According to Series in Periodic Table (mg/kg) [a]

| Periodic group | Series 4 | Series 5 | Series 6 |
|---|---|---|---|
| IIA | Beryllium, 4 [b] | Strontium, 123 | Barium, 8 |
| IVB | Titanium, slight | Zirconium, 175–4100 | Hafnium, slight? |
| VB | Vanadium, 4–5 | Niobium, 14 | Tantalum, 38 |
| VIB | Chromium, 400 | Molybdenum, 115 | Tungsten, 116 |
| VIIB | Manganese, 210 | Technetium— | Rhenium, slight |
| VIII | Iron, slight | Ruthenium, slight | Osmium, slight |
| VIII | Cobalt, 20 | Rhodium, slight | Iridium, slight |
| VIII | Nickel, 180 | Palladium, 18.6 | Platinum, 20 |
| IB | Copper, 20 | Silver, slight | Gold, slight |
| IIB | Zinc, 57 | Cadmium, 0.3–6 | Mercury, 16 |
| IIIA | Gallium, 200 | Indium, 10 | Thallium, 15–25 |
| IVA | Germanium, 1200 | Tin, 100 | Lead, 50 |
| VA | Arsenic, 40 | Antimony, 11 | Bismuth ? |
| VIA | Selenium, 3.5 | Tellurium, 2.5 | Polonium— |

[a] Data from E. Browning. (1969). "Toxicity of Industrial Metals," 2nd ed. Butterworth, London.

[b] Numbers refer to minimal lethal doses parenterally.

crust. Among those of lowest abundance are the most toxic (Table I). During the evolutionary development of higher organisms, there was need for the development of mechanisms to handle elements with high abundances, several of which were used in biological processes. There was little need for homeostatic mechanisms to handle elements of low abundances in the hydrosphere and geosphere.

Figure 2 illustrates three hypothetical curves of toxicity of nonessential trace elements, showing no beneficial activity. As concentration increases, toxicity begins to appear.

## A. Cellular Toxicity

Table XXXI shows the cellular toxicities of 42 trace elements.

When an element is injected. intestinal homeostatic mechanisms are bypassed. Renal and biliary excretion, and in a few cases, pulmonary excretion, are left for removing the substance from contact with cells. When urinary excretion of an element is inefficient, the element is likely to be toxic by injection.

The bulk elements, sodium, potassium, magnesium, calcium, chlorine,

TABLE XXXII

CARCINOGENICITY OF METALS IN EXPERIMENTAL ANIMALS ACCORDING TO ROUTE OF ADMINISTRATION[a]

| Metal | Oral | Parenteral | Inhalation |
|---|---|---|---|
| Beryllium | 0 | Osteosarcoma | Carcinoma, lung (also Man) |
| Cadmium | 0 | Sarcoma, teratoma | — |
| Chromium (VI) | 0 | Sarcoma | Carcinoma, lung (also Man) |
| Cobalt | 0 | Sarcoma | — |
| Fe-dextrans | — | Sarcoma | — |
| Lead | Renal carcinoma | Renal carcinoma | — |
| Nickel | 0 | Sarcoma | Carcinoma, lung (also Man) |
| Zinc (chicks) | 0 | Teratoma (intratesticular) | — |
| Selenium | Sarcoma, hepatoma | — | — |
| Arsenic | 0 (Carcinoma-Man) | — | — |
| Titanium | 0 | Carcinoma | — |
| Rhodium | Lymphoma, carcinoma | — | — |
| Palladium | Lymphoma, carcinoma | — | — |

[a] From F. W. Sunderman, Jr. (1971). Metal carcinogenesis in experimental animals. *Fd. Cosmet. Toxicol.* **9**, 105, and personal observations.

sulfur, and phosphorus, in their physiological states, have very low orders of toxicity. What toxicity may occur is conditioned by electrolyte imbalance or large excesses influencing electrochemical functions. In essence they are innately inert from a toxicological aspect, performing essential biochemical reactions and acting as integral structures. Those taking part in structures of living things are calcium, fluorine, magnesium, nitrogen, phosphorus, sulfur, silicon, strontium, and barium. Those with electrochemical properties are calcium, chlorine, potassium, magnesium, nitrogen, sodium, phosphorus, and sulfur. In elemental states, however, most of them are toxic, as they form strong bases or acids.

The table shows that, although cellular toxicity, as judged from the minimal lethal dose by intravenous or intraperitoneal injection in experimental animals, varies considerably, it is quite similar for many heavier elements, with the exception of cadmium, selenium, and tellurium. Furthermore, cellular toxicity increases with atomic weight within a group in the chromium, manganese, nickel, copper, zinc, gallium, germanium, arsenic, and selenium groups, but decreases in the vanadium. Cellular toxicity bears little relationship to abundance in the earth's crust, and probably is a function of the atomic structure of the element and its affinity for cellular ligands.

One form of cellular toxicity is expressed in the property of a metal to cause tumors. This property is illustrated in Table XXXII. Nine metals produced malignant tumors when injected into experimental animals, but only one of these was effective orally. Four other elements were orally carcinogenic, but probably not parenterally so. Lung cancers were caused by three of the metals effective parenterally.

## B. Oral Toxicity

In Table XXXIII are the oral toxicities of the same elements, along with their concentrations in crustal rocks. The toxic doses are very different, and in general decrease with decreasing crustal abundance. The elements occurring naturally in high concentrations are not toxic to mammals except in very high doses.

When the gene or genes governing homeostasis of an essential metal are absent or weak, the metal accumulates in the body during life. Accumulation of copper occurs in hereditary cuprism—hepatolenticular degeneration, or Wilson's disease—which is usually fatal before the third decade unless carefully treated. Hereditary ferrism, or hemochromatosis, causes accumulation of iron, which may not be fatal until the fifth to seventh decades. These two diseases illustrate Bertrand's law. There may ex-

TABLE XXXIII

CHRONIC MINIMAL ORAL TOXICITIES OF TRACE ELEMENTS IN EXPERIMENTAL ANIMALS ACCORDING TO SERIES IN PERIODIC TABLES AND CONCENTRATION IN EARTH'S CRUST, DIET (MG/KG), AND CRUSTAL ROCKS (PPM)[a]

| Periodic group | Series 4 | | Series 5 | | Series 6 | |
|---|---|---|---|---|---|---|
| | Diet (mg/kg) | Crust (ppm) | Diet (mg/kg) | Crust (ppm) | Diet (mg/kg) | Crust (ppm) |
| IIA | Beryllium 20 | 3 | Strontium >1500 | 400 | Barium >500 | 450 |
| IIB | Titanium 5000 | 5700 | Zirconium >10 | 165 | Hafnium ? | 3 |
| VB | Vanadium 100 | 135 | Niobium 50 | 20 | Tantalum 8000 | 2 |
| VIB | Chromium 10,000 | 100 | Molybdenum 125 | 2 | Tungsten 1000 | 2 |
| VIIB | Manganese 5000 | 1,000 | Technetium — | — | Rhenium ? | 0.005 |
| VIII | Iron 5000 | 56,300 | Ruthenium ? | 0.001 | Osmium ? | 0.0015 |
| VIII | Cobalt 200 | 25 | Rhodium 5 | 0.01 | Iridium ? | 0.001 |
| VIII | Nickel 1000 | 75 | Palladium ? | 0.01 | Platinum ? | 0.005 |

| | | | | | | |
|---|---|---|---|---|---|---|
| IB | 400 | Copper | 55 | Silver | 0.07 | Gold | 0.004 |
| IIB | 4000 | Zinc | 70 | Cadmium | 0.2 | Mercury | 0.1 |
| IIIA | >1000 | Gallium | 15 | Indium | 0.1 | Thallium | 0.5 |
| IVA | 100 | Germanium | 5 | Tin | 2 | Lead | 12 |
| VA | 20 | Arsenic | 2 | Antimony | 0.2 | Bismuth | 0.2 |
| VIA | 8 | Selenium | 0.05 | Tellurium | 0.001 | Polonium | $2 \times 10^{-10}$ |

[a] Data from E. Browning (1969). "Toxicity of Industrial Metals," 2nd ed. Butterworth, London.

ist hereditary manganism, causing Parkinson's disease, but this has not been proved.

## C. Accumulation with Age during Constant Oral Exposure

As might be expected, those elements which accumulate in the tissues of mammals including man with constant exposure, are toxic, whereas those not accumulating are not. This statement applies to relatively small doses, for as stated previously, homeostasis can be broken down by excesses. In Table XXXIV are the elements found by experiment to accumulate in rat, mouse, or human tissue, in the estimated order of overall recondite toxicity. The first six are well known. Cadmium is the most toxic, because it probably remains in tissues for life, unlike mercury, which leaves the body quite rapidly. Lead's innate toxicity is relatively low, but exposures in the modern environment are high and stores in human bone offer potential hazards if released. Beryllium also is poorly excreted, but most exposures are very low at present. The last six elements show minor or few toxic manifestations.

TABLE XXXIV

Elements Which Accumulate in Mammalian Tissues with Age and Constant Exposures to Oral or Inhaled doses, in Order of Recondite Toxicity

| Element | Tissue affinity of element | Rat | Mouse | Man | Remarks, principal manifestation |
|---|---|---|---|---|---|
| Cadmium | Kidney, liver, arteries, prostate | 880 | 300+ | 300+ | Hypertension, emphysema |
| Beryllium | Lung, all organs | + | + | + | Beryllosis |
| Antimony | All | 100+ | 100+ | ? | Heart lesions |
| Mercury | Kidney, brain | 5 | 5 | + | Erythrism |
| Lead | Bone, brain, prostate | 5 | 3 | 20 | Mental effects |
| Arsenic | All | 70–200 | 2 | + | Keratotic cancers |
| Niobium | Spleen | 0 | 9 | ? | Liver degeneration |
| Germanium | All | 2–3 | 30 | ? | Short life-span |
| Tin | Spleen, heart, lung, prostate, bladder | 2 | 2 | 8 | Unknown |
| Selenium | Kidney | 3 | 3 | + | Cancer in rats |
| Titanium | Heart, lung | — | 4–25 | + | Unknown |
| Fluorine | Bone | 50 | 50 | + | Osteosclerosis |
| Barium | Bladder, bone | ? | ? | + | Unknown |
| Strontium | Kidney, bone | ? | ? | + | Unknown |
| Aluminum | Lung | ? | ? | + | Unknown |
| Chromium | Lung | ? | ? | + | Unknown |
| Vanadium | Lung, fat | ? | ? | + | Unknown |

Column header: Order of accumulation × controls

3. RECONDITE TOXICITY OF TRACE ELEMENTS 163

When one compares these first six elements in the table with their concentrations on the earth's crust and in the seawater, one finds that crust contains less than 3 ppm of all but lead (12 ppm), and that seawater has less than 0.4 ppb and usually less than 0.1 ppb.

### D. Accumulation from Respiratory Exposures

Homeostasis of cobalt, selenium, molybdenum, iodine, and fluorine is largely accomplished by the kidney; 50–88% of the amount ingested is excreted in the urine. These elements are absorbed from inspired air by the lungs and then enter the body to be excreted. Renal excretory mechanisms are poor, however, for vanadium, chromium, manganese, iron, copper, nickel, and zinc; only 2–8% of the intake is so excreted. In addition, this route of excretion is poor for the abnormal metals lead, cadmium, beryllium, zirconium, tin, strontium, and barium—with 0.6–14% found in urine—and mediocre for arsenic, whereas it is good for mercury, antimony, tellurium, titanium, niobium, and boron.

The elements which accumulate in human lung with age are aluminum, beryllium, chromium, iron, tin, strontium, titanium, and vanadium. The elements absorbed from human lung into other tissues are barium, beryllium, cadmium, chromium, manganese, nickel, lead, tin, and strontium. Therefore, under conditions of heavy exposure from mine dusts or badly polluted air, metals which are absorbed from the lung and poorly excreted by the kidney—in the main, these are the ones with intestinal homeostatic mechanisms—could accumulate in the body. They are beryllium, cadmium, lead, tin, chromium, barium, nickel, manganese, and strontium. The first three are toxic: manganese causes Parkinsonism in miners (illustrating Bertrand's law); chromium and nickel cause lung cancers in exposed workers; and barium causes baritosis. Some metals entering the body from air thus may accumulate, for there is no way to get rid of them easily.

### E. Prediction of Toxicity of an Element

Because marine animals have mediocre-to-poor homeostatic mechanisms for elements, and because marine plants probably have few or none, it is obvious that any element in seawater is nontoxic at seawater concentrations. This rule applies to the bulk elements and to boron, bromine, fluorine, silicon, and strontium, all of which occur in the 1.3–65 ppm range. Seawater precipitates all metals entering the oceans by way of rivers, except sodium, a little magnesium, potassium and strontium, and seawater contains little dissolved chromium (0.05 ppb), manganese (2 ppb), iron (10 ppb), cobalt (0.27 ppb), copper (3 ppb), zinc (10 ppb), and molybdenum (10 ppb), but enough to sustain life. In very small concentrations (less than 0.1 ppb) are silver, gold, beryllium, bismuth, cadmium, gallium, germanium, mercury, indium, lanthanum, niobium, lead, antimony, scandium, selenium, tantalum, thorium, thallium, tungsten, yttrium, and zirconium, most of which show more or less recondite toxicity to mammals. Between 10 ppb and 0.1 ppb are the elements aluminum, barium, iodine, tin, titanium, uranium, and vanadium, some of which are active and some of which are inactive biologically. Lithium at 180 ppb and arsenic at 3 ppb are also nontoxic (Table I). Therefore, one can predict whether or not an element is toxic to living cells with reasonable accuracy from its concentration in sea water, provided its atomic structure is such as to combine readily with organic ligands in tissues.

One can also predict recondite toxicity from the concentration of an element on the earth's crust (Table I). It is those elements with naturally low concentrations that man has concentrated and put into his environment that give us concern.

### F. Interactions of Trace Elements

A major mechanism for toxicity is probably the interaction of one element with another. When an essential element is a cofactor of an enzyme, and another element of the same periodic group is introduced in similar concentrations—or smaller ones—the enzyme may not be able to distinguish between the two. The second element is larger, but its outer shell is similar in the number of electrons. It is as if a key fitted a lock but does not turn, although the right key fits and turns.

These interactions can occur between elements of the same periodic group, between elements contiguous on the periodic table, or between elements with similar atomic radii. They also occur according to the Laws of Chelation, which depend upon the affinities of ligands for specific elements. The stability constants of chelates of metals of the transition series increase according to atomic number up to the group containing nickel or copper, and decline with that containing zinc. Thus, an element with a higher stability constant can displace one with a lower. Although stability constants of metalloenzyme complexes are largely unknown, the complexes can act the same way toward abnormal metals as do simple chelates.

To complicate the situation further, in metal-activated enzymes the metal is loosely bound to the enzyme, acting as a bridge between enzyme and substrate. It is readily displaced. In metalloenzymes, the metal is tightly bound; to displace it the displacing metal must become more tightly bound. In addition, an element may form an insoluble salt with a metal, thus removing it from its site on enzymes.

Therefore, there are five possible mechanisms of interaction to explain toxicity of elements:

1. Displacement of an essential trace element by the heavier one in the same periodic group, e.g., zinc by cadmium, copper by silver, phosphorus by arsenic.

2. Displacement of an essential trace element by a similar one in a contiguous group, e.g., copper by cadmium, zinc by copper, copper by nickel.

3. Displacement of an essential trace element by one with a similar atomic radius (theoretical).

TABLE XXXV

POSSIBLE INHIBITIONS OF SOME METAL-ACTIVATED ENZYMES AND METALLOENZYMES BY ABNORMAL TRACE METALS

| Enzyme | Metal | Inhibitor | System |
|---|---|---|---|
| Tyrosinase | Copper | Nickel, molybdenum | Pigmentation |
| Cytochrome oxidase | Copper | Nickel | Cytochrome |
| Monoamine oxidase | Copper | — | Collagen synthesis |
| Dopamine-$\beta$-hydroxylase | Copper | — | Amine oxidation |
| Ceruloplasmin | Copper | — | Oxidation |
| $\delta$-Aminolevulinic acid dehydrase | Copper | Lead | Porphyrin synthesis |
| Carboxypeptidase | Zinc | Cadmium | Protein catabolism |
| Carbonic anhydrase | Zinc | Cobolt, Cadmium | $CO_2$ formation |
| Alkaline phosphatase | Zinc | Molybdenum | — |
| Alcohol dehydrogenase | Zinc | Cadmium? | Alcohol catabolism |
| Lactic dehydrogenase | Zinc | Cadmium? | — |
| Glutamic dehydrogenase | Zinc | Cadmium? | — |
| Xanthine oxidase | Iron, molybdenum | Tungsten | Uric acid synthesis |
| Aldehyde dehydrogenase | Iron, molybdenum | — | — |
| Mevalonic kinase | Manganese | Vanadium, Chromium? | Squalene synthesis |
| Pyruvate carboxylase | Manganese | — | Glucose metabolism |
| Farnesyl pyrophosphatase | Manganese | Vanadium | Cholesterol synthesis |
| Succinic dehydrogenase | ? | Niobium | Succinic acid catabolism |
| 1-Aromatic amino acid decarboxylase | Zinc? | Cadmium | Amino acid oxidation |

TABLE XXXVI

ELEMENTS LIKELY TO COMPETE WITH EACH OTHER ON BIOLOGICAL SITES[a]

| Element | Competing element | Preferred ligand | Probable mode of action (see text) | Example |
|---|---|---|---|---|
| Vanadium | Niobium, manganese | ? | 1 | Oxidation of 5-OH tryptophane |
| Chromium | Zirconium, molybdenum | Insulin? | 3? | Aortic plaques |
| Manganese | Magnesium, iron | $PO_4$ | 3? | — |
| Iron | Cadmium, zinc, copper manganese | Porphyrin | 2 | Anemia |
| Cobalt | Lead, iodine | Porphyrin | 4 | — |
| Nickel | Copper | O-N | 4 | Tyrosinase |
| Copper | Molybdenum, silver, nickel, cadmium, zinc, mercury | SH | 1,2 | Tyrosinase |
| Zinc | Cadmium | SH | 1 | Carboxypeptidase inhibition |
| Molybdenum | Copper, $SO_4$, tungsten | Flavin | 3,4,5 | Tungsten inhibition of xanthine oxidase |
| Selenium | Sulfur, arsenic, cadmium, mercury, tellurium | SH | 1,5 | Displacement in keratin |
| Phosphorus | Arsenic | $PO_4$ | 1 | Arsenolecithin |
| Magnesium | Beryllium | $PO_4$ | 1,4 | Rickets |
| Calcium | Strontium | $PO_4$ | 1 | Rickets |

[a] Data from E. J. Underwood. (1971). "Trace Elements in Human and Animal Nutrition," 3rd ed. Academic Press, New York, and C. H. Hill and G. Matrone. (1970). Chemical parameters in the study of in vivo and in vitro interactions of transition elements. Fed. Proc. 29, 1474.

4. Displacement of an essential metal on a metalloprotein by one with a greater affinity for the protein's ligands, e.g., cobalt by lead, copper by lead, copper by mercury.

5. The competing element may bind the essential element in a firm complex, e.g., cadmium selenate or beryllium phosphate.

In Tables XXXV–XXXVII we have attempted to show examples of these types of interactions. When they occur, the activity of the enzyme may be (a) inhibited, (b) enhanced, or (c) partly inhibited and partly enhanced when the enzyme acts on two substrates. In Table XXXV are shown a list of some enzymes possibly inhibited by trace elements; the list is incomplete. Elements likely to compete are listed in Table XXXVI, and examples from experiments in mice given selenium in Table XXXVII. Zinc and cadmium bind selenium directly, whereas arsenic appears to displace selenium.

One can obtain an idea of the strength of a displacing element by analyzing organs of rats and mice for the element and for the essential trace metals. Nickel is a weak displacing metal, not accumulating to any extent in tissues. In Table XXXVIII are shown the effects of feeding nickel on nickel, manganese, copper, and zinc in five organs of rats. The experiments were for life. There was more manganese in kidney and less in spleen in the nickel-fed group than in the controls, less copper in lung and spleen, less zinc in lung, and less nickel in liver. Also shown are the effects of 50 ppm molybdenum on copper; copper was increased in all organs but kidney, the source being the diet. In mice (Table XXXIX), the nickel-fed group had more manganese and zinc in liver and more nickel in kidney.

TABLE XXXVII

INTERRELATIONSHIPS OF SELENIUM AND TRACE ELEMENTS IN RATS. APPROXIMATE CHANGE IN EXECRETION OR BLOOD LEVELS OF SELENIUM AS AFFECTED BY TRACE ELEMENTS

| Element | Respiratory | Urine | Feces | Blood | Molar ratio Se:M | Binding at injection site |
|---------|-------------|-------|-------|-------|------------------|--------------------------|
| Zinc | – – – – | – | – | – – – | 1:12 | + |
| Cadmium | – – – – | – – | – | – – | 1:4 | + |
| Arsenate | – – – | 0 | + + + + | – | 1:5 | 0 |
| Tellurite | – | 0 | + | – | 1:10 | 0 |
| Sulfate | 0 | 0 | 0 | 0 | 1:48 | 0 |

Note: Selenium and an element were injected together, intramuscularly, and [75]Se measured in air, urine, feces, and blood. Zinc and cadmium depressed excretion of selenium by all routes, and arsenic increased fecal excretion. Selenium was in the form of selenite. From K. P. McConnell and D. M. Carpenter. (1971). Interrelationships between selenium and specific trace elements. *Proc. Soc. Exp. Biol. Med.* **137,** 996.

Cadmium is a strong displacing agent. In Table XL are the effects on tissue zinc of feeding 10 ppm cadmium. Zinc doubled in kidney and tripled in liver, as well as increasing in heart and lung, but not in spleen. Cadmium increased markedly, 700 times in liver and 1800 times in kidney. The table also shows the very low cadmium concentrations obtained with our low-cadmium diet, and the predilection of cadmium for liver and kidney. With this pronounced displacement of zinc, some biochemical ef-

TABLE XXXVIII
Effect of Feeding 5 ppm Nickel on Essential Trace Metals in Rat Tissues and 50 ppm Molybdenum in Plain Water on Copper. Significant Differences Only ($\mu$g/gm) Dry Weight

| Element | Heart | Lung | Liver | Kidney | Spleen |
|---|---|---|---|---|---|
| Manganese | | | | | |
| Control | — | — | — | 2.2±0.52 | 3.2±0.59 |
| Nickel-fed | — | — | — | 4.2±0.79 | 1.8±0.40 |
| $p$ | — | — | — | <0.025 | <0.025 |
| Copper | | | | | |
| Control | — | 15.2±1.28 | — | — | 24.2±2.75 |
| Nickel-fed | — | 9.8±0.97 | — | — | 16.3±2.24 |
| $p$ | — | <0.01 | — | — | <0.025 |
| Zinc | | | | | |
| Control | — | 80±5.4 | — | — | — |
| Nickel-fed | — | 60±5.7 | — | — | — |
| $p$ | — | <0.05 | — | — | — |
| Nickel | | | | | |
| Control | — | — | 2.0±0.34 | — | — |
| Nickel-fed | — | — | 0.9±0.15 | — | — |
| $p$ | — | — | <0.005 | — | — |
| Nickel in diet and water (ppm) | | | | | |
| Control | 0.44 | | | | |
| Nickel-fed | 5.44 | | | | |
| Copper | | | | | |
| Control | 20.3±1.30 | 6.9±0.29 | 8.6±0.41 | — | 6.8±0.49 |
| Molybdenum-fed | 31.5±0.92 | 15.1±2.64 | 14.0±2.80 | — | 17.7±1.63 |
| $p$ | <0.005 | <0.005 | <0.01 | — | <0.001 |
| Molybdenum in diet and water (ppm) | | | | | |
| Control | 0.25 | | | | |
| Molybdenum-fed | 50.25 | | | | |

Note: There were 56 controls, 61 molybdenum-fed, and 64 nickel-fed rats. Differences in heart were not significant. There was no copper in molybdenum water or in controls for this group.

## TABLE XXXIX
### Effect of Feeding Nickel (5 ppm) on Tissue Concentrations of Essential Trace Elements in Mice, Significant Values Only ($\mu$g/gm) Dry Weight

| Element | Kidney | Liver |
|---|---|---|
| Manganese | | |
| Control | — | 3.3±0.27 |
| Nickel-fed | — | 4.4±0.37 |
| $p$ | — | <0.05 |
| Zinc | | |
| Control | — | 118±8.7 |
| nickel-fed | — | 139±6.4 |
| $p$ | — | <0.05 |
| Nickel | | |
| Control | 4.3±0.55 | — |
| Nickel-fed | 10.7±1.25 | — |
| $p$ | <0.01 | — |

Note: There were 47 control and 59 nickel-fed mice. No significant differences appeared in heart, lung or spleen, nor was copper altered in any organ.


## TABLE XL
### Effect of Feeding Cadmium (10 ppm) on Zinc and Cadmium Concentrations in the Organs of Rats ($\mu$g/gm) Wet Weight

| Element | Heart | Lung | Kidney | Liver | Spleen |
|---|---|---|---|---|---|
| Zinc | | | | | |
| Control | 15.4±0.95 | 12.3±1.59 | 13.4±1.37 | 12.7±2.88 | 21.4±1.46 |
| Cadmium-fed | 20.3±0.85 | 16.8±1.46 | 28.1±1.28 | 39.3±3.41 | 19.8±1.27 |
| $p$ | <0.005 | <0.05 | <0.005 | <0.0005 | N.S. |
| Cadmium | | | | | |
| Control | 0.02±0.001 | 0.06±0.018 | 0.03±0.002 | 0.03±0.008 | 0.06±0.016 |
| Cadmium-fed | 3.6±0.37 | 3.1±0.39 | 54.7±4.82 | 20.9±3.91 | 5.4±1.54 |
| $p$ | <0.0005 | <0.0005 | <0.0005 | <0.0005 | <0.0005 |
| Molar value of differences | | | | | |
| Zinc | 4.9 | 4.5 | 14.7 | 26.6 | −1.6 |
| Cadmium[a] | 2.1 | 1.8 | 31.8 | 12.1 | 3.9 |
| Molar ratio, cadmium:zinc | 0.43 | 0.40 | 2.6 | 0.45 | (2.43) |

[a] 58% of differences in cadmium between controls and cadmium-fed values.
Note: There were 58 control and 28 cadmium-fed rats.

TABLE XLI

Concentrations of Manganese, Copper, Zinc, and Nickel in Rats Given Plain Water or Water Containing These Metals for Life (μg/gm) Dry Weight. Significant Differences Only

| Element | Heart | Lung | Kidney | Liver | Spleen | Diet and water (ppm) |
|---|---|---|---|---|---|---|
| Manganese |  |  |  |  |  |  |
| Plain water | 1.9±0.16 | 1.0±0.05 | — | — | 1.9±0.22 | 12.7 |
| Basic water | 2.7±0.46 | 2.8±0.33 | — | — | 3.2±0.59 | 22.7 |
| p | <0.05 | <0.005 | — | — | <0.025 | — |
| Copper |  |  |  |  |  |  |
| Plain water | — | 6.9±0.29 | — | 8.6±0.41 | 6.8±0.49 | 1.36 |
| Basic water | — | 15.2±1.28 | — | 22.8±4.28 | 24.2±2.75 | 6.36 |
| p | — | <0.0005 | — | <0.001 | <0.0005 | — |
| Zinc |  |  |  |  |  |  |
| Plain water | 61±3.2 | 45±1.5 | 60±2.1 | 64±4.4 | 70±3.4 | 22.3 |
| Basic water | 117±11.0 | 80±5.4 | 108±9.2 | 142±12.8 | 124±11.7 | 72.3 |
| p | <0.0005 | <0.0005 | <0.0005 | <0.0005 | <0.0005 | — |
| Nickel |  |  |  |  |  |  |
| Plain water | — | — | — | 1.1±0.26 | — | 0.44 |
| Basic water | — | — | — | 2.0±0.34 | — | 0.44 |
| p | — | — | — | <0.05 | — | — |
| Plain water | 11.8±2.66 | — | — | — | 15.1±3.20 | 0.44 |
| Nickel-fed | 3.7±0.56 | — | — | — | 4.9±0.87 | 5.44 |
| p | <0.01 | — | — | — | <0.01 | — |

Note: In the basic water were zinc (50 ppm), manganese (10 ppm), copper (5 ppm), no nickel. Concentrations in starch diet shown in Table XXIV.

fects should be expected, in spite of accumulation of zinc. The molar ratios of the differences of cadmium and zinc show that only in the kidney is there more cadmium than zinc, which is where effects should be expected and where they appear.

Before feeding animals an abnormal trace element which could displace an essential one, it is necessary to know whether or not the tissues of the animals are saturated with the essential ones. Obviously, if they are not saturated, with every binding site filled and stores replete, less of the abnormal element will be needed to cause the toxic effects of displacement. Thus, the elemental content of the diet is most important, both for experimental animals and man. We have already shown that chromium protects against the toxicity of lead (Table X). A diet marginal in essential trace elements predisposes to toxicity, even though it may be adequate for growth.

In Table XLI are given the differences between the concentrations of manganese, copper, and zinc, as well as nickel, in the organs of rats receiving plain water and in those given our basic water containing luxus amounts of these essential trace metals. No accumulation with age occurred. It is clear that the starch diet was marginal in copper and zinc, and contained not enough manganese. Growth of the rats on plain water, however, was not depressed, and the diet was adequate in this respect.

This study also showed that there was significantly more nickel in the hearts and spleens of rats fed plain water than in those given the trace metals plus nickel, indicating that the other metals inhibit the absorption and/or retention of nickel. Therefore, the organs had space for more essential trace metals than the diet supplied, except nickel, and presumably would be more susceptible to unnatural metals competing for ligands on or in cells. These experiments illustrate the necessity of an adequate diet in any study of toxicity in animals.

## G. Other Mechanisms of Toxicity

Not many metallic inhibitors to metalloenzymes acting by displacement are known (Table XXXV). There are, however, many examples of enzyme poisonings by metals which bind amino, imino, and sulfhydryl groups on proteins, such groups being reactive sites which chelate metals (3). Copper, mercury, cadmium, and silver are examples. The order of stability of sulfur chelates of metals is $Hg > Cu > Ni > Pb > Co = Cd > Zn > Fe > Mn > Mg > Ca$. Toxicity of metals partly depends on electronegativity, and the order of decreasing electronegativity of divalent metals is as follows: $Hg > Cu > Sn > Pb > Ni > Co > Fe > Cd > Zn > Mn > Cr > Mg > Ca > Sr > Ba$. The last seven metals have low orders of toxicity and are essential. Incidently, crustal abundances also follow a somewhat similar order: Be < Hg < Ag < Cd < Sn < Pb < Co < Cu < Zn < Ni < Cr < Sr < Ba < Mn < Mg < Ca < Fe, the first six being toxic and most of the last 11 being essential.

Other electronegative metals such as silver, molybdenum, antimony, tellurium, and tungsten also form insoluble sulfides and are enzyme poisons *(3)*.

Arsenate and chlorate behave as antimetabolites for phosphate and nitrate, respectively. Probably borate, bromate, permanganate, antimonate, selenate, tellurate, tungstate, and beryllilum can also act as antimetabolites *(3)*.

Some metals form stable precipitates or chelates with essential metabolites, such as when aluminum, beryllium, scandium, titanium, yttrium, and zirconium react with phosphate, barium with sulfate, and iron with ATP.

Some metals catalyze the decomposition of essential metabolites, such as lanthanum and its series decomposing ATP.

Some metals combine with cell membranes, affecting permeability, such as gold, cadmium, copper, mercury, lead, uranium or free halogens $F_2$, $Cl_2$, $Br_2$, and $I_2$. These elements affect cellular transport systems for sodium, potassium, or chloride, or rupture the membrane *(3)*.

Some elements replace electrochemically or structurally essential elements but fail to function; examples include lithuim replacing sodium, rubidium replacing potassium, cesium replacing potassium, and bromine replacing chlorine. Toxicity depends on the degree of divergence from the neon or argon structure as follows *(3)*:

$$Li > Na = K < Rb < Cs$$
$$Be > Mg = Ca < Sr < Ba$$
$$F > Cl < Br < I$$

Metal–organic compounds are either more toxic than metal ions or less so. For example, alkyl lead, tin, and mercury are highly toxic, as are most of the carbonyls, whereas the chelates are much less toxic.

The valence state of the element which occurs in nature is always the least toxic form, e.g., tetravalent carbon, silicon, germanium, tin, lead, vanadium; pentavalent nitrogen, phosphorus, arsenic, antimony, bismuth: hexavalent sulfur (also divalent), selenium, tellurium, molybdenum; trivalent chromium. The mammalian body usually has the ability to oxidize or reduce elements into the form required by the body, e.g.,

$$Mn^{2+} \longrightarrow Mn^{3+}, Cr^{6+} \longrightarrow Cr^{3+}, Fe^{2+} \rightleftarrows Fe^{3+}, Cu^{+} \rightleftarrows Cu^{2+}, Mo^{6+} \longrightarrow Mo^{5+} \longleftarrow Mo^{3+}$$

and probably $V^{5+} \longrightarrow V^{4+} \longleftarrow V^{3+}$. Manganese is trivalent in blood, molybdenum is pentavalent in molybdoflavin enzymes.

The mammalian body responds to one toxic metal by synthesizing a protein which binds it. Metallothionein is synthesized by a number of tissues in response to feeding or injecting cadmium *(35a)*. This protein is unusual in that it has a high component of sulfur-containing amino acids, which bind cadmium, mercury, copper, zinc, and lead. Synthesis of the protein, however, is not induced by any known metal but cadmium. Whether or not tolerance to a toxic element depends upon similar processes is not known, but cadmium may be unique in this respect because of its low order of abundance on the earth's crust and the lack of need for detoxifying mechanisms during evolutionary development.

TABLE XLII

EFFECTS OF CADMIUM IN FOOD AND WATER ON SYSTOLIC BLOOD PRESSURE OF RATS[a]

| Age (months) | Cd (0.07 ppm) | Cd (0.63 ppm) | Cd (5.1 ppm) | $p$[b] |
|---|---|---|---|---|
| | | *Females* | | |
| 3 | 85±2.2 | 109±3.2 | — | <0.001 |
| 4 | 87±4.4 | 110±3.7 | — | <0.001 |
| 5 | 81±2.2 | 112±6.1 | — | <0.001 |
| 7 | — | 115±4.0 | — | <0.001 |
| 12 | 84±5.8 | — | 211±8.3 | <0.001 |
| 13 | 82±3.4 | — | — | — |
| 17 | 92±4.9 | — | 182±12.6 | <0.001 |
| 24 | 84±3.8 | — | 205±10.9 | <0.001 |
| 30 | 99±4.2 | — | 229±12.9 | <0.001 |
| | | *Males* | | |
| 12 | 106±5.7 | — | 124±5.6 | <0.025 |
| 17 | 94±3.8 | — | 122±4.5 | <0.001 |
| 24 | 79±3.6 | — | 137±6.2 | <0.001 |
| 30 | 93±5.1 | — | 198±7.9 | <0.001 |
| | | *Females*, 17 | | |
| Calcium in water | | | 92[c] | |
| No calcium | | | 253[d] | <0.001 |
| Renal cadmium (ppm) | 0.03±0.002 | 0.76±0.060 | 54.7±4.82 | <0.0001 |
| Hepatic cadmium (ppm) | 0.03±0.008 | 0.58±0.160 | 20.9±3.91 | <0.0001 |

[a] In all groups but three given calcium, there were 16–24 rats. In the third column, cadmium (5.0 ppm) was given in water. Data from Kanisawa and Schroeder *(27)*. Blood pressure in mm Hg.
[b] $p$ is significance of the difference between the two groups shown.
[c] 8 rats normotensive, 2 hypertensive (260 mm Hg).
[d] All of 10 rats were hypertensive.

## XII. PRODUCTION OF CHRONIC DISEASES SIMULATING HUMAN DISORDERS

Two common cardiovascular diseases can be reproduced in rats by inducing trace metal imbalances. These disorders mimic the physiological, biochemical, and pathological changes which characterize the human condition.

### A. Cadmium Hypertension

The most subtle action of cadmium yet discovered is the effect on blood pressure. Even small increments in food raised the blood pressures of rats. In Table XLII are shown the mean systolic blood pressures of rats given our low-cadmium diet (0.07 ppm cadmium), and a commercial diet (0.63 ppm cadmium). Pressures were taken on warmed, anaesthesized rats and were basal. Those fed the commercial diet had significantly higher pressures than those fed the low-cadmium diet, and their kidneys contained 25 times as much cadmium. There was also 20 times as much cadmium in their livers. This experiment not only illustrates the subtle action of cadmium on normal blood pressure but points out that earlier experimental studies of hypertension have been made in the presence of varying concentrations of renal and hepatic cadmium coming from commercial diets.

When 5 ppm cadmium was given in water, all rats became hypertensive at 2 years of age. This condition was associated with the following changes: (a) hypertrophy and thickening of renal arterioles (Table XIX) and in other arteries. (b) left ventricular hypertrophy (6), and (c) increased deposition of lipid plaques in the aorta. These changes are characteristic of human hypertension. Many deaths were caused by internal hemorrhage, and life-span was shortened.

The same accumulation of cadmium and the same changes in cadmium : zinc ratios occur in human hypertension (Table XLIII).

Cadmium accumulates in the walls of arteries, changing their reactivity to vasoconstrictor substances *(36–38)*. Injected cadmium has produced hypertension in the rat *(39,40)*, rabbit *(41)*, and dog *(42)*, when given intraperitoneally.

The cadmium can be partly removed from kidney, liver, and, presumably, blood vessels, by injecting a chelating agent which has a higher affinity for cadmium than for zinc *(43)*. Such an agent must have a high stability constant for both metals, higher than those in tissues, and be relatively nontoxic. We can assume that much zinc in the mammalian body is more loosely bound than are many other metals, for ethylenediaminetetraacetic acid (EDTA) injected in man causes zincuria of 6 to 12 times normal, with only a doubling of the excretion of other metals *(44)*, and the drug can induce zinc deficiency. In order to save zinc, and deposit it in places from which cadmium was removed, a zinc-loaded chelate is required. Sodium zinc cyclohexanediaminotetraacetic acid (CDTA) was found to be efficient in this respect, causing reversal of hypertension for many months, removing cadmium from kidney and liver and leaving zinc *(43)*. It appears to work similarly in man. Oral doses are ineffective in rats.

Cadmium can have other subtle effects. In Table XLIV is shown recondite toxicity of only 1 ppm added to drinking water, in terms of inhibition of two serum enzymes, serum glucose level ovarian weight, fertility, and viability of offspring of rats. These changes occurred in 240 days *(45)*. We have confirmed effects on reproduction *(31)*. Oxygen consumption of rats was also increased.

TABLE XLIII

RENAL CADMIUM (PPM ASH) AND CADMIUM/ZINC RATIOS (+SEM) IN HUMAN KIDNEYS ACCORDING TO MAJOR CAUSE OF DEATH[a]

| Cause of death | No. cases | Cd (mean µg/gm) | $p$[b] | Cd/Zn (mean µg/gm) | $p$[b] |
|---|---|---|---|---|---|
| United States mainland | | | | | |
| Hypertension | 17 | 4220 | — | 0.77 | — |
| Accidents | 117 | 2940 | <0.0005 | 0.62 | <0.01 |
| Arteriosclerotic heart disease | 27 | 2660 | <0.0005 | 0.62 | <0.01 |
| Miscellaneous | 26 | 3380 | N.S. | 0.58 | <0.01 |
| Foreign | | | | | |
| Hypertension | 17 | 5080 | — | 0.94 | — |
| Accidents | 23 | 3170 | <0.025 | 0.66 | <0.005 |
| Arteriosclerotic heart disease | 12 | 2430 | <0.01 | 0.49 | <0.005 |
| All cases | | | | | |
| Cerebral vascular accident | 23 | 4266 | — | 0.80 | — |
| Traumatic accident | 140 | 2980 | <0.0005 | 0.62 | <0.005 |

[a] Data from Schroeder *(35)*.
[b] $p$ is significance of differences of mean from hypertension or cerebral vascular accident.

TABLE XLIV

EFFECTS OF CADMIUM (1 PPM) IN DRINKING WATER ON VARIOUS FUNCTIONS OF RATS. CHANGES FROM CONTROLS [a]

| Function | Change (%) | $p$ [b] |
|---|---|---|
| SGOT | −14.0 | <0.05 |
| Glucose, serum | −14.7 | <0.04 |
| Aldolase | −23.8 | <0.001 |
| Succinic oxidase | −60 | >0.05 |
| Phosphorylase, hepatic | | |
| Total | −12.5 | — |
| a | +21.2 | — |
| b | −16.6 | — |
| Oxidative phosphorylation by hepatic mitochondria | +7.4 | — |
| Oxygen consumption | | |
| Males | +33.9 | <0.02 |
| Females | +48.8 | <0.01 |
| Ovarian weight | −40.7 | |
| Fertility of females | −14 | |
| Viability of progeny | −26–37 | |

[a] From Sporn et al. (1970). *Igeina* **19**, 729–739.
[b] $p$ is significance of change from control values.

Injected cadmium produces another hypertensive manifestation, toxemia of pregnancy in rats *(46)*. It also causes sterility and induces sodium retention *(47)*. These effects can be ameliorated or prevented by surplus zinc.

It is very likely that human hypertension is a sign of recondite cadmium toxicity. Both the renal cadmium and zinc changes, and the finding of 40 times as much urinary cadmium in hypertensive persons as in normal ones reinforces this theory. There is a significant correlation of deaths from hypertensive heart disease and airborne cadmium in this country *(48)*.

The evidence, therefore, for cadmium being a causal factor in human hypertension can be summarized as follows:

1. Higher renal cadmium or cadmium : zinc ratios in persons dying of hypertensive causes *without severe renal damage*. Cadmium is lost from the kidney when the kidney degenerates *(35)*. Lener *(49)* has confirmed our findings in 22 patients. Morgan *(50)*, on the other hand, found little difference in renal cadmium in Negroes dying in the hospital from hypertension or other causes; perhaps their kidneys were damaged.

2. High urinary cadmium in patients with severe hypertension, presumably with damaged kidneys.

3. General correlation of the incidence of hypertension with renal cadmium in various areas of the world *(35)*.
4. Reduction of blood pressure by Na$_2$Zn CDTA in preliminary experiments, with removal of cadmium.
5. Accumulation of cadmium by arteries.
6. Reproduction of the disease by feeding cadmium to rats, and its reversal by the zinc chelate, which removes cadmium. Reproduction of human renal and hepatic cadmium levels in rats. The extreme sensitivity of the blood pressure to cadmium. Our observations have been confirmed *(51)*. Induction of the release of renin by cadmium *(40)* as well as retention of sodium *(47)*.

Persons in Japan severely poisoned by cadmium from a zinc and copper mine apparently did not have excessive hypertension. They showed very high hepatic, bone, and tissue cadmium and low renal cadmium probably associated with renal failure. The disease was characterized by severe osteomalacia and there was heavy accumulation of lead and loss of calcium. Postmenopausal women were mainly affected and many died of *"itai-itai"* or ouch-ouch disease *(52,53)*.

## B. Overt Cadmium Toxicity

Demonstrable toxicity from cadmium in exposed workers is not accompanied by hypertension. There is proteinuria, renal damage, and pulmonary emphysema, coming from cadmium in inspired air. This reversal of effect with increasing dose was demonstrated in rats *(37)* by intraarterial injections; small doses were pressor, large doses were depressor. Therefore, the dose of cadmium is all-important in determining effects. So is the route of administration; intravenous cadmium is irregularly pressor and depressor *(54)*, but intraperitoneal cadmium is always pressor and pulmonary cadmium may be pressor only locally.

Therefore, cadmium is toxic at all but the very smallest levels of intake, and the manifestations of its toxicity in mammals change with increasing doses.

## C. Atherosclerosis in Rats

This very common human disorder was studied in several ways. In man, it is characterized by subintimal deposits of lipid material forming in areas of degeneration of mucopolysaccharides, which build up to produce plaques. In the coronaries the plaque may occlude the arterial lumen, or lose its intima and constitute the focus of a clot. In the aorta, plaques only occasionally do serious harm, but in the legs and cerebral arteries they may cause ischemic gangrene or infarcts, preceded by ischemia. With the disease go abnormal glucose tolerance or mild diabetes mellitus, and a lipid metabolic disorder characterized by elevated serum cholesterol and fats (triglycerides). The basic abnormality of the disease is probably a factor causing serum lipids to rise with age and glucose metabolism to be depressed.

That trace elements may influence these functions in rats has been partly documented. In Table XLV are recorded microscopic findings of focal myocardial fibrosis, the probable result of occlusion of coronary arteries, as influenced by eight trace elements in drinking water. There were few such scars in the control, selenate, tellurite, and nickel groups, whereas there was a moderately significant increase in the niobium, zirconium, and lead groups, and a more significant increase in the vanadium, cadmium, and antimony groups. Niobium and vanadium, and zirconium and chromium interact, and chromium protects against lead intoxication; these interactions may explain the lesions. Vanadium, zirconium, antimony, and niobium affect lipid metabolism, as does chromium.

TABLE XLV

INTERSTITIAL FOCAL MYOCARDIAL FIBROSIS IN RATS FED VARIOUS TRACE ELEMENTS FOR LIFE IN DRINKING WATER

| Element | Dose (ppm) | No. rats | Fibrosis No. | % | $p^a$ | Myocarditis, focal | Chromium in water (ppm) |
|---|---|---|---|---|---|---|---|
| Controls | — | 61 | 1 | 1.6 | — | — | 1 |
| Controls | — | 52 | 0 | 0 | — | — | 5 |
| Selenate | 3 | 65 | 2 | 3.0 | N.S. | — | 5 |
| Tellurite | 2 | 36 | 2 | 5.6 | N.S. | — | 5 |
| Nickel | 5 | 30 | 4 | 13.3 | <0.01 | — | 5 |
| Niobium | 5 | 78 | 12 | 15.4 | <0.0005 | 1 | 1 |
| Zirconium | 5 | 63 | 12 | 19.0 | <0.0005 | 1 | 1 |
| Lead[b,c] | 25 | 31 | 8 | 25.8 | <0.0001 | — | 1 |
| Vanadium | 5 | 27 | 7 | 25.9 | <0.0001 | — | 1 |
| Cadmium[c] | 5 | 23 | 6 | 26.1 | <0.0001 | — | 5 |
| Antimony[c] | 5 | 60 | 23 | 38.3 | <0.0001 | — | 1 |

[a] $p$ is difference from controls by chi-square analysis.
[b] Males only.
[c] Recondite toxicity in terms of longevity.

Note: These sections of heart were all read by J. B. Blennerhassett, M.D., of the Department of Pathology, Massachusetts General Hospital, Boston, Massachusetts.

## D. Aortic Lipids and Plaques

The feeding of certain trace elements induces plaques in the aortas of rats. These lesions can be considered a sign of recondite toxicity. In Tables XLVI and XLVII are the differences from the controls. Plaques can be visualized readily by examining the aortas under ultraviolet light, and graded + to 4+ in this way (55).

The total fluorescent score was calculated by assigning 0.5 to ±, 1 to +, and 4 to 4+, and dividing by the number of aortas. The controls given chromium had low values, and the number with 2+ to 4+ was small. However, male rats fed zirconium, niobium, vanadium, antimony, lead

TABLE XLVI
Fluorescent Scores on Aortas of Male Rats

| Element | No. | Score[a] | 2+ to 4+ No. | Total score | % | $p$[b] | Chromium in water (ppm) |
|---|---|---|---|---|---|---|---|
| Control-1 | 27 | 1.60 | 14 | 49 | 51.8 | — | 0 |
| Control-2 | 45 | 1.14 | 13 | 35 | 29.0 | — | 1 |
| Control-3 | 48 | 1.15 | 15 | 39 | 31.2 | — | 5 |
| Tin | 43 | 1.15 | 10 | 31 | 22.8 | — | 1 |
| Germanium | 55 | 1.36 | 24 | 62 | 43.6 | <0.01 | 1 |
| Arsenic | 48 | 1.39 | 21 | 55 | 43.8 | — | 1 |
| Chromium | 24 | 1.40 | 2 | 5 | 8.3 | <0.01 | 5 |
| Zirconium | 46 | 1.70 | 24 | 65 | 52.2 | <0.0005 | 1 |
| Vanadium | 32 | 1.81 | 19 | 51 | 59.3 | <0.0005 | 1 |
| Antimony | 47 | 1.82 | 26 | 77 | 55.2 | <0.0005 | 1 |
| Lead-1 | 30 | 2.00 | 21 | 52 | 70.0 | — | 0 |
| Lead-2 | 42 | 2.13 | 30 | 83 | 71.4 | <0.0005 | 1 |
| Niobium | 45 | 2.34 | 33 | 97 | 72.7 | <0.0005 | 1 |
| Tellurite | 28 | 2.34 | 22 | 61 | 78.6 | <0.0001 | 5 |
| Cadmium | 25 | 2.70 | 23 | 58 | 92.2 | <0.0001 | 0 |
| Selenite | 11 | 2.73 | 10 | 29 | 90.9 | <0.0005 | 5 |
| Selenate | 27 | 2.83 | 23 | 73 | 85.3 | <0.0001 | 5 |
| *Young rats—torula diet* | | | | | | | |
| Control | 13 | 1.27 | 6 | 13 | 46.1 | — | 0 |
| Chromium | 8 | 0.69 | 1 | 2 | 12.5 | — | 5 |
| Vanadium | 12 | 0.87 | 4 | 10 | 33.3 | — | 0 |
| Vanadium + Chromium | 12 | 0.67 | 1 | 2 | 8.3 | <0.025 | 5 |

[a] Score calculated by assigning 0.5 to ±, 1 to +, 2 to ++, 3 to +++, and 4 to ++++, and dividing by number of aortas.
[b] $p$ is significance of difference from comparable control value of 2+ to 4+ scores by chi-square analysis.

## TABLE XLVII
### FLUORESCENT SCORES ON AORTAS OF FEMALE RATS

| Element | No. | Score[a] | 2+ to 4+ No. | Total score | Percentage | $p^a$ | Chromium in water (ppm) |
|---|---|---|---|---|---|---|---|
| Control-1 | 20 | 1.70 | 7 | 19 | 35.0 | — | 0 |
| Control-2 | 44 | 1.00 | 12 | 32 | 27.2 | — | 1 |
| Control-3 | 45 | 0.87 | 10 | 27 | 22.2 | — | 5 |
| Tin | 50 | 1.21 | 20 | 51 | 40.0 | — | 1 |
| Germanium | 42 | 1.27 | 16 | 40 | 38.2 | — | 1 |
| Chromium | 19 | 1.40 | 1 | 3 | 5.3 | <0.001 | 5 |
| Arsenic | 50 | 1.67 | 29 | 77 | 58.0 | <0.01 | 1 |
| Zirconium | 51 | 1.74 | 25 | 70 | 49.0 | — | 1 |
| Vanadium | 39 | 1.93 | 22 | 63 | 56.3 | <0.001 | 1 |
| Lead | 20 | 1.94 | 13 | 28 | 65.0 | — | 0 |
| Antimony | 46 | 2.10 | 27 | 80 | 58.6 | <0.0005 | 1 |
| Niobium | 50 | 2.30 | 34 | 101 | 68.0 | <0.0005 | 1 |
| Selenite | 17 | 2.41 | 15 | 40 | 87.9 | <0.0001 | 5 |
| Cadmium | 26 | 2.60 | 24 | 54 | 92.3 | <0.001 | 0 |
| Tellurite | 30 | 2.78 | 26 | 81 | 86.7 | <0.0001 | 5 |
| Selenate | 30 | 3.25 | 27 | 95 | 90.0 | <0.0001 | 5 |
| Cadmium, injected with Zn CDTA | 11 | 0 | 0 | 0 | 0 | <0.0001 | 0 |

[a] Score calculated by assigning 0.5 to ±, 1 to +, 2 to ++, 3 to +++, and 4 to ++++, and dividing by number of aortas.

[b] $p$ is significance of difference from comparable control value of 2+ to 4+ scores by chi-square analysis.

—the elements which produced myocardial scars—and cadmium had significantly increased scores, with high percentages of 2+ to 4+. Unlike the situation with myocardial scars, tellurium and selenium had high scores, many with 2+ to 4+. In females, the same elements, except zirconium, gave high scores.

Eleven cadmium-fed hypertensive female rats were injected with $Na_2Zn$ CDTA in one dose. Aortic fluorescence 2 weeks later was wiped out, although a high score was expected, and there were no plaques. Forty-four young rats aged 4 to 5 months were weaned on the torula yeast diet. They were given chromium, vanadium, and the two together. Fluorescent scores were low, and there were only two plaques in those fed chromium, both small. Young rats naturally have low scores, but the difference from controls was significant in this experiment.

Fluorescence was caused by lipids, for it could be removed by lipid solvents and the dissolved material continued to fluoresce, while the aorta did not. These data, therefore, show that certain trace elements cause lipid deposition and plaques in the aorta, whereas chromium reduces the plaques and the lipids.

There was a significant correlation of serum cholesterol levels in male rats with aortic plaques and fluorescence scores ($r = 0.59$, $p < 0.01$) but not in females.

Therefore, the disease atherosclerosis was reproduced in rats by chromium deficiency. It mimicked the human disease in all of its basic essentials: Pathological lesions, elevated serum cholesterol, glucose intolerance, and occlusions of coronary arteries.

### E. Human Atherosclerosis

A number of trace elements have been implicated in atherosclerosis by experiments on animals (56). These are listed in Table XLVIII, along with others implicated in secondary changes. Aside from chromium, manganese and vanadium affect lipid metabolism in rats and are theoretically protective. Excesses of copper in the diet of experimental animals increased the tendency to atherosclerosis (57,58). Copper in human aorta, however, decreases with age and, presumably, with increasing severity of atherosclerosis.

We can examine the aortic concentrations of 20 elements according to geographical area (59). In Table XLIX are the data on males; they can be interpreted in the light of the variable incidence of atherosclerosis, which is low in the Near and Far East, in Africa, and in Switzerland, and highest in the United States. These variations are reflected in the calcium and ash values. In terms of wet weight, ash increases with age regularly from the first to the eighth decade 3.5 times, calcium 5 times, and magnesium 5.6 times; these changes are undoubtedly secondary to the disease (60).

TABLE XLVIII
TRACE ELEMENTS CONSIDERED INVOLVED EXPERIMENTALLY IN CARDIOVASCULAR DISEASES[a]

| Disease | Protective | Inductive |
| --- | --- | --- |
| Atherosclerosis | Chromium, manganese, vanadium, cobalt | Cobalt (injected), copper, chromium deficiency |
| Hypertension | Zinc | Cadmium, zinc deficiency |
| Aortic calcification | Fluorine, magnesium | Fluorine deficiency |
| Elasticity of arteries | Lithium, copper | |
| Focal myocardial necrosis | Selenium | Arsenic |

[a] Adapted from Masironi (56).

### TABLE XLIX
Significant Differences in Elemental Content of Aorta in Five Areas of World, Males, Aged 20–59 (ppm Ash) Median Values[a]

| Element | United States | Africa | Near East | Far East | Switzerland |
|---|---|---|---|---|---|
| Essential | | | | | |
| Chromium | 1.9 | 5.5 | 11[b] | 15[b] | 30[b] |
| Manganese | 8 | 13[b] | 18[b] | 22[b] | 9 |
| Iron | 2900 | 2800 | 4600 | 5600[b] | 2300 |
| Copper[c] | 91 | 110 | 180[b] | 160[b] | 110 |
| Nonessential | | | | | |
| Aluminum | 28 | 840[b] | 1000[b] | 450[b] | 69 |
| Barium | 7 | 14[b] | 19[b] | 19[b] | 17[b] |
| Nickel | <5 | 7 | 24 | 21[b] | 13[b] |
| Silver | 0.1 | <0.1 | 1.4[b] | 1.0[b] | <0.1[b] |
| Titanium | <5 | 20[b] | 59[b] | 20[b] | 12[b] |
| Bulk | | | | | |
| Calcium (%)[d] | 5.0 | 3.3 | 2.9 | 2.4[b] | 6.6 |
| Phosphorus (%) | 7 | 6 | 13[b] | 10[b] | 8 |
| Ash (% of dry wt.)[e] | 3.8 | 4.4 | 3.0 | 2.6[b] | 4.6 |

[a] Data from Tipton et al. (59). There were no significant differences in aortic cadmium, lead, magnesium, molybdenum, potassium, strontium, tin, vanadium, or zinc.
[b] Differs from United States value, $p < 0.001$.
[c] Decreases with age, $p < 0.001$, $r = -0.51$, United States values only.
[d] Increases with age, $p < 0.001$, $r = +0.43$.
[e] Increases with age, $p < 0.001$, $r = +0.51$.

Note: The incidence of atherosclerotic heart disease is very high in the United States and very low in Switzerland, Japan, and Thailand. It is moderately low in Taiwan, Manila, Hong Kong, India, and Africa [personal observations and "Atherosclerosis," Vol. 1, DHEW Publ. No. (NIH) 72-137, 1971].

On viewing these data on a possible etiological basis, one can suspect chromium, manganese, and copper are among the essential trace elements which are protective, and aluminum, barium, nickel, and titanium among the abnormal ones, which are also "protective." Of these, chromium and manganese appear as "protective" in Table XLVIII. In no case could one of these elements be considered as "inductive," except calcium.

Table L lists the elements involved as secondary to atherosclerosis and myocardial infarction. Silver was said to be increased in the aorta; in the geographical data it was decreased, if anything. Copper, manganese, and chromium were decreased, which fits the geographical data.

In order to obtain further clues, we can examine the heart from the geographical data (Table LI). Chromium is the only element which fits Table XLVIII and that not too well.

A breakdown of the data (Table LII) indicates high aortic chromium

TABLE L

SECONDARY CHANGES IN TRACE ELEMENTS IN ATHEROSCLEROSIS AND MYOCARDIAL INFARCTION[a]

|  | Increase | Decrease |
|---|---|---|
| Atherosclerosis |  |  |
| Aorta | Iron, molybdenum, cobalt, lead, silver, zinc | Copper, lithium, manganese, chromium |
| Heart | Cobalt, copper, zinc | Manganese |
| Plasma, or blood | Manganese | Zinc |
| Myocardial infarction |  |  |
| Injured tissue, heart | Barium, bromine, antimony | Manganese, molybdenum, aluminum, rubidium cobalt, cesium, zinc |
| Serum | Copper, nickel, manganese, boron, molybdenum, calcium | Zinc, iron |
| Urine | Copper |  |

[a] Adapted from Masironi (56).

in Honolulu, Anchorage, the Far East, Switzerland, and two cities in India; intermediate levels in most of Africa and Delhi; and low levels in the United States. There levels were reasonably well correlated with the prevalence of coronary occlusion in the several cities.

TABLE LI

SIGNIFICANT DIFFERENCES IN ELEMENTAL CONTENT OF HEART MUSCLE IN FIVE AREAS OF THE WORLD, MALES, AGED 20–59 (PPM ASH), MEDIAN VALUES[a]

| Element | United States | Africa | Near East | Far East | Switzerland |
|---|---|---|---|---|---|
| Essential |  |  |  |  |  |
| Chromium | 1.6 | 0.9 | 4.0 | 6.3[b] | 4.6 |
| Iron | 4700 | 4700 | 4500 | 7000[b] | 5100 |
| Nonessential |  |  |  |  |  |
| Aluminum | 20 | 250[b] | 190[b] | 180[b] | 22 |
| Barium | 0.7 | 5.0[b] | 7.4[b] | 3.5[b] | 3.6[b] |
| Lead | 5 | 5 | 21 | 21[b] | 14 |
| Silver | <0.1 | <0.1 | 0.5[b] | 0.3[b] | <0.1 |
| Titanium | <5 | <5 | 19[b] | 10[b] | <5 |
| Bulk |  |  |  |  |  |
| Phosphorus | 15 | 15 | 16 | 19[b] | 14 |

[a] Data from Tipton et al. (59). There were no significant differences in cardiac cadmium, calcium, copper, magnesium, manganese, molybdenum, nickel, potassium, strontium, tin, vanadium, or zinc.
[b] Differs from United States values, $p < 0.001$.

## TABLE LII
AORTIC CHROMIUM FROM VARIOUS GEOGRAPHICAL AREAS ($\mu$g/gm ASH) [a]

| Geographical area | No. cases | Mean ± SEM ($\mu$g/gm) | Prevalence of coronary heart disease (% of cases) |
|---|---|---|---|
| United States, 9 cities | 64[b] | 1.9 | |
|  | 103[c] | 4.4±0.5 | 11.0 |
| San Francisco | 27 | 2.6±1.1 | 64.3 |
| Honolulu | 12 | 14±4.3 | 0.0 |
| Anchorage | 2 | 13±9.7 | 0.0 |
| Far East | 35[b] | 15[d] | 7.5 |
| Japan | 28 | 15±2.9 | 7.1 |
| Taipei | 10 | 26±10 | 0.0 |
| Manila | 10 | 37±11 | 0.0 |
| Bangkok | 10 | 44±24 | 0.0 |
| Hong Kong | 10 | 7.6±1.9 | 30.0 |
| Africa | 13[b] | 5.5 | 0.0 |
| Caucasoid | 13 | 4.3±1.4 | |
| Negroid | 41 | 7.5±2.8 | |
| Addis Ababa | 5 | 3.7±1.8 | |
| Lagos | 17 | 3.7±1.1 | |
| Cairo | 8 | 6.0±2.1 | |
| Welkom | 5 | 25±6.5 | |
| Bern, Switzerland | 9[b] | 30±23 | 20.0 |
| India | 9[b] | 11[d] | 0.0 |
| Delhi | 8 | 6.0±1.9 | |
| Lucknow | 4 | 22±11 | |
| Bombay | 8 | 71±55 | |

[a] Data from Schroeder et al. (61).
[b] Males 20–59 years old, only.
[c] Accidental or sudden deaths only.
[d] Differs from United States value, $p < 0.001$.

Analysis of aortas of people dying of coronary heart disease showed virtually no aortic chromium, and 64.6% had no detectable chromium at all, whereas of people dying of accidents 80–100% showed aortic chromium (Table LIII), and the differences in concentration were significant. No other trace metal showed imbalance in aortas of subjects with coronary heart disease (61). This deficiency was specific for coronary disease, although subjects with other cardiovascular diseases had intermediate values of aortic chromium.

Therefore, two common human cardiovascular diseases can be reproduced in rats by trace metal imbalances. Their similarities are shown in Table LIV.

## TABLE LIII
Chromium in Aortas of Subjects Dying from Atherosclerotic Heart Disease (AHD), Other Cardiovascular Diseases (CVD), and Accidents ($\mu$g/gm Dry Weight)[a]

| Location | No. of cases | Aortic chromium ($\mu$g/gm) | Prevalence (%) | p |
|---|---|---|---|---|
| San Francisco | | | | |
| AHD | 15 | 0.05±0.009 | 13.3 | — |
| AHD-moderate | 3 | 0.03±0.003 | 0 | — |
| Accidents | 10 | 0.23±0.076 | 80 | <0.005 |
| United States, 9 cities | | | | |
| AHD | 13 | 0.05±0.088 | 46.2 | — |
| CVD | 15 | 0.20±0.090 | 60 | — |
| Accidents | 103 | 0.26±0.067 | 87.4 | <0.005 |
| Africa | | | | |
| CVD | 2 | 0.12±0.026 | 100 | — |
| Other | 11 | 0.19±0.025 | 90.9 | <0.025 |
| Mid-East | | | | |
| CVD | 3 | 0.22±0.084 | 66.7 | — |
| Other | 11 | 1.28±0.831 | 100 | — |
| Far East | | | | |
| AHD | 5 | 0.25±0.132 | 100 | — |
| CVD | 20 | 0.31±0.073 | 85 | — |
| Accidents | 8 | 0.97±0.532 | 100 | — |

[a] Data from Schroeder et al. (59).

## TABLE LIV
Experimental Counterparts of Human Cardiovascular Diseases. Trace Metal Imbalances

| Abnormality | Rats | Human beings |
|---|---|---|
| Atherosclerosis, Chromium deficiency | | |
| Glucose tolerance | Reduced | Reduced |
| Response to chromium | Normal | Normal in 40–50% |
| Serum cholesterol | Elevated | Elevated |
| Response to chromium | Reduced | Moderately reduced in 40–50% |
| Aortic plaques | Induced | ? Induced |
| Response to chromium | Prevented | ? |
| Status of tissue chromium | Deficient | Deficient, especially aorta |
| Hypertension, Cadmium excess | | |
| Blood pressure | Elevated | Elevated |
| Response to zinc chelate | Lowered | Moderately lowered |
| Renal arteriolar sclerosis | Present | Present |
| Cardiac enlargement | Present | Present |
| Renal cadmium | 40–60 ppm | 40–80 ppm |
| Renal cadmium: zinc ratio | >0.58 | >0.70 |
| Atherosclerosis | Increased | Increased |

On the surface it may not appear justifiable to include a deficiency disease as an example of recondite toxicity. As we have stated, however, deficiency opens the way to toxicity, and chromium deficiency has all the stigmata of toxicity. One cannot consider trace element imbalances without considering deficiencies as well as excesses.

## XIII. RECONDITE TOXICITY OF OTHER METALS OR ELEMENTS IN MAN

In Table I we find five toxic metals: cadmium, lead, mercury, antimony, and beryllium. Of these, two, cadmium and lead, are found in the human body in abnormally large amounts, a result of abnormal industrial exposures. We have shown that the smallest amount of cadmium exerts some effect, which, if amplified could be considered toxic.

Lead, as we have shown, shortens median life-span, reduces maximal longevity, and inhibits reproduction; in man, the smallest amount of lead exerts an effect which, if amplified, could be considered toxic. The enzyme $\delta$-aminolevulinic acid dehydrase (62) is inhibited at all levels of exposure in proportion to blood lead levels. Therefore, no person living today in industrialized societies where lead from motor vehicle exhausts is widespread is free of the recondite toxicological effects of lead. The fact that such a disturbance does no visible or detectable "harm" in terms of health does not invalidate a warning of what could happen with larger doses. Thus, cadmium and lead have very low thresholds of recondite toxicity.

Mercury does not appear to have a low threshold of activity, or at least one has not been detected. People exposed to mercury in dental amalgams, laboratories, or industry apparently can tolerate much higher levels of mercury than of cadmium. Judging by hair levels, human beings remain healthy with one third to one half of the concentration deemed toxic, and 10 times the normal concentrations of cadmium. Mercury is less toxic in a chronic frame of reference than cadmium, because it is quite readily excreted from the mammalian body, whereas cadmium is not.

Mercury accumulates only moderately in kidney and liver, probably bound to metallothionein. It is also widely distributed in other tissues, and a balance at normal environmental exposures appears to be achieved, so that output equals intake.

When mercury is alkylated, its behavior changes radically; the same is found for lead and tin. It becomes lipotropic. Thus, tetramethyl and tetraethyl lead and tin, triethyl tin, and ethyl and methyl mercury all share this property, entering the brain, being stored there, and causing damage to nerve cells. In the case of alkyl mercury, the damage is permanent, of lead semipermanent, and of tin transient. These alkyl compounds must not be confused with their inorganic precursors. It is claimed that 80–100% of the mercury in all animal products is methyl mercury *(63)*.

Antimony is fairly toxic of itself, but we do not know the threshold levels or the earliest change from the smallest dose. Beryllium is probably the most toxic of all the elements, causing cancer in animals and granulomata in animals and man.

TABLE LV

CORRELATION COEFFICIENTS ($r$) OF SOME WATERBORNE TRACE ELEMENTS AND DEATH RATES FROM HYPERTENSIVE HEART DISEASE (HHD) AND ATHEROSCLEROTIC HEART DISEASE (AHD), UNITED STATES DATA, WHITE MALES AGED 45–64 YEARS[a]

| Element | River water (HHD) $r$ | $p$ | Municipal water (AHD) $r$ | $p$ |
|---|---|---|---|---|
| *Potassium* | — | — | −0.48 | <0.0005 |
| *Magnesium* | — | — | −0.40 | <0.0005 |
| Hardness | −0.44 | <0.01 | −0.41 | <0.0005 |
| *Silicon* | — | — | −0.34 | <0.0005 |
| *Sodium* | — | — | −0.27 | <0.01 |
| *Calcium* | — | — | −0.23 | <0.02 |
| *Vanadium* | −0.41 | <0.01 | −0.34 | <0.0005 |
| *Chromium* | −0.34 | <0.01 | — | N.S. |
| Barium | −0.26 | N.S. | −0.34 | <0.0005 |
| *Zinc* | −0.43 | <0.01 | — | N.S. |
| *Copper* | +0.11 | N.S. | +0.29 | <0.005 |
| Strontium | — | — | −0.29 | <0.005 |
| Fluorine | −0.53 | <0.01 | — | N.S. |
| Lithium | — | — | −0.28 | <0.005 |
| *Manganese* | −0.35 | <0.05 | +0.26 | <0.01 |
| α-Radioactivity | −0.42 | <0.01 | | |
| β-Radioactivity | −0.52 | <0.001 | −0.21 | <0.025 |
| Boron | −0.34 | <0.05 | — | N.S. |
| Lead | −0.46 | <0.01 | — | N.S. |
| Nickel | −0.36 | <0.05 | — | N.S. |
| *Molybdenum* | −0.36 | <0.05 | — | N.S. |

[a] Data from Masironi *(64)* and Schroeder *(65–67)*. Essential elements in italics. N.S. = Not significant, $r$ being low.

Note: Hardness of municipal water showed the following negative correlations: with HHD, −0.57; with vascular lesions of the central nervous system, −0.34.

## XIV. INNATE TOXICITY FROM WATER

Drinking water is one variable to which all populations are exposed. It contains the soluble elements in the soil which it leaches. Surface waters are usually soft; well waters are hard with calcium and magnesium salts. River waters vary considerably in hardness. There were significant positive correlations of hardness of United States river water and concentra-

TABLE LVI

SUMMARY OF WATER QUALITY AND CARDIOVASCULAR DEATH RATES; HYPERTENSIVE HEART DISEASE (HHD), CEREBROVASCULAR DISEASE (CVD), AND ARTERIOSCLEROTIC HEART DISEASE (AHD), WHITE MALES 45–64. COEFFICIENTS OF CORRELATION $(r)$ [a]

| Area | Type of water | Water quality | Disease | $r$ | Ref. |
|---|---|---|---|---|---|
| Japan | R[b] | $SO^{2-}_4/HCO_3-$ | CVD | + High | (71) |
| United States | M[c] | Hardness | HHD | −0.57 | (65, 66) |
| | | | CVD | −0.34 | |
| | | | AHD | −0.48 | |
| United States | M | Trace metals Hardness | HHD | −0.42 | (67) |
| | | | CVD | −0.25 | |
| | | | AHD | −0.51 | |
| Great Britain | M | Hardness | HHD | −0.22 | (68) |
| | | | CVD | −0.42 | |
| | | | AHD | −0.39 | |
| Great Britain | M | Hardness | CVD | −0.56 | (71a) |
| | | | AHD | −0.52 | |
| United States | R | Hardness Trace metals Radioactivity | HHD | −0.44 | (64) |
| | | | AHD | −0.13 | |
| Ontario | M | Hardness | AHD | −High | (70) (sudden deaths) |
| Sweden | M | Hardness | Other HD | −High | (69) |
| South America | M | Hardness | HHD | −High | (64) (71b) |
| Netherlands | M | Hardness | All heart | −High women | (71c) |

[a] Data from references 64–71 including 71a, 71b, and 71c.
[b] R = River water.
[c] M = Municipal water.

tions of the following trace elements; (r values from 0.95 to 0.90) in this order: Bi, Sb, Sn, Co, Cd, Cr, V, Ni, Mo, Zn; (0.87 to 0.65) Pb, B, Mn; (0.57 to 0.44) F, Be, Ag, Ba; (0.30 to 0.21) Fe, Cu. There were significant negative correlations of trace elements in river water and deaths from hypertensive heart disease in persons living in areas drained by these rivers as follows: $r > -0.50$ for fluorine; $r = -0.50$ to $0.40$ for vanadium, zinc, lead, and tin; $r = -0.40$ to $0.30$ for bismuth, antimony, cobalt, nickel, cadmium, chromium, molybdenum, manganese, boron,

TABLE LVII

Uptake of Cadmium from Pipes by Soft Water[a]

| Area | Cadmium (µg/gm) | Zinc (µg/gm) | Hardness (ppm) | pH |
|---|---|---|---|---|
| Brattleboro, Vermont | | | | |
| Inlet to reservoir | 2.1 | 3.5 | 18.5 | 6.5 |
| Reservoir | 2.5 | 3.5 | — | — |
| Water main after 5 miles of flow | 14.0–21.0 | — | — | — |
| Hospital tap, galvanized | | | | |
| Cold running | 8.3 | 160 | — | — |
| Stagnant 24 hours | 15.0–77.0 | 1830 | — | — |
| Hot running | 21.0 | — | — | — |
| Institution, cold running, brass pipe | 1.0 | — | 18.5 | 6.5 |
| Bridgeport, Connecticut | | | | |
| Tap | 14.0 | — | 25 | 6.6 |
| White Plains, New York | | | | |
| Tap | 14.0 | — | 72 | 7.0 |
| Bangor (Roseto), Pennsylvania | 0.0 | — | 110 | 7.6 |
| Deep well, Vermont | | | | |
| Iron pipe | 1.1 | 100 | Hard | — |
| Iron pipe | 3.5 | 2160 | Hard | — |
| Artesian well, Vermont | | | | |
| Copper and plastic pipe | 12.0 | 219 | Hard | — |
| Spring, Vermont | | | | |
| Iron pipe | 3.5 | — | Soft | — |
| Copper pipe | 8.3 | 770 | Soft | — |
| Iron pipe | 3.8 | 660 | Soft | — |
| South Carolina | | | | |
| Iron pipe | 12.3 | 219 | Soft | — |
| Arkansas | | | | |
| Bottled | <0.3 | <0.3 | Hard | — |
| Distilled, glass still | 0.5 | 6 | — | — |
| Deionized | 0 | 0 | — | — |
| Snow, moderate traffic, suburban | 1.5 | 1380 | — | — |
| Hilltop | 0.35 | 45 | — | — |
| Hilltop | 0.38 | 8 | — | — |

[a] Data from Schroeder et al. (75).

and silver. Poor correlations were found for barium, beryllium, iron, and copper. For hardness, $r = -0.44$, and for radioactivity, $r = -0.52$ to $-0.42$. All correlations were negative—that is, the softer the water and the more dilute the element, the higher the death rate. Coronary heart disease was poorly correlated with these constituents of water *(64)*.

One half or more of cases of coronary heart disease have mild or moderate hypertension, one of the "risk factors." Perhaps this is the reason. Death rates from this disease are correlated in respect to the constituents of municipal water listed in Table LV. Both hypertensive heart disease and coronary heart disease are thus correlated with something in hard water or its absence in soft water *(65–67)*.

This relationship has been shown in Great Britain *(68)*, Sweden *(69)*, Canada *(70)*, South America *(64)*, Washington State *(64)*, and The Netherlands *(64)*. In Japan, the relationship was between acidity of river water and cerebral hemorrhage, all waters being soft *(71)*. A summary is shown in Table LVI.

From published reports it appears that water quality does not influence mortality from atherosclerosis, except insofar as its effect on hypertension is concerned. A comparative autopsy study from cities in the Americas, Asia, South Africa, and Norway *(64)* showed no relationship with atherosclerosis, nor did one appear in London and Glasgow *(72)*, although myocardial scars and old occlusions were more prevalent in Glasgow (soft water) than in London (hard water). Cities which had softened their water during the last 30 years, however, had a significant increase in cardiovascular death rates *(73)*.

Therefore, the inference is strong that hypertension is a disorder effected by soft water, and in Japan by acid water. Soft waters are usually acid, and as such corrode water pipes. In fact, most of the galvanized iron plumbing in our soft water area has corroded and has been replaced with copper. The galvanizing grade of zinc contains considerable cadmium, which can enter the water, especially stagnant water. Any water with a pH of less than 8.0 is said to be corrosive and certainly is with a pH of 7.0 or less. The uptake of cadmium from pipes in a municipal supply is illustrated in Table LVII. It is likely that the increment of soluble cadmium in water influences the incidence of hypertension in the populations supplied by soft, acid waters. It is also likely that cadmium in water is more easily absorbed from the intestine than is cadmium in food.

It is unlikely that elements other than cadmium in water influence the death rate from hypertension. In the first place, all trace elements but cobalt, fluorine, molybdenum, boron, lithium, and titanium are poorly absorbed from the gastrointestinal tract—less than 10% of the intake. Of those well absorbed, fluorine, molybdenum, and boron have significant

TABLE LVIII

INCREMENT OF BULK AND TRACE ELEMENTS IN DRINKING WATER TO TOTAL DAILY INTAKES[a]

| Elements | Intake from water Median (mg/day) | Intake from water Maximum[b] (mg/day) | Average intake from food and water (mg/day) | Proportion of total intake from water Median (%) | Proportion of total intake from water Maximum (%) |
|---|---|---|---|---|---|
| **Essential** | | | | | |
| Calcium | 52 | 100 | 800 | 6.5 | 11.8 |
| Magnesium | 12.5 | 40 | 210 | 5.9 | 16.8 |
| Sodium | 24 | 100 | 4400 | 0.5 | 2.2 |
| Potassium | 3.2 | 10 | 3300 | 0.09 | 0.3 |
| Vanadium | <0.008 | 0.02 | 2 | 0.6 | 1.0[d] |
| Chromium | 0.001 | 0.01 | 0.1 | 1.0 | 9.2[d] |
| Manganese | 0.01 | 0.2 | 3 | 0.3 | 6.3[d] |
| Iron | 0.09 | 0.3 | 15 | 0.6 | 2.0[d] |
| Cobalt | 0.006 | 0.01 | 0.3 | 2.0 | 3.3 |
| Nickel[c] | 0.005 | 0.02 | 0.4 | 1.3 | 4.8[d] |
| Copper | 0.02 | 0.2 | 2.5 | 0.8 | 7.5[d] |
| Zinc | 0.5 | 2.1 | 13 | 3.8 | 14.4[d] |
| Selenium | <0.02 | — | 0.15 | <13.3 | — |
| Fluorine | 0.4 | 1.0 | 1.8 | 22.2 | 41.7 |
| Molybdenum | 0.003 | 0.02 | 0.34 | 0.9 | 5.6 |
| **Nonessential** | | | | | |
| Silicon | 14.2 | 60 | >20 | <71.0 | <90.0[d] |
| Aluminum | 0.1 | 1.0 | 45 | 0.2 | 2.2[d] |
| Barium | 0.09 | 0.76 | 1.24 | 7.3 | 39.8[d] |
| Strontium | 0.22 | 1.0 | 2 | 11.0 | 40.0[d] |
| Boron | 0.06 | 0.2 | 1.0 | 6.0 | 17.5 |
| Bismuth | Trace | — | 0.002 | —[d] | — |
| Beryllium | Trace | — | 0.00001 | —[d] | — |
| Antimony | Trace | — | <1.0 | —[d] | — |
| Lead | 0.007 | 0.02 | 0.41 | 1.7 | 4.7[d] |
| Lithium | 0.004 | 0.1 | 2.0 | 0.2 | 4.7 |
| Silver | 0.0005 | 0.001 | 0.07 | 0.7 | 1.4[d] |
| Tin | 0.002 | 0.005 | 4.0 | 0.05 | 0.1[d] |
| Titanium | <0.003 | 0.01 | 0.3 | 0.1 | 3.2 |
| Uranium | 0.0003 | 0.004 | 1.4 | 0.02 | 0.3[d] |
| Cadmium | 0.005 | 0.04 | 0.07 | 7.1 | 38.1[d] |

[a] Data from Durfor and Becker (76), Howell (77), and Schroeder (74) at 2 liters of water per day.

[b] Maximum value for 87-98% of cities. Individual values can be much higher in areas with very hard water.

[c] Nickel is possibly essential for mammals, but unproven.

[d] Elements poorly absorbed by the gastrointestinal tract, i.e., <10%.

negative correlations with cardiovascular disease in river water but not in municipal water; lithium correlated in municipal water, but its concentration was very low as was that of cobalt, molybdenum, and boron (Table LVIII). Second, the increment supplied by water is usually small compared to the daily amount ingested in food (Table LVIII). No other metal in small amounts produces hypertension experimentally. In more than 90% of 100 United States cities, water supplies, or can supply, a sizeable increment of fluorine, silicon, strontium, and cadmium, and in hard water areas, can also supply extra chromium, magnesium, calcium, and boron. Over half the dietary content of cadmium could come from water, probably soft water running through pipes. Fluorine, magnesium, and calcium are reasonably well absorbed, and fluorine could be implicated in cardiovascular disease (Table XLVIII) as a protective influence on aortic calcification, although we found no significant correlation with hypertensive or atherosclerotic heart disease.

Hypertension is largely a disease of civilization; and the first step of modern civilization is to have running water in houses. Most houses built since World War II have copper pipes, but before that time galvanized iron was used almost universally. Although copper costs more than iron, the high labor costs of pipe-fitters, who must cut and thread each pipe, makes copper, which is easily soldered, cheaper overall. Although at first glance the argument may seem specious, one reason for the very high incidence of hypertension in American Negroes (it is not high in Virgin Island Negroes) may lie in the fact that most Negroes in the United States live in old houses which have galvanized pipes. When the water is soft, it may dissolve enough cadmium to influence death rates from this cause. In some Caribbean islands, rain water is collected from galvanized iron roofs, and undoubtedly it contains cadmium, which may account for the excess incidence of hypertension in those islands.

**Other Diseases Caused by Recondite Toxicity**

No examples of recondite toxicity caused by trace elements are known in man, other than those discussed. They may exist, and probably do, and for disclosure require constant search. Deficiency of zinc, as found by plasma analyses, occurs in a variety of conditions and in normal older persons, pregnant women, and women taking contraceptives. Giving zinc salts orally has increased healing of wounds and of indolent ulcers of the legs, and improved circulation in ischemic areas. That zinc deficiency increases toxicity of cadmium is possible, but speculative. Likewise, deficiencies of manganese, copper, fluorine, and chromium occur in other conditions *(74)*.

## XV. SUMMARY AND CONCLUSIONS

Recondite toxicity of trace elements, that is, subtle metabolic changes consistent with reasonable survival, has been evaluated from a number of parameters and is summarized in Table LIX.

Toxicity varies inversely with the concentration of the element in sea water and on the earth's crust. Elements in sea water at concentrations of less than 1 ppb are chromium, selenium, cobalt, lead, antimony, beryllium, cadmium, mercury, bismuth, tungsten, germanium, zirconium, silver, and niobium. Elements with concentrations on the earth's crust of 10 ppm or less are molybdenum, selenium, lead, antimony, beryllium, cadmium, mercury, tin, arsenic, tungsten, germanium, uranium, bismuth, tellurium, palladium, rhodium, silver, and boron. When land and sea are considered together, elements of low abundance in both are selenium, lead, antimony, beryllium, cadmium, mercury, tungsten, germanium, bismuth, tellurium, palladium, rhodium, and silver. All show recondite toxicity, and only selenium has a known biological function.

In contrast, the other essential trace elements occur in sea water in concentrations of 2–1300 ppb, and in the earth's crust at 23–50,000 ppm. Therefore, they were available for use during the evolution of living things.

Although all elements—in fact, all substances, even water—are toxic in large amounts, mammalian homeostatic mechanisms repel or excrete excesses by way of the gut, liver, or kidney and handle amounts liable to be encountered in food and water. These mechanisms probably exist to some extent in all land animals and in marine vertebrates, and apply to the 17 essential bulk and trace elements in the body.

No such mechanisms appear to exist for the elements found in low concentrations in the environment, for they accumulate in mammalian tissues with age and exposure. The natures of some metals, however, are such that a form of homeostasis exists, e.g., rapid renal excretion or chemical precipitation in the intestine.

Cadmium is the metal with the lowest threshold of recondite toxicity, elevation of blood pressure being caused by as little as 0.5 ppm in the

TABLE LIX

SUMMARY OF RECONDITE TOXIC EFFECTS OF ABNORMAL TRACE ELEMENTS IN RATS AND MICE[a]

| Element | Longevity or life-span | Growth | Reproduction | Liver lesions | Serum glucose elevated | Cholesterol elevated | Aortic lipids | Myocardial fibrosis | Tumors | Urine protein | Glycosuria | Other signs |
|---|---|---|---|---|---|---|---|---|---|---|---|---|
| **Rats and mice** | | | | | | | | | | | | |
| Cadmium | ++[b] | 0 | +++++ | 0 | + | + | ++++ | + | 0 | ++++ | ++ | Hypertension, renal vascular disease |
| Lead | +++ | 0 | +++++ | 0 | ++ | 0 | +++++ | +++++ | 0 | +++++ | +++++ | Susceptibility to infections |
| Antimony | +++ | ± | N.D. | 0 | ++ | ++ | +++++ | +++++ | 0 | +++ | 0 | Highly toxic |
| Selenium (IV) | +++++ | +++++ | +++++ | ++++ | + | ++ | +++++ | 0 | ++++(VI) | 0 | 0 | Series incomplete |
| Beryllium | N.D.[c] | ++ | N.D. | N.D. | 0 | N.D. | N.D. | N.D. | N.D. | 0 | 0 | |
| Tin | + | 0 | + | +++ | + | 0 | 0 | 0 | 0 | 0 | 0 | |
| Nickel | ++ | 0 | N.D. | + | 0 | 0 | 0 | 0 | 0 | 0 | 0 | Series incomplete |
| Aluminum | N.D. | 0 | 0 | N.D. | 0 | 0 | N.D. | N.D. | N.D. | 0 | 0 | |
| Arsenic | ± | 0 | N.D. | 0 | 0 | + | 0 | 0 | 0 | 0 | + | Sl. suppression of tumors |
| Germanium | + | 0 | N.D. | +++ | 0 | 0 | + | 0 | 0 | + | 0 | Sl. suppression of tumors |
| Tellurium (IV) | + | 0 | N.D. | 0 | ++ | ++ | +++++ | 0 | 0 | 0 | ++++ | |
| Niobium | + | 0 | N.D. | ++ | 0 | 0 | +++++ | ++ | 0 | 0 | 0 | Series incomplete |
| Barium | N.D. | 0 | N.D. | N.D. | 0 | + | N.D. | N.D. | N.D. | 0 | 0 | Series incomplete |
| Tungsten | N.D. | 0 | N.D. | N.D. | +++ | ++ | N.D. | N.D. | N.D. | 0 | + | Series incomplete |
| **Mice** | | | | | | | | | | | | |
| Mercury, methyl | +++++ | +++++ | +++++ | N.D. | | | | | N.D. | | | 5 ppm (1 ppm tolerated) |
| Palladium | 0 | ++ | N.D. | 0 | | | | | + | | | |
| Rhodium | 0 | ++ | N.D. | 0 | | | | | + | | | |
| Chromium (IV) | 0 | + | N.D. | 0 | | | | | 0 | | | |
| Yttrium | 0 | +++ | N.D. | 0 | | | | | 0 | | | |
| Gallium | + | ++ | N.D. | 0 | | | | | 0 | | | |

[a] Table is necessarily incomplete because of work in progress.
[b] The + signs indicate the degree of adverse effects found.
[c] N.D.-Not yet determined.

diet. Lead also has a low threshold, and beryllium probably has a low one too. Mercury and antimony have moderately low thresholds. Thresholds are higher for most other elements and very high for almost all of the essential trace elements.

Effects of an abnormal element on growth are not necessarily consistent with its effects on longevity, nor are effects on longevity always consistent with effects on fertility and the viability of offspring. Signs of recondite toxicity can be bizarre and unexpected, and include hypertension, atherosclerosis, diabetes mellitus, coronary artery occlusion, and malignant tumors, as well as alterations in carbohydrate and lipid metabolism, glycosuria, proteinuria, shortened longevity, reproductive abnormalities, and weight loss in older animals.

It is very likely that modern exposures to industrial elements with recondite toxicity contribute to some of the chronic diseases of modern man.

### REFERENCES

1. 1967 Mineral Facts and Problems. (1970). US Dept. of the Interior, Bureau of Mines, US Gov't. Printing Office, Washington, D.C.
2. Tipton, I. H. Gross and Elementary Composition of Reference Man. In ICRP Report of Subcommittee II on Permissible Dose for Internal Radiation, Chapter 2. Pergamon, Oxford (in press).
3. Bowen, H. J. M. (1966). "Trace Elements in Biochemistry." Academic Press, New York.
4. Schroeder, H. A., Vinton, W. H., Jr., and Balassa, J. J. (1963). Effect of chromium, cadmium and other trace metals on the growth and survival of mice. J. Nutr. 80, 39.
5. Schroeder, H. A., Vinton, W. H., Jr., and Balassa, J. J. (1963). Effects of chromium, cadmium and lead on the growth and survival of rats. J. Nutr. 80, 48.
6. Schroeder, H. A., Balassa, J. J., and Vinton, W. H., Jr. (1965). Chromium, cadmium and lead in rats: Effects on life span, tumors and tissue levels. J. Nutr. 86: 51.
7. Schroeder, H. A., and Balassa, J. J. (1961). Abnormal trace metals in man: Lead. J. Chronic Dis. 14, 408.
8. Schroeder, H. A. (1966). Chromium deficiency in rats: A syndrome simulating diabetes mellitus with retarded growth. J. Nutr. 88, 439.
9. Schroeder, H. A., Mitchener, M., and Nason, A. P. (1970). Zirconium, niobium, antiomony, vanadium and lead in rats: Life term studies. J. Nutr. 100, 59.
10. Schroeder, H. A. (1967). Effects of selenate, selenite and tellurite on the growth and early survival of mice and rats. J. Nutr. 92, 334.
11. Schroeder, H. A., Kanisawa, M., Frost, D. V., and Mitchener M. (1968). Germanium, tin and arsenic in rats. Effects on growth, survival, pathological lesions and life span. J. Nutr. 96, 37.
12. Schwarz, K., and Milne D. B. (1971). Growth effects of vanadium in the rat. Science 174, 426.
13. Schroeder, H. A., and Mitchener, M. (1972). Selenium and tellurium in mice: Effects on growth, reproduction, survival and tumors. Arch. Environ. Health 24, 66.
14. Schroeder, H. A., and Mitchener, M. (1971). Scandium, chromium (VI), gallium

yttrium, rhodium, palladium, indium in mice: Effects on growth and life span. *J. Nutr.* **101**, 1431.
15. Schroeder, H. A., Mitchener, M., Balassa, J. J., Kanisawa, M., and Nason, A. P. (1968). Zirconium, niobium, antimony and fluorine in mice. Effects on growth, survival and tissue levels. *J. Nutr.* **95**, 95.
16. Schroeder, H. A., and Balassa, J. J. (1967). Arsenic, germanium, tin and vanadium in mice. Effects on growth, survival and tissue levels. *J. Nutr.* **92**, 245.
17. Schroeder, H. A., Balassa, J. J., and Vinton, W. H. Jr. (1964). Chromium, lead, cadmium, nickel and titanium in mice: Effect on mortality, tumors and tissue levels. *J. Nutr.* **83**, 239.
18. Schroeder, H. A., and Mitchener, M. (1971). Selenium and tellurium in rats: Effects on growth, survival and tumors. *J. Nutr.* **101**, 1531.
19. Nelson, A. A., Fitzhugh, O. G., and Clavery, H. O. (1943). Liver tumors following cirrhosis caused by selenium in rats. *Cancer Res.* **3**, 230.
20. Volgarev, M. N., and Tscherkes, L. A. (1967). Further studies in tissue changes associated with sodium selenate. *In* "Selenium in Biomedicine" (O. H. Muth, J. E. Oldfield, and P. H. Weswig, eds.), AVI Publ., Westport, Connecticut.
21. McCay, C. M., Spurling, G., and Barnes L. L. (1943). Growth, ageing, chronic diseases and life span in rats. *Arch Biochem* **2**, 469.
22. Jones, D. C., and Kimmelsdorf, D. J. (1963). Lifespan measurements in the male rat. *J. Gerontol.* **18**, 318.
23. Berg, B. M., and Harmison, C. R. J. (1963). Growth, disease and ageing in the rat. *J. Gerontol.* **12**, 370.
24. Verzár, F. (1959). *In* "The Lifespan of Animals" (G. E. Wolstenholme and M. O'Connor, eds.), Ciba Found. Colloq. Ageing, Vol. 5, p. 82. Little, Brown, Boston, Massachusetts.
25. Gilbert C. and Gilman, J. (1958). Spontaneous neoplasms in the albino rat. *S. Afr. J. Med. Sci.* **23**, 257.
26. Kibler, H. H., Silsby, H. D., and Johnson, H. D. (1963). Metabolic trends and life span of rats living at 9°C and 28°C. *J. Gerontol.* **18**, 235.
27. Kanisawa, M., and Schroeder, H. A. (1969). Renal arteriolar changes in hypertensive rats given cadmium in drinking water. *J. Exp. Mol. Pathol.* **10**, 81.
28. Curran, G. L. (1954). Effect of certain transition group elements on hepatic synthesis of cholesterol in the rat. *J. Biol. Chem.* **210**, 765.
29. Schroeder, H. A., Mitchener, M., and Nason, A. P. (1971). Influence of various sugars, chromium and other trace metals on serum cholesterol and glucose of rats. *J. Nutr.* **101**, 247.
30. Mertz, W., and Roginski, E. E. (1969). Effects of chromium (III) supplementation on growth and survival under stress in rats fed low protein diets. *J. Nutr.* **97**, 531.
31. Schroeder, H. A., and Mitchener, M. (1971). Toxic effects of trace elements on the reproduction of mice and rats. *Arch. Environ. Health* **23**, 102.
32. Ferm, V. H. (1972). Teratogenic effects of metals on mammalian embryos. *Advan. Teratol.* **2**, 51–75.
32a. Ferm, V. H., and Carpenter, S. J. (1967). Developmental malformations resulting from the administration of lead salts. *Exp. Mol. Pathol.* **7**, 208.
33. Ferm, V. H., and Carpenter, S. J. (1968). Malformations induced by sodium arsenate. *J. Reprod. Fert.* **17**, 199.

33a. Ferm, V. H., and Carpenter, S. J. (1970). Teratogenic and embryopathic effects of indium, gallium, and germanium. *Toxicol. Appl. Pharmacol.* **16**, 166.
34. Weinberg, E. D. (1964). Manganese requirements for sporulation and other secondary biosynthetic processes of Bacillus. *Appl. Microbiol.* **12**, 436.
35. Schroeder, H. A. (1965). Cadmium as a factor in hypertension. *J. Chronic. Dis.* **18**, 647.
35a. Shaikh, Z. A. (1971). The fate of cadmium in the mammalian organism. Ph.D. thesis, Dalhousie Univ. Halifax, Nova Scotia.
36. Schroeder, H. A., Baker, J. T., Hansen, N. M., Size, J. G., and Wise, R. A. (1970). Vascular reactivity of rats altered by cadmium and a zinc chelate. *Arch. Environ. Health* **21**, 609.
37. Perry, H. M., Jr., Erlanger, M., Yunice, A., and Perry, E. F. (1967). Mechanism of the acute hypertensive effect of intra-arterial cadmium and mercury in anaesthetized rats. *J. Lab. Clin. Med.* **70**, 963.
38. Thind, G. S., Stephan, K. T., and Blakemore, W. S. (1970). Inhibition of vasopressor responses by cadmium. *Amer. J. Physiol.* **219**, 577.
39. Schroeder, H. A., Kroll, S S., Little, J. W., Livingston, P. O., and Myers, M. A. G. (1966). Hypertension in rats from injection of cadmium. *Arch. Environ. Health* **13**, 788.
40. Perry, H. M., Jr., and Erlanger, M. W. (1970). Elevated peripheral renin activity in cadmium-induced hypertension. *J. Lab. Clin. Med.* **76**, 852.
41. Thind, G. S., Karreman, G., Stephan, K. F., and Blakemore, W. S (1970). Vascular reactivity and mechanical properties of normal and cadmium-hypertensive rabbits. *J. Lab. Clin. Med.* **76**, 560.
42. Thind, G. S., Biery, D. N., Bovee, K. C., and Zinsser, H. F. (1972). Production of arterial hypertension by cadmium. *Amer. J. Cardiol.* **29**, 299.
43. Schroeder, H. A., and Buckman, J. (1967). Cadmium hypertension. Its reversal in rats by a zinc chelate. *Arch. Environ. Health* **14**, 693.
44. Perry, H. M., Jr., and Perry, E. F. (1959). Normal concentrations of some trace metals in human urine: Changes produced by ethylenediamine-tetraacetate. *J. Clin. Invest.* **38**, 1452.
45. Sporn, A., Cirstea, A., Ghizelea, G., Dinu, I., Boghianu, L., Ozeranschi, L., and Botescu, E. (1970). Contributions to the study of the chronic toxicity of cadmium. *Igiena* **19** (12), 729.
46. Parizek, J. (1957). The destructive effect of cadmium ion on testicular tissue and its prevention by zinc. *J. Endocrinol.* **15**, 56.
47. Perry, H. M., Jr., Perry, E. F. and Purifoy, J. E. (1971). Anti-natriuretic effect of intramuscular cadmium in rats. *Proc. Soc. Exp. Biol. Med.* **136**, 1240.
48. Carroll, R. E. (1966). The relationship of cadmium in the air to cardiovascular disease death rates. *J. Amer. Med. Ass.* **198**, 267.
49. Lener, J. and Bibr, B. (1972). Cadmium and hypertension. *Lancet* **1**, 970.
50. Morgan, J. M., Burch, H. B., and Watkins, J. B. (1971). Tissue cadmium and zinc content in emphysema and bronchogenic carcinoma. *J. Chronic. Dis.* **24**, 107.
51. Perry, H. M., Jr., and Erlanger, M. (1971). Hypertension and tissue metal levels after intraperitoneal cadmium, mercury and zinc. *Amer. J. Physiol.* **220**, 808.

52. Kobayashi, J. (1971). Relation between the "itai-itai" disease and the pollution of river water by cadmium from a mine. In "Fifth International Water Pollution Research Conference." Pergamon, Oxford.
53. Tsuchiya, K. (1969). Causation of ouch-ouch disease. An introductory review. *Keio J. Med.* **18**, 181.
54. Schroeder, H. A., and Perry, H. M., Jr. (1955). Anti-hypertensive effects of metal binding agents. *J. Lab. Clin. Med.* **46**, 416.
55. Schroeder, H. A., and Balassa, J. J. (1965). Influence of chromium, cadmium, and lead on rat aortic lipids and circulating cholesterol. *Amer. J. Physiol.* **209**, 433.
56. Masironi, R. (1969). Trace elements and cardiovascular diseases. *Bull. W. H. O.* **40**, 305.
57. Harman, D. (1963). Role of serum copper in coronary atherosclerosis. *Circulation* **28**, 658.
58. Harman, D. (1968). Atherogenesis in minipigs: Effect of dietary fat unsaturation and of copper. *Circulation, Suppl. VI* **38**, 8.
59. Tipton, I. H., Schroeder, H. A., Perry, H. M., Jr., and Cook, M. J. (1965). Trace elements in human tissue. III. Subjects from Africa, the Near and Far East and Europe. *Health Phys.* **11**, 403.
60. Schroeder, H. A., Nason, A. P., and Tipton, I. H. (1968). Essential metals in man: Magnesium. *J. Chronic Dis.* **21**, 815.
61. Schroeder, H. A., Nason, A. P., and Tipton, I. H. (1970). Chromium deficiency as a factor in atherosclerosis. *J. Chronic Dis.* **23**, 123.
62. Hernberg, S., Nikkanen, J., Mellin, G., and Lilus, H. (1970). Delta-aminol-levulinic acid dehydrase as a measure of lead exposure. *Arch. Environ. Health* **21**, 140.
63. Westöö, G. (1967). Determination of methyl mercury compounds in foodstuffs. II. Determination of methylmercury in fish, egg, meat and liver. *Acta Chem. Scand.* **21**, 1790.
64. Masironi, R. (1970). Cardiovascular mortality in relation to radioactivity and hardness of local water supplies in the USA. *Bull. W. H. O.* **43**, 687.
65. Schroeder, H. A. (1960). Relation between mortality from cardiovascular disease and treated water supplies. Variations in states and 163 largest municipalities in The United States. *J. Amer. Med. Ass.* **172**, 1902.
66. Schroeder, H. A. (1960). Relations between hardness of water and death rates from certain chronic and degenerative diseases in the U.S. *J. Chronic Dis.* **12**, 586.
67. Schroeder, H. A. (1966). Municipal drinking water and cardiovascular death rates. *J. Amer. Med. Ass.* **195**, 81.
68. Morris, J. M., Crawford, M. D., and Heady, J. A. (1961). Hardness of local water supplies and mortality from cardiovascular disease in country boroughs of England and Wales. *Lancet* **1**, 860.
69. Biörck, G., Bostrom, H., and Widstrom, A. (1965). On relationship between water hardness and death rate from cardiovascular disease. *Acta Med. Scand.* **178**, 239.
70. Anderson, T. W., LeRiche, W. H., and MacKay J. S. (1969). Sudden death: Correlation with hardness of water supply. *New Engl. J. Med.* **280**, 805.
71. Kobayashi, J. (1957). Geological relationship between chemical nature of river water and death-rate from apoplexy: preliminary report. *Ber. Ohara Inst. Landwirt. Biol.* **11**, 12.
71a. Crawford, M. D., Gardner, M. J., and Morris, J. N. (1968). Mortality and hardness of local water supplies. *Lancet* **1**, 827.
71b. Puffer, R. R., and Griffith, G. W. (1967). "Patterns of Urban Mortality." Pan American Health Organization, Sci. Publ. No. 151, Washington, D. C.

71c. Biersteker, K. (1967). Hardness of drinking water and mortality. T. Soc. Geneeska **24**, 658.
72. Crawford, T., and Crawford, M. D. (1967). Prevalence and pathological changes of ischemic heart disease in a hard-water and in a soft-water area. *Lancet* **1**, 229.
73. Crawford, M., Gardner, M., and Morris, J. (1971). Changes in water hardness and local death-rates. *Lancet* **2**, 327.
74. Schroeder, H. A., and Nason, A. P. (1971). Trace element analysis in clinical chemistry. *Clin. Chem.* **17**, 461.
75. Schroeder, H. A., Nason, A. P., Tipton, I. H., and Balassa, J. J. (1967). Essential trace metals in man: Zinc. Relation to environmental cadmium. *J. Chronic Dis.* **20**, 179.
76. Durfor, C. N., and Becker, E. (1962). Public water supplies of the 100 largest cities in the United States, 1962. *Geol. Surv. Water Supply Paper* **1812**.
77. Howell, G. P. Elemental Intake, Output and Balances of Reference Man. *In* "ICRP Report of Subcommittee II on Permissible Dose for Internal Radiation, Chapter 3. Pergamon, Oxford (in press).

# Author Index

Numbers in parentheses are reference numbers and indicate that an author's work is referred to although his name is not cited in the text. Numbers in italics show the page on which the complete reference is listed.

## A

Adler, T. K., 12 (48), 17 (62), 18, 20 (62), 21, 22, 23 (89), 39 (89), 40, *51*, *52*, *53*, *56*
Adrian, E. D., 67 (23), *103*
Agurell, S., 47 (162), 48 (162), *57*
Aldridge, W. N., 60 (7), 61 (7, 8), 67, 69, 73 (35), 75 (27), 100 (35), *102*, *103*
Alsleben, B., 4 (6), *49*
Anders, M. W., 35 (119), *55*
Anderson, H. H., 18 (72), 43 (150), *53*, *56*
Anderson, T. W., 188 (70), 190 (70), *198*
Andres, V., Jr., 77 (37), *103*
Aronow, L., 9 (41), *51*
Asami, T., 21 (85), 22 (85), *53*
Asatoor, A. M., 28, *54*
Asghar, K., 39, *56*
Aull, J. L., 99 (61), *105*
Axelrod, J., 18, 19, *53*

## B

Baker, B. R., 59, 60, *102*
Baker, E. M., 21 (85, 86), 22 (85, 86), *53*
Baker, J. T., 174 (36), *197*
Baker, W. P., 27, *54*
Balassa, J. J., 112 (4, 5, 6), 113 (6, 7), 114 (4), 116 (4, 5, 6), 119 (15, 16, 17), 120 (4), 124 (4, 6, 15, 16, 17), 137 (17), 179 (55), 189 (75), *195*, *196*, *198*, *199*
Barnes, L. L., 130 (21), *196*

Barry, H., III, 48, *57*
Baselt, R. C., 29, *54*
Baucum, F. G., 7 (21), *50*
Becker, E., 191, *199*
Beckett, A. H., 18, 29, *52*, *53*, *54*
Belleau, B., 20 (80), *53*
Berg, B. M., 130 (23), *196*
Bergmann, F., 61 (11), *102*
Berjerot, N., 2, *49*
Bernstein, E., 9 (39), *51*
Bibr, B., 176 (49), *197*
Biersteker, K., 188 (71c), *199*
Biery, D. N., 174 (42), *197*
Biörck, G., 188 (69), 190 (69), *198*
Blakemore, W. S., 174 (38, 41), *197*
Blane, G. F., 19 (79), 40 (79), 43, *53*, *56*
Blumberg, H., 25, *54*
Bodansky, O., 66, 70, *103*
Boegli, G., 47 (164), *57*
Boghianu, L., 175 (45), *197*
Bostrom, H., 188 (69), 190 (69), *198*
Botescu, E., 175 (45), *197*
Boura, A. L. A., 19 (79), 40 (79), *53*
Boursnell, J. C., 67, *103*
Bovee, K. C., 174 (42), *197*
Bowen, H. J. M., 111 (3), 171 (3), 172 (3), *195*
Boyer, R. N., 29 (103), *54*
Braid, P. E., 71 (30), 101 (64), *103*, *105*
Brauer, R. W., 45, *57*

201

Brazda, F. G., 6, 7 (19, 20, 21, 22), *50*
Breckenridge, A., 8 (34), *51*
Brine, D. R., 47 (163, 164), 48 (163), *57*
Brine, G. A., 47 (163), 48 (163), *57*
Brodeur, J., 8, *51*
Brodie, B. B., 4, 6 (15), 9 (39), *49, 50, 51*
Brons, D., 61 (14), *102*
Buckman, I., 174 (43), 175 (43), *197*
Burch, H. B., 176 (50), *197*
Burns, J. J., 5 (11), 6 (11), 35 (11), *50*
Butler, T. C., 9, 10, *51*

## C

Cafruny, E. J., 27, 29, 33 (106), *54*
Carchman, R. A., 23 (90), 25 (90), *53*
Carpenter, S. J., 156 (32a, 33, 33a), *196, 197*
Carroll, R. E., 176 (48), *197*
Casarett, L. J., 29, *54*
Casy, A. F., 18 (69, 70), 29 (104), *52, 53, 54*
Chernov, H. I., 22 (92), 45 (92), *54*
Chiesara, E., 8 (25), *50*
Chiu, Y. C., 101 (65), *105*
Christensen, H. D., 47 (163, 164), 48 (163), *57*
Cirstea, A., 175 (45), *197*
Claussen, U., 47 (160), *57*
Clavery, H. O., 128 (19), *196*
Clouet, D. H., 18 (67), 20 (67), 40, *52*
Clowes, G. H. A., *51*
Cochin, J., 44 (151), *56*
Cohen, J. A., 99 (51), *104*
Conner, E. H., 9 (40), *51*
Conney, A. H., 5 (11), 6 (11, 13), 35 (11), *50*
Cook, M. J., 181 (59), 182 (59), 183 (59), 185 (59), *198*
Cosmides, G. J., 6 (13), *50*
Costa, E., 48, *57*
Costley, E. C., 43 (147), *56*
Coulson, R. A., 6 (17), *50*
Courtney, D. K., 77 (37), *103*
Craig, A. L., 40 (138), *56*
Crawford, M. A., 10 (43), 28 (101), *51, 54*
Crawford, M. D., 188 (68, 71a), 190 (68, 72, 73), *198, 199*

Crawford, T., 190 (72), *198*
Curran, G. L., 144 (28), *196*

## D

Dauterman, W. C., 71 (31, 32, 33), 79 (33), 90 (33), 91, 94 (33, 47), 101 (32, 65), *103, 104, 105*
Davies, D. R., 99 (59), *105*
Davies, D. S., 8 (34), *51*
Davis, M. M., 18, *53*
Davison, A. N., 61 (8), *102*
Davson, H., 39 (133), *55*
Dayton, H. B., 25, *54*
Dayton, P. G., 8 (33), *51*
DeJong, L. P. A., 90 (46), 91 (46), 94, *104*
Dessaur, H. C., 7 (19), *50*
Dinu, I., 175 (45), *197*
Dixon, A. C., 21 (85), 22 (85), *53*
Dixon, M., 65, 70 (20), 99, *103*
Dobbs, H. E., 40, 43, 45, *56*
Dole, V. P., 39, *55*
Donnelly, R. A., 11, 29 (46), *51*
Downs, C. E., 97, *104*
Durfor, C. N., 191, *199*

## E

Easson, L. H., 64, *102*
Ebert, A. G., 9, *51*
Eddy, N. B., 2 (1), 17 (61), *49, 52*
Edery, H., 47 (161), 48 (165), *57*
Eglitis, I., 39 (131), *55*
Eich, W. F., 8 (26), *50*
Elison, C., 18 (66), 19, *52, 53*
Elliott, H. W., 18 (66), 19, 20, 39, 43, 44, *52, 53, 55, 56*
Ellman, G. L., 77, *103*
Erlanger, M., 174 (37), 177 (37, 51), *197*
Erlanger, M. W., 174 (40), 177 (40), *197*
Estabrook, R. W., 6 (13), *50*
Eyring, H., 99, *104*

## F

Fahrney, D., 84 (41), 98 (41), *104*
Featherstone, R. M., 77 (37), *103*
Feldberg, W., 67 (23), *103*

# AUTHOR INDEX

Ferm, V. H., 156 (32, 32a, 33, 33a), *196, 197*
Fitzgerald, A. E., 19 (79), 40 (79), *53*
Fitzhugh, O. G., 128 (19), *196*
Flesher, J. W., 40 (142), *56*
Foster, W. R., 7 (20), *50*
Fouts, J. R., 6 (13), *50*
Freudenthal, R. I., 47 (163, 164), 48 (163), *57*
Friberg, L., 176 (49), *197*
Frost, D. V., 116 (11), 119 (11), 124 (11), *195*
Fujimoto, J. M., 7, 8 (23, 24, 27, 28), 11, 17 (54, 55), 21 (86), 22 (54, 86, 91, 93, 94, 95), 23 (91), 24, 25, 26, 31 (107, 112), 32 (114), 33 (93, 114, 115), 34 (93, 115, 116), 35 (117, 120, 121), 36 (127), 37, 46 (158), 49 (170), *50, 51, 52, 53, 54, 55, 57*

## G

Gaddum, J. H., 64 (15), *102*
Gardner, M. J., 188 (71a), 190 (73), *199*
Ghizelea, G., 175 (45), *197*
Gidley, J. T., 47 (164), *57*
Gilbert, C., 130 (25), 134 (25), 137 (25), *196*
Gillette, J. R., 6 (13, 15), *50*
Gilman, J., 130 (25), 134 (25), 137 (25), *196*
Ginsburg, S., 61 (9), 70, 84 (9), 90 (45), *102, 104*
Gold, A. M., 84 (41), 98 (41), *104*
Goldstein, A., 9 (41), *51*, 65 (17, 18), 66, *102*
Gorodetzsky, C. W., 47 (160), *57*
Grasetti, D. R., 12 (51), 14 (51), *52*
Green, A. L., 70, 99 (29, 59), *103, 105*
Greenfeld, Y., 47 (161), *57*
Griffith, G. W., 188 (71b), *199*
Grunfeld, Y., 48 (165), *57*

## H

Haarstad, V. B., 22 (93), 33 (93), 34 (93), *54*
Haggart, J., 44 (151), *56*
Hakim, R., 34 (116), 35 (120, 121), *55*
Halbach, H., 2 (1), *49*
Halberg, F., 11 (47), *51*
Hall, J. M., 45 (152), *56*
Hamilton, H., 18 (72), *53*
Hansen, N. M., 174 (36), *197*
Harbison, R. D., 48, *57*
Harman, D., 181 (57, 58), *198*
Harmison, C. R. J., 130 (23), *196*
Harper, N. J., 18 (69, 70), *52, 53*
Harrison, M. A., 90 (45), 99 (52), *104*
Hartley, B. S., 99 (56), *104*
Hassan, M. M. A., 29 (104), *54*
Hastings, F. L., 90 (44), 99 (53), 101 (44, 66), *104, 105*
Hatch, M. A., 61 (9), 70, 84 (9), *102*
Heady, J. A., 188 (68), 190 (68), *198*
Hellenbrand, K., 89 (42), *104*
Hernberg, S., 186 (62), *198*
Hodgson, E., 6 (12), *50*
Holmstedt, B., 67 (22), *103*
Howell, G. P., 191, *199*
Hudingsfelder, S., 7 (22), *50*
Hugg, C. C., Jr., 29, 33, 39, *54, 56*
Hunter, A., 97, *104*

## I

Ida, S., 17 (58, 64), 18 (58, 64), *52*
Indindoli, L., 19 (78), 25 (78), *53*
Inturrisi, C. E., 32 (114), 33 (114), *55*
Isbell, H., 2 (1), 47 (160), *49, 57*
Iverson, F., 60 (6), 72 (6), 73 (6), 76 (6) 77 (6), 86 (6), 90 (44), 99, 101 (44, 62), *102, 104, 105*

## J

Jansz, H. S., 61 (14), *102*
Janz, F. B., 99 (51), *104*
Jasinski, D., 47 (160), *57*
Johnson, H. D., 130 (26), *196*
Jones, D. C., 130 (22), *196*

## K

Kamata, O., 17 (64), 18 (64) *52*
Kanisawa, M., 116 (11), 119 (11, 15), 124 (11, 15), 137 (27), 173, *195, 196*
Karreman, G., 174 (41), *197*

## Author Index

Kato, R., 8 (25), *50*
Keltch, A. K., *51*
Kemp, A., Jr., 61 (12), 69, *102*
Kemp, J., 12 (50), *51*
Kibler, H. H., 130 (26), *196*
Kilby, B. A., 67 (23), *103*
Kim, W. K., 39 (131), *55*
Kimmelsdorf, D. J., 130 (22), *196*
Kirsten, I., 9, *51*
Klaassen, C. D., 8, *50*, *51*
Kobayashi, J., 177 (52), 188 (71), 190 (71), *198*
Korte, F., 47 (160), *57*
Kovnot, P. J., 9 (40), *51*
Krahl, M. E., *51*
Kroll, S. S., 174 (39), *197*
Krueger, H., 17 (61), *52*
Kupferberg, H. J., 15, 16, 45, *52*, *57*

### L

La Du, B. N., 6 (15, 16), *50*
La Motta, R. V., 81 (40), 99 (40), *104*
Lener, 176, *197*
LeRiche, W. H., 188 (70), 190 (70), *198*
Levine, L., 36 (124), *55*
Lilus, H., 186 (62), *198*
Lister, R. E., 19 (79), 40 (79), *53*
Little, J. W., 174 (39), *197*
Livingston, P. O., 174 (39), *197*
Lockett, M. F., 18, *53*
London, D. R., 28 (102), *54*

### M

McCay, C. M., 130, *196*
McComb, R. B., 81 (40), 99 (40), *104*
McIvor, R. A., 99 (54), 101 (54), *104*
MacKay, J. S., 188 (70), 190 (70), *198*
Mackworth, J. F., 66, 67, 70, 72, *103*
McMillan, D. E., 23 (90), 25, *53*
McNay, J. L., 8 (33), *51*
Main, A. R., 60 (5, 6), 70 (5), 71 (5, 30, 31, 32, 33), 72 (6, 34), 73 (6), 76, 77 (6) 79 (33, 36), 81 (34), 82 (34), 86 (6, 34), 90 (33, 44), 91, 94 (33, 47), 98 (50), 99 (6, 53, 61, 62), 100 (34), 101 (32, 34, 44, 62, 65, 66), *102*, *103*, *104*, *105*
Mandel, H. G., 6 (16), *50*
Mannering, G. J., 6, 21, 22, *50*, *53*

March, C. H., 20, 44, *53*
Marchand, C., 8, *51*
Mark, L. C., 9 (39), *51*
Martin, M., 7 (22), *50*
Martin, W. R., 19 (77), 23 (77), *53*
Marx, G. F., 41 (145), 42, *56*
Masironi, R., 181, 183, 187, 188 (64), 190 (64), *198*
Matilla-Plata, B., 48, *57*
May, D. G., 32 (114), 33 (114, 115), 34 (115), *55*
Mazur, A., 66, 70, *103*
Mechoulam, R., 47 (161), 48 (166), *57*
Mellett, L. B., 22 (87), 23 (87), 29, 33 (106), 40 (141), *53*, *54*, *56*
Mellin, G., 186 (62), *198*
Mertz, W., 145 (30), *196*
Metcalf, R. L., 89, *104*
Miller, J. W., 18, 39, *53*, *55*
Milne, D. B., 119 (12), *195*
Milne, M. D., 10, 28, *51*, *54*
Milthers, K., 19, *53*
Mintz, M., 19 (78), 25 (78), *53*
Misra, A. L., 18 (65), 20, 21, *52*, *53*
Mitchell, C. L., 21, 21 (81), *53*
Mitchener, M., 116 (9, 11, 18), 117 (9), 119 (9, 11, 13, 14, 15), 120 (13), 124 (9, 11, 13, 14, 15), 128 (14, 18), 145 (29), 151 (31), 175 (31), *195*, *196*
Miya, T. S., 9, *51*
Morgan, J. M., 176, *197*
Mori, M., 17 (60), 18 (60), *52*
Morris, J. N., 188 (68 71a), 190 (68, 73), *198*, *199*
Muehlenbeck, H. E., 22 (87), 23 (87), *53*
Mulé, S. J., 17 (63), 40 (140, 141, 142), *52*, *56*
Muraki, T., 40 (139), *56*
Myers, D. K., 61 (12, 13), 65 (19), 69, 99 (19), *102*, *103*
Myers, M. A. G., 174 (39), *197*

### N

Nachmansohn, D., 61 (11), *102*
Nakazawa, K., 48, *57*
Nason, A. P., 116 (9), 117 (9), 119 (9, 15), 124 (9, 15), 145 (29), 181 (60), 184 (61), 189 (75), 191 (74), 192 (74), *195*, *196*, *198*, *199*
Nelson, A. A., 128 (19), *196*

## AUTHOR INDEX

Nichols, H. R., 8 (26), *50*
Nikkanen, J., 186 (62), *198*
Nilsson, I. M., 47, 48 (162), *57*
Nilsson, J. L. G., 47 (162), 48 (162), *57*
Nitze, H. R., 9, *51*
Nix, M., 101 (64), *105*
Noll, C. R., Jr., 81 (40), 99 (40), *104*
Nordberg, G., 176 (49), *197*

### O

Ober, K., 22 (95), *54*
Oberst, F. W., 43, *56*
O'Brien, R. D., 60 (3), 69, 70 (28), 80 (28), 99, *102, 103, 104*
O'Dea, R. F., 40 (138), *56*
Oguri, K., 17 (58, 59, 60, 64), 18 (58, 59, 60, 64), 22 (59), *52*
Ohlsson, A., 47 (162), 48 (162), *57*
Ohnhaus, E. E., 8, *51*
Oka, T., 17 (57), *52*
Ooms, A. J. J., 77 (38), 80, 99 (38), *103*
Oosterbaan, R. A., 99 (51), *104*
Ozeranschi, L., 175 (45), *197*

### P

Parizek, J., 176 (46), *197*
Perry, E. F., 174 (37), 175 (44), 176 (47), 177 (37, 47), *197*
Perry, H. M., Jr., 174 (37, 40), 175 (44), 176 (47), 177 (37, 40, 47, 51, 54), 181 (59), 182 (59), 183 (59), 185 (59), *197, 198*
Peters, L., 27, *54*
Peterson, R. E., 46, 47, *57*
Pfeffer, M., 19 (78), 25 (78), *53*
Phillips, P. M., 18 (69), *52*
Piscator, M., 176 (49), *197*
Pitt, C. G., 47 (163, 164), 48 (163), *57*
Plaa, G. L., 8, 45, *50, 51, 57*
Price, H. L., 9 (40), *51*
Price, M. L., 9 (40), *51*
Puffer, R. R., 188 (71b), *199*
Purdie, J. E., 99 (54), 101 (54), *104*
Purifoy, J. E., 176 (47), 177 (47), *197*

### Q

Quame, B. A., 38, *55*
Quebbemann, A. J., 35, *55*

### R

Redman, C. M., 40 (142), *56*
Reinberg, A., 11 (47), *51*
Reiner, E., 73 (35), 100 (35), *103*
Remmer, H., 4, 6, 9, *49, 50, 51*
Rennick, B. R., 35, *55*
Roberts, R. J., 8 (28), *50*
Roginski, E. E., 145 (30), *196*
Rosenfeld, R., 47 (164), *57*

### S

Safer, J. N., 9 (40), *51*
Sandberg, F., 47 (162), 48 (162), *57*
Sanner, J. H., 41, 43, *56*
Schanker, L. S., 10 (45), 45, *51, 56, 57*
Schor, J. M., 19 (78), 25 (78), *53*
Schroeder, H. A., 112 (4, 5, 6), 113 (6, 7), 114 (4), 116 (4, 5, 6, 8, 9, 10, 11, 18), 117 (8, 9, 10), 119 (9, 10, 11, 13, 14, 15, 16, 17), 120 (4, 13), 124 (4, 6, 9, 11, 13, 14, 15, 16, 17), 128 (14, 18), 137 (17, 27), 139 (8), 145 (8, 29), 151 (31), 173, 174 (36, 39, 43), 175 (35), 177 (35, 54), 179 (55), 181 (59, 60), 182 (59), 183 (59), 184, 185, 187, 188 (65, 66, 67), 189, 190 (65, 66, 67), 191, 192 (74), *195, 196, 197, 198, 199*
Schwarz, K., 119 (12), *195*
Scribner, B. H., 10 (43), 28 (101), *51, 54*
Seevers, M. H., 2 (1), 44 (151), *49, 56*
Serrone, D. M., 7, 8 (23, 24), *50*
Shaikh, Z. A., 173 (35a), *197*
Shani, A., 47 (161), *57*
Shaw, E., 98, *104*
Shaw, F. H., 21, *53*
Shimomura, K., 17 (64), 18 (64), *52*
Siegert, M., 4 (10), 9, *50, 51*
Silsby, H. D., 130 (26), *196*
Simenhoff, M. L., 28 (102), *54*
Size, J. G., 174 (36), *197*
Smith, A. A., 20 (82), *53*
Smith, D. S., 46 (158), *57*
Smith, H. J., 70, 99 (29), *103*
Sofia, R. D., 48, *57*
Soucie, W. G., 99 (61), *105*
Spector, S., 36 (123), *55*
Sperber, I., 31, 32, 35 (111), 45, *54, 56*
Sporn, A., 175 (45), *197*
Spulak, F. V., 47 (160), *57*

Spurling, G., 130 (21), *196*
Stedman, E., 64, *102*
Steiger, B., 45 (152), *56*
Stenwick, M. W., 39, *56*
Stephan, K. F., 174 (38, 41), *197*
Stowe, C. M., 45, *57*
Straus, O. H., 65 (18), 66, *102*
Sumwalt, M., 17 (61), *52*
Svensmark, O., 81 (39), *104*

**T**

Takemori, A. E., 39, 40 (138), *56*
Tarkan, E., 99 (61), *105*
Taylor, J. F., 29 (104), 36 (126), 39, *54*, *55*
Testino, L., 47 (164), *57*
Thind, G. S., 174 (38, 41, 42), *197*
Thorzeirsson, S. S., 8 (34), *51*
Tipton, I. H., 111 (2), 181 (59, 60), 182, 183, 184 (61), 185 (59), 189 (75), *195*, *198*, *199*
Tolbert, B. M., 43 (150), *56*
Tscherkes, L. A., 128 (20), *196*
Tsuchiya, K., 177 (53), *198*
Tsukamoto, H., 17 (58, 59, 60, 64), 18 (58, 59, 60, 64), 22 (59), *52*
Tucker, G. T., 29 (103), *54*

**U**

Ueki, S., 17 (64), 18 (64), *52*

**V**

Vassanelli, P., 8 (25), *50*
Verzár, F., 130 (24), *196*
Vinton, W. H., Jr., 112 (4, 5, 6), 113 (6), 114 (4), 116 (4, 5, 6), 119 (17), 120 (4), 124 (4, 6, 17), 137 (17), *195*, *196*
Volgarev, M. N., 128 (20), *196*
Von Vunakis, H., 36 (124), *55*

**W**

Waddell, W. J., 10, *51*
Wahlquist, M., 47 (162), 48 (162), *57*
Wall, M. E., 47, 48 (163), *57*

Wang, R. I. H., 36 (127), 37, *55*
Warringa, M. G. P. J., 61 (14), 99 (51), *102*, *104*
Wasserman, E., 36 (124), *55*
Watkins, J. B., 176 (50), *197*
Watrous, W. M., 32, 33, 34, 35 (117), *55*
Way, E. L., 6 (16), 12, 14, 15, 16, 17 (54, 55, 62), 18, 20 (62), 21 (86), 22 (54, 62, 86), 31 (107), 39, 40, 43, *50*, *51*, *52*, *53*, *54*, *56*
Way, W. L., 43, *56*
Webb, E. C., 65, 66, 67, 70, 72, 99, *103*
Weinberg, E. D., 157, *197*
Weiner, I. M., 27, *54*
Weinstein, S. H., 19, 25, *53*
Westöö, G., 187 (63), *198*
Whitsett, T. L., 8 (33), *51*
Widstrom, A., 188 (69), 190 (69), *198*
Williams, R. T., 2, *49*
Wilson, I. B., 61 (9, 10, 11), 70, 84 (9), 90, 99 (52, 60), 101 (60), *102*, *104*, *105*
Wise, R. A., 174 (36), *197*
Wolf, P. S., 23 (90), 25 (90), *53*
Woods, L. A., 17 (56), 18 (65), 19 (76), 20, 21 (81), 22 (87, 92), 23 (87, 88), 27, 40 (141, 143), 41, 43, 44, 45 (92), *52*, *53*, *54*, *56*
Wright, C. I., 12, *51*
Wuepper, K. D., 40, *56*

**Y**

Yeh, S. Y., 18 (65), 22 (92), 23 (88), 40 (143), 45 (92), *52*, *53*, *54*, *56*
Yim, G. K. W., 9, *51*
Yoshimura, H., 17 (58, 59, 60, 64), 18 (58, 59, 60, 64), 22 (59), *52*
Young, J. M., 12 (50, 51), *51*, *52*
Yunice, A., 174 (37), 177 (37), *197*

**Z**

Zamiatowski, R., 35 (121), *55*
Zinsser, H. F., 174 (42), *197*

# Subject Index

## A

Acetylcholinesterase, inhibition kinetics of, 68
Alcohol dehydrogenase, metal inhibition of, 165
Aldehyde dehydrogenase, metal inhibition of, 165
Alkaline phosphatase, metal inhibition of, 165
N-Allylnormorphine, see Nalorphine
Aluminum
  abundance and annual consumption of, 111
  in aorta, 182
  toxicity of, 164, 172, 194–195
    oral, 162
    respiratory, 163
Amberlite XAD–12, morphine separation on, 37
p-Aminohippuric acid, uinary excretion of, 30, 32, 34
δ-Aminolevulinic acid dehydrase, metal inhibition of, 165
Amphetamines, urinary monitoring of, 36, 38
Amyloidosis, trace element effect on, 132–133
Antimony
  abundance and annual consumption of, 110
  effects on
    atherosclerosis, 178–181
    fats in body, 134
    growth, 117, 119–123
    infection, 135–137
    serum constituents, 139, 141, 143
    survival and longevity, 124, 126, 129
    teeth, 138
    tumors, 127
    urinary abnormalities, 138
  toxicity of, 164, 172, 187, 194–195
    cellular, 157
    oral, 161, 162
    respiratory, 163
  as trace element, 109
Apparent tubular excretion fraction (ATEF), calculation of, in drug excretion, 32–33
Argyria, from excess silver, 111
1-Aromatic amino acid decarboxylase, metal inhibition of, 165
Arsenic
  abundance and annual consumption of, 110
  as carcinogen, 158
  effects on
    atherosclerosis, 179–181
    fats in body, 134
    growth, 119–123
    kidney lesions, 137
    longevity, 129, 131
    reproduction, 151, 153, 156
    serum constituents, 139, 140, 142, 144, 145
    tumors, 127, 128
    urinary abnormalities
  toxicity of, 165–167, 172, 194–195
    cellular, 157, 159
    oral, 161, 162

207

respiratory, 163
as trace element, 109
Active-site-directed irreversible inhibition
  kinetics of, 59–105
    covalent bond formation, 84
    first-order, 67–69
    inhibitory power, 66–67
    inhibition progress curves, 73
    stoichiometry and early studies 64–66
Arteriolar disease, of kidneys, trace element effects on, 137
Atherosclerosis, trace elements affecting, 177–178
ATP, metal chelation of, 172
Azaserine, as active-site-directed irreversible inhibitor, kinetics of, action, 60

## B

Barbital, tolerance to, 9
Baritosis, from excess barium, 111
Barbiturates
  distribution, to CNS, 8–9
  metabolism of, 2
    enzyme inhibitor effect on, 8
    nikethamide effects on, 7
  tolerance to, relation to metabolism of, 3–8
  urinary excretion of, 9–11
  urinary monitoring of, 36, 38
Baritosis, from barium, 163
Barium
  abundance and annual consumption of, 111
  effects on
    atherosclerosis, 182
    growth, 117, 120
    infection, 136
    serum constituents, 139, 141, 143
  toxicity of, 164, 172, 194–195
    cellular, 157
    oral, 160, 161
    respiratory, 163
Benzomethamine, excretion of, 45
Bertrand's law of optimal nutritive concentration, of trace element, 155, 157, 159, 163
Beryllium
  abundance and annual consumption of, 110
  as carcinogen, 158, 187
  effects on
    growth, 116, 117, 118, 120, 194
    infection, 136
    serum constituents, 139, 141, 143, 144
  toxicity of, 164, 166, 167, 172, 187, 194–195
    cellular, 157
    oral, 160, 162
    respiratory, 163
Beryllosis, from excess beryllium, 110
Bile
  flow of, barbiturate effects on, 8
  morphine excretion by, 43–47
Bismuth
  abundance and annual consumption of, 111
  toxicity of, 164, 172
    cellular, 157
    oral, 161
Blood-brain barrier, to morphine, 16, 40
Blood pressure, cadmium effects on, 173–177
Body weight, trace element effects on, 124
Boron
  abundance and annual consumption of, 111
  in seawater, 163
  toxicity of, 163
Brain, drug transport of, 39–41
Bromine
  in seawater, 163
  toxicity of, 172
Bromosulfophthalein, excretion of, 45
Butallylonal, in studies on barbiturate tolerance, 6

## C

Cadmium
  abundance and annual consumption of, 110
  as carcinogen, 158
  effects on
    atherosclerosis, 178–182, 185
    fats in body, 134
    growth, 117, 120–123
    hypertension, 192, 193
    infection, 135
    reproduction, 151, 152, 155, 156

SUBJECT INDEX

serum constituents, 139, 140, 143, 144
survival and longevity, 124–126
teeth, 138
tumors, 127, 128
urinary abnormalities, 138
in human body, 186
hypertension from, 173–177
toxicity of, 164, 165–169, 171–173
  cellular, 157, 159
  oral, 160, 162
  overt, 177
  respiratory, 163
as trace element, 109
Calcium
  uptake from pipes by water, 189
  abundance and annual consumption of, 110
  in aorta, 182
  toxicity of, 158, 159, 167
Cancer, from excess chromium, nickel, or selenium, 110
Carbamate cholinesterase inhibitors, kinetics of action of, 60–102
Carbon, toxicity of, 172
Carbonic anhydrase, metal inhibition of, 165
Carboxypeptidase, metal inhibition of, 165
Carcinogens, trace metals as, 158, 159, 163
Catechol, in studies of drug excretion, 35
Cellular toxicity, of trace elements, 157–159
Central nervous system (CNS), barbiturate distribution to, 8–9
Ceruloplasmin, metal inhibition of, 165
Cesium, toxicity of, 172
Chelation, in toxicity of trace elements, 164
Chicken, morphine transport and metabolism in, 31–35
Chlorine, toxicity of, 158, 172
Chlorothiazide, excretion of, 45
Cholesterol, in serum, trace element effects on, 146, 148–151
Cholinesterase inhibitors, kinetics of action of, 60–102
Choroid plexus, morphine concentration by, 39
Chromium
  in aorta, 184
  as carcinogen, 158

effects on
  amyloidosis, 133
  atherosclerosis, 179–183, 185
  fats in body, 133, 134
  growth, 116–124
  infection, 135–137
  kidney lesions, 137
  serum constituents, 139–151
  survival and longevity, 124–126, 129
  teeth, 133, 138
  tumors, 127, 128
  urinary abnormalities, 138, 139
toxicity of, 165, 167, 172, 194–195
  cellular, 157, 159
  oral, 160, 162
  respiratory, 163
in seawater, 164
as trace element, essentiality, 109
Circadian rhythm, in drug excretion, 10–11
Cobalt
  abundance and annual consumption of, 110
  as carcinogen, 158
  effects on, atherosclerosis, 181–183
  in seawater, 164
  toxicity of, 165–167
    cellular, 157
    oral, 160
    respiratory, 163
  as trace element essentiality, 109
Cocaine, cross tolerance to morphine of, 20
Codeine
  dealkylation of, 18, 19
  demethylation of, 23
  morphine from metabolism of, 2
    pathway of, 21–23
  as morphine metabolite, 18
  urinary monitoring of, 36, 38
Copper
  abundance and annual consumption of, 110
  effects on
    atherosclerosis, 181–183
    serum constituents, 149–151
  hereditary disease involving, 159
Copper
  in seawater, 164
  toxicity of, 165–168, 170–173

cellular, 157, 159
oral, 160
respiratory, 163
as trace element, essentiality, 109
Cuprism, copper accumulation in, 110, 159
Cyprenorphine, brain transport of, 40–41
Cytochrome oxidase, metal inhibition of, 165
Cytochrome $P_{450}$ in barbiturate metabolism, 6

## D

Demethylation, in morphine drug metabolism, 19–20
DFP
  chemical name of, 62
  as cholinesterase inhibitor, kinetics of, 60, 71–72
Diabetes mellitus, chromium induction of, 139
Diets
  for metalfree experiments, 113–115
  trace metals in, 144
O,O-Diethyl S-2-diethylaminoethyl phosphorothiolate, see Tetram
Diethyl p-nitrophenyl phosphate, see Paraoxon
Dihydromorphine
  placental transfer of, 41–43
  urinary excretion of, 29–31
Diethylaminoethanol, as blocker of morphine transport, 35
Diisopropyl phosphorofluoridate, see DFP
Dopamine β-hydroxylase, metal inhibition of, 165
Drug abuse, urine monitoring for, 35–39
Drug dependence, 1–57
  to barbiturates, 1–11
Drugs
  fate of, in drug dependence, 1–57
  transport of, in brain, 39–41

## E

Emphysema, from excess cadmium, 110
EN 2265, as naloxone metabolite, 24–26
Enzymes
  role in drug tolerance, 8–9

trace element inhibitors of, 166, 167, 171, 172
Eserine, chemical name of, 63
Ethobromide, excretion of, 45
Etorphine
  biliary excretion of, 45
  brain transport of, 40, 43
  metabolism of, 19

## F

Farnesyl pyrophosphate, metal inhibition of, 165
Ferrism, hereditary, 159
Fertility, trace element effects on, 151–156
Fluorine
  abundance and annual consumption of, 110
  effects on
    atherosclerosis, 181
    fats in body, 134
    growth, 118, 119, 122
    tumors, 127
  in seawater, 163
  toxicity of, 159, 172
    oral, 162
    respiratory, 163
  as trace element, essentiality, 109
Fluorosis, from excess fluorine, 110
FRAT technique, for drug monitoring, 36–37
Fujimoto-Wang methods, for drug detection, 37–38

## G

Gallium
  effects on
    amyloidosis, 132–133
    growth, 119, 122, 194
    survival and longevity, 124, 131, 194
    tumors, 127, 195
  toxicity of, 164, 194–195
    cellular, 157, 159
    oral, 160
Germanium
  abundance and annual consumption of, 111
  effects on
    atherosclerosis, 179–180

# SUBJECT INDEX

fat in body, 133, 134
growth, 119–123
kidney lesions, 137
longevity, 129
serum constituents, 139, 140, 142
tumors, 127, 129
urinary abnormalities, 138
toxicity of, 164, 172
  cellular, 157, 159
  oral, 161, 162
Glomerular filtration, of drugs and metabolites, 27
Glucuronides
  of morphine, 17, 22
  of naloxone, 22–24
Glucose, in serum, trace element effects on, 139–143
Glutamic dehydrogenase, metal inhibition of, 165
Glycosuria, trace element effects on, 138–139
Gold
  toxicity of, 164, 172
    cellular, 157
    oral, 160

## H

Hafnium
  toxicity of
    cellular, 157
    oral, 160
Heart disease
  from excess antimony, 110
  waterborne trace elements and, 187–188
Heart muscle, trace elements in, 183
Hemochromatosis, from excess iron, 110
Hepatolenticular degeneration, see Cuprism
Heroin
  metabolic pathways of, 13
  morphine from metabolism of, 2, 12–16
  placental transfer of, 42
  potency relative to morphine, 12–
  toxicity of, 16–17
Hexobarbital
  metabolism of, nikethamide effects on, 7
  oxidation of, 4–5
11-Hydroxy-$\Delta^9$-tetrahydrocannabinol, as marihuana metabolite, 47–49

Hypertension, from cadmium, 110, 173–177, 192, 193

## I

Indium
  effects on
    amyloidosis, 133
    growth, 120, 122, 124
    longevity, 131
    teeth, 133
    tumors, 127
  toxicity of, 164
    cellular, 157
    oral, 160
Indocyanine green, clearance, after drug use, 8
Infection, trace element effects on, 135–137
Iodine
  abundance and annual consumption of, 110
  toxicity of, 163–167
Iridium
  toxicity of
    cellular, 157
    oral, 160
Iron
  abundance and annual consumption of, 110
  as carcinogen, 158
  effects on atherosclerosis, 182
  excess consumption of, disease from, 110
  hereditary disease involving, 159–160
Iron
  in seawater, 164
  toxicity of, 165, 167
    cellular, 157
    oral, 160
    respiratory, 163
  as trace element, essentiality, 109
Itai-itai disease, 177

## K

Kidney disease, from excess uranium, 111
Kidneys
  arteriolar disease of, trace element effects on, 137
  barbiturate excretion by, 9–11

fatty changes in, trace element effects on, 133–136
Kinetics, of active-site-directed irreversible inhibition, 59–105

## L

Lanthanum, toxicity of, 164, 172
Lactic dehydrogenase, metal inhibition of, 165
Lead
　abundance and annual consumption of, 110
　as carcinogen, 158
　effects on
　　atherosclerosis, 178–181
　　growth, 120–123
　　infection, 135–137
　　reproduction, 151, 152, 154, 155
　　kidney lesions, 137
　　serum constituents, 139, 141, 143–145, 156
　　survival and longevity, 126
　　teeth, 138
　　tumors, 127, 128
　　urinary abnormalities, 138
　in human body, 186
　toxicity of, 164, 165, 167, 172, 194–195
　　cellular, 157
　　oral, 161, 162, 163
　　respiratory, 163
　as trace element, 109
Levorphanol, urinary excretion of, 28
Lilly 18947, as blocker of morphine transport, 35
Lipids, in aorta, trace element effect on, 179
Lithium
　abundance and annual consumption of, 111
　effects on atherosclerosis, 181
　toxicity of, 164, 172
Liver
　fatty changes in, trace element effects on, 133–136
　role in drug metabolism, 2, 3
　　barbiturates, 5, 7, 8
　　morphine compounds, 19–20
Longevity, trace element effects on, 124–126, 129–132

Lung cancer, from trace metals, 163

## M

Magnesium
　abundance and annual consumption of, 110
　in seawater, 163
　toxicity of, 158, 159
Malaoxon
　chemical name of, 62
　as cholinesterase inhibitor, kinetics of, 71–102
Malathion, as cholinesterase inhibitor, kinetics of, 71
Manganese
　abundance and annual consumption of, 110
　effects on
　　atherosclerosis, 181
　　serum constituents, 149–151
　in seawater, 164
　toxicity of, 165–171
　　cellular, 157, 159
　　oral, 160
　　respiratory, 163
　as trace element, essentiality, 109
Manganism
　from excess iron, 110
　hereditary, 162, 163
Marihuana, metabolites of, 47–49
Mepiperphenidol
　excretion of, 45
　in studies of drug excretion, 34
Meperidine
　dealkylation of, 18, 19
　placental transfer of, 42–43
　urinary excretion of, 28–29
Mercury
　abundance and annual consumption of, 110
　effects on
　　growth, 120
　　reproduction, 151, 155, 156
　in human body, 186–187
　toxicity of, 164, 166, 167, 171–173
　　cellular, 157
　　oral, 160, 162
　　respiratory, 163
　as trace element, 109

SUBJECT INDEX 213

Metalloenzymes, trace elements in, 164–165
  inhibitors of, 171
Metallothionein, as metal-binding protein, 173
Metals, trace amounts, see Trace elements
Methadone
  dealkylation of, 18
  transport of, 43
  urinary excretion of, 28, 29
$N$-Methylpipyridyldiphenylcarbamate (MPDC)
  as blocker of morphine transport, 35
  effect on barbiturate metabolism, 8
Mevalonic kinase metal inhibition of, 165
Molybdenum
  abundance and annual consumption of, 110
  effects on
    growth, 116, 120, 121
    reproduction, 151, 153, 155, 156
    serum constituents, 139, 140, 142–144, 148, 151
    survival and longevity, 124–125
  in seawater, 164
  toxicity of, 165, 166, 168, 172
    cellular, 157
    oral, 160
    respiratory, 163
  as trace element, essentiality, 109
6-Monoacetylmorphine
  as heroin metabolite, 14–16
  potency relative to morphine, 14–15
  toxicity of, 14
Monoamine oxidase, metal inhibition of, 165
Morphine
  biliary excretion of, 43–47
  blood-brain barrier to, 16–17, 40
  codeine as metabolite of, 18
    metabolic pathway for, 21–2
  dealkylation of, 18, 19
  Fujimoto-Wang method of detection, 37–38
  glucuronides of, 17–18
  as heroin metabolite, 14–16
  metabolism of, 17–21
    unidentified metabolites, 20–21
  placental transfer of, 42–43
  potency relative to morphine, 12
  sulfate detoxication metabolites of, 22
  toxicity of, 16
  transport and metabolism of
    in brain, 39–41
    in chicken, 31–35
Morphine-3-ethereal sulfate
  biliary excretion of, 46–47
  excretion of, 33–35
Morphine-3-glucuronide, biliary excretion of, 44–45, 46

N

Nalorphine
  brain transport of, 40
  dealkylation of, 18, 19
Naloxone
  dealkylation of, 19
  formulas of, 24
  glucuronide of, 22–26
  metabolism of, 23–26
  pharmacology of, 25–26
Narcotic analgesics
  cerebral transport of, 40
  placental transfer of, 43
  urinary excretion of, 29–31
  urinary monitoring of, 36, 38
Narcotics
  excretion in urine, 26–39
Neostigmine, chemical name of, 63
Nickel
  abundance and annual consumption of, 110
  as carcinogen, 158
  effects on
    atherosclerosis, 178, 182, 183
    growth, 116, 117, 120–122
    infection, 136
    reproduction, 154, 155, 156
    serum constituents, 139–142, 145, 148
    survival and longevity, 124, 125, 129
    tumors, 127, 128
  toxicity of, 165–171
    cellular, 157, 159
    oral, 160
    respiratory, 163
Nikethamide, effect on barbiturate metabolism, 6–8
Niobium
  abundance and annual consumption of, 111

effects on
  atherosclerosis, 178–181
  fats in body, 133, 134
  growth, 117, 119–123
  infection, 135
  serum constituents, 140–142, 144
  survival and longevity, 125, 129
  teeth, 138
  tumors, 127
  urinary abnormalities, 138
toxicity of, 164, 165, 167
  cellular, 157
  oral, 160, 162
  respiratory, 163
Nitrogen, toxicity of, 158, 159, 172
NOR compounds, as narcotic analgesic metabolites, 18
Normeperidine, urinary excretion of, 28–29
Normorphine
  as drug metabolite, 2
  narcotic action of, 18–19

## O

Obstetrics, morphine use compared to meperine in, 42–43
Organophosphate cholinesterase inhibitors, kinetics of action of, 60–102
Organosulfate cholinesterase inhibitors, kinetics of action of, 60–61
Osmium toxicity of
  cellular, 157
  oral, 160
Oxidase, microsomal, role in barbiturate metabolism, 6

## P

Palladium
  abundance and annual consumption of, 111
  as carcinogen, 158
  effects on
    amyloidosis, 133
    growth, 119, 122, 124
    survival and longevity, 125
  teeth, 133
  toxicity of
    cellular, 157
    oral, 160
    tumors, 127

Paraoxon
  chemical name of, 62
  as cholinesterase inhibitor, kinetics of, 101
Parkinson's disease, hereditary manganism and, 162, 163
Pentobarbital
  oxidation of, 4
  tolerance related to, 4–6
Phenobarbital
  effects on biliary morphine excretion, 47
  effect on marihuana excretion, 49
  in studies on barbiturate tolerance, 6
  urinary excretion of, 10–11
Phenol red, excretion of, 45
Phosphorus, toxicity of, 158, 159, 165, 166, 172
Physostigmine, see Eserine
Placenta, drug transfer of, 41–43
Platinum
  toxicity of
    cellular, 157
    oral, 160
Plumbism, from excess lead, 110
Pneumonia, trace element effects on, 135–137
Pollution, trace elements from, 163
Polonium
  toxicity of, cellular, 151
Potassium
  abundance and annual consumption of, 110
  in seawater, 163
Probenecid, in studies of drug excretion, 34
Procainamide, excretion of, 45
n-Propyl paraoxon, as cholinesterase inhibitor, kinetics of, 68
Prostigmine, see Neostigmine
Proteinuria, trace element effects on, 138–139
Pyruvate carboxylase, metal inhibition of, 165

## R

Reproduction, trace element effects on, 151–156
Rhenium, toxicity of, cellular, 157

SUBJECT INDEX 215

oral, 160
Rhodium
　abundance and annual consumption of, 111
　as carcinogen, 158
　effects on
　　amyloidosis, 133
　　growth, 119, 122, 124
　　longevity, 131
　　teeth, 133
　　tumors, 127
　toxicity of
　　cellular, 157
　　oral, 160
Rocks (igneous), metal distribution in, 110–111
Rubidium, toxicity of, 172
Ruthenium toxicity of,
　cellular, 157
　oral, 160

S

Scandium
　effects on
　　amyloidosis, 133
　　growth, 118, 122
　　teeth, 133
　　tumors, 127
　toxicity of, 164, 172
Seawater, metals distribution in, 110–111, 163
Selenium
　abundance and annual consumption of, 110
　as carcinogen, 158
　effects on
　　atherosclerosis, 178–182
　　amyloidosis, 133
　　fats in body, 133, 134
　　growth, 116, 117, 119–121, 124
　　infection, 135
　　serum constituents, 139–142, 144
　　survival and longevity, 124, 125, 129, 131, 132
　　reproduction, 151, 152, 155, 156
　　teeth, 133, 138
　　tumors, 127, 128
　　urinary abnormalities, 138
　toxicity of, 164, 166, 167
　　cellular, 157, 159
　　oral, 161, 162
　　respiratory, 163
　as trace element
　　essentiality, 109
Serum, constituents of, trace element effects on, 139–148
Silicon
　in seawater, 163
　toxicity of, 158, 172
Silver
　abundance and annual consumption of, 111
　effects on, atherosclerosis, 182, 183
　toxicity of, 164–165, 171, 172
　　cellular, 157
　　oral, 160
SKF 525A
　as blocker of morphine transport, 35
　effects on
　　barbiturate metabolism, 48–49
　　tetrahydrocannabinol metabolism, 48–49
Sodium
　abundance and annual consumption of, 110
　toxicity of, 158, 159, 172
Strontium
　abundance and annual consumption of, 110
　in seawater
　toxicity of, 158
　　cellular, 157
　　oral, 160, 162
　　respiratory, 163
Succinic dehydrogenase, metal inhibition of, 165
Sulfobromophthalein, clearance, after drug use, 8
Sulfur, toxicity of, 158, 159, 166, 172

T

Tantalum,
　toxicity of, 164
　　cellular, 157
　　oral, 160
Technetium
　toxicity of
　　cellular, 157

oral, 160
Teeth, trace element effect on, 133, 138, 139
Tellurium
  abundance and annual consumption of, 111
  effects on
    amyloidosis, 133
    atherosclerosis, 178–181
    growth, 119–121, 123, 124
    infection, 135
    serum constituents, 139, 141, 143, 144, 148
    survival and longevity, 124, 129, 131, 132
    teeth, 133, 138
    tumors, 127, 128, 129
    urinary abnormalities, 138
  toxicity of, 166, 167, 172
    cellular, 157, 159
    oral, 161
    respiratory, 163
Tetraethylammonium (TEA), in studies of drug excretion, 32
Δ⁹-Tetrahydrocannabinol, metabolism of, 47–49
Tetram, chemical name of, 63
Thallium, toxicity of, 164
  cellular, 157
  oral, 160
Thin-layer chromatography, use in drug detection, 38–39
Thiopenthal
  in studies on barbiturate tolerance, 6
  tolerance to, 6, 9
Thorium, toxicity of, 164
Tin
  abundance and annual consumption of, 111
  effects on
    atherosclerosis, 179–181
    fats in body, 133, 134
    growth, 121–122, 124
    kidney lesions, 137
    longevity, 129
    teeth
    tumors, 127
    serum constituents, 139, 140, 143, 144
    urinary abnormalities, 138
  toxicity of, 164, 172

cellular, 157
oral, 161, 162
respiratory, 163
as trace element, 109
Titanium
  abundance and annual consumption of, 111
  as carcinogen, 158
  effects on
    atherosclerosis, 182, 183
    growth, 118, 122, 123
    infection, 136
    reproduction, 154, 155, 156
    tumors, 127
  toxicity of, 164, 172
    cellular, 157
    oral, 160, 162
    respiratory, 163
Tolerance, to barbiturates, relation to metabolism of, 3–8
Toxicity, of trace elements, 156–173
TPCK
  as active-site-directed irreversible inhibitor, kinetics of action, 60
  chemical name of, 63
Trace elements
  abundance and annual consumption of, 110–111
  effects on
    amyloidosis, 132–133
    atherosclerosis, 177–186, 195
    body weights, 124
    fats in body, 133–137
    growth, 115–124, 194
    infection, 135–137
    kidney lesions, 137
    reproduction, 151–156, 194
    serum constituents, 139–148, 194
    survival and longevity, 124–126, 194
    teeth, 133, 138, 139
    tumors, 129–129, 195
    urinary abnormalities, 138–139, 195
  laboratory study plan, 109–110
    diet for, 113–115
    metalfree environment for, 112–113
  toxicity of, 156–173
    cellular, 157, 158–159
    growth effects
    interactions, 164–171
    mechanisms, 156–173

# SUBJECT INDEX

oral, 162–163
prediction, 163–164
respiratory, 163
waterborne, heart disease and, 187
3-Trimethylaminophenyl-*N*,*N*-dimethyl carbamate, see Neostigmine
Tumors, trace element effects on, 126–129
Tungsten
  abundance and annual consumption of, 111
  effects on
    growth, 119
    infection, 136
    serum constituents, 139, 141, 143, 144, 148
    toxicity of, 164–166, 172
    cellular, 157
    oral, 160
Tyrosinase, metal inhibition of, 165

## U

Uranium
  abundance and annual consumption of, 111
  toxicity of, 164, 172
Uric acid, in serum, trace element effects on, 148
Urine
  abnormalities of
    trace element effects on, 138–139
    monitoring of, for drug abuse, 35–39
    narcotic excretion by, 26–39
      by glomerular filtration, 27
      pH effects on, 27–29

## V

Vanadium
  abundance and annual consumption of, 110
  effects on
    atherosclerosis, 178–181
    fats in body, 134
    growth, 118–129
    infection, 135, 137
    longevity, 129, 131
    teeth, 138
    tumors, 127, 128
    urinary abnormalities, 138

serum constituents, 139–142, 144, 148
toxicity of, 164–166, 172
  cellular, 157
  oral, 160, 162
  respiratory, 163
Vitamin E, effects on, glycosuria, 138, 139, 147

## W

Water
  basic, metals in, effects on serum glucose and cholesterol, 148–151
  drinking, trace elements in, 191
  toxicity of, 157
  trace elements in, heart disease and, 187–188
Weinberg's principle, 155, 157
Wilson's disease, see Cuprism

## X

Xanthine oxidase, 148
  metal inhibition of, 165

## Y

Yttrium
  effects on
    amyloidosis, 133
    growth, 119, 123, 124
    survival and longevity, 125
    teeth, 133
    tumors, 127
    toxicity of, 164, 172
Yttrium
  toxicity of, 164, 172

## Z

Zinc
  abundance and annual consumption of, 110
  in cadmium hypertension, 175, 177
  as carcinogen, 158
  effects on
    atherosclerosis, 181, 183
    cadmium deficiency, 192
  in seawater, 164
  toxicity of, 165–171

cellular, 157, 159
oral, 160
respiratory, 163
as trace element, essentiality, 109
Zirconium
abundance and annual consumption of, 111
effects on
atherosclerosis, 178–181
fats in body, 134
growth, 117, 119–122
infection, 135, 137
longevity, 129
serum constituents, 139–142, 149–151
teeth, 138
tumors, 127, 128
urinary abnormalities, 138
toxicity of, 164, 166, 172
cellular, 157
oral, 160
respiratory, 163